Immunology

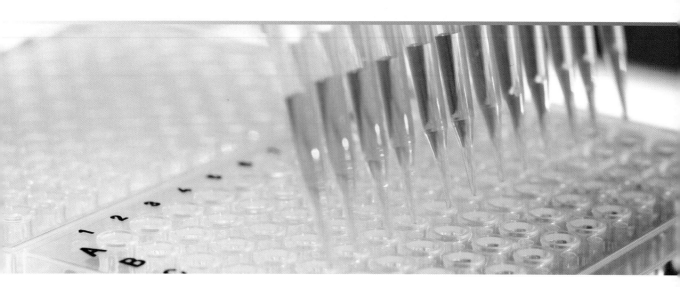

Edited by

Angela Hall
*Department of Immunology, Imperial College
Healthcare NHS Trust*

Christine Yates
*Immunology Department, Hull and East Yorkshire
Hospitals NHS Trust*

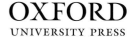
OXFORD
UNIVERSITY PRESS

OXFORD
UNIVERSITY PRESS

Great Clarendon Street, Oxford OX2 6DP

Oxford University Press is a department of the University of Oxford.
It furthers the University's objective of excellence in research, scholarship,
and education by publishing worldwide in

Oxford   New York

Auckland Cape Town Dar es Salaam Hong Kong Karachi
Kuala Lumpur Madrid Melbourne Mexico City Nairobi
New Delhi Shanghai Taipei Toronto

With offices in

Argentina Austria Brazil Chile Czech Republic France Greece
Guatemala Hungary Italy Japan Poland Portugal Singapore
South Korea Switzerland Thailand Turkey Ukraine Vietnam

Oxford is a registered trade mark of Oxford University Press
in the UK and in certain other countries

Published in the United States
by Oxford University Press Inc., New York

British Library Cataloguing in Publication Data

Data available

Library of Congress Cataloging in Publication Data

Data available

Typeset by MPS Limited, A Macmillan Company
Printed in Italy on acid-free paper by
LEGO SpA – Lavis TN

ISBN 978-0-19-953496-8

1 3 5 7 9 10 8 6 4 2

Books are to be returned on or before
the last date below.

LIBREX—

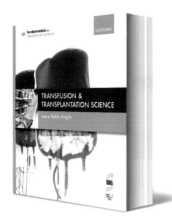

TRANSFUSION & TRANSPLANTATION SCIENCE

EDITED BY Robin Knight

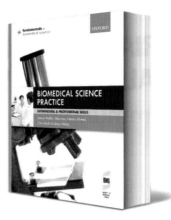

BIOMEDICAL SCIENCE PRACTICE

EXPERIMENTAL & PROFESSIONAL SKILLS

EDITED BY Nadia Glencross, Nessar Ahmed, Chris Smith & Qiuyu Wang

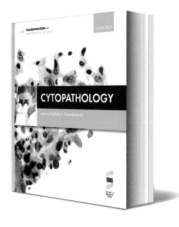

CYTOPATHOLOGY

EDITED BY Behdad Shambayati

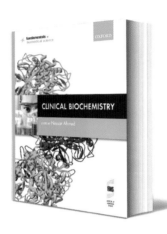

CLINICAL BIOCHEMISTRY

EDITED BY Nessar Ahmed

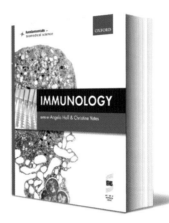

IMMUNOLOGY

EDITED BY Angela Hall & Christine Yates

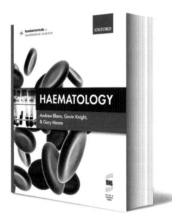

HAEMATOLOGY

Andrew Blann, Gavin Knight, & Gary Moore

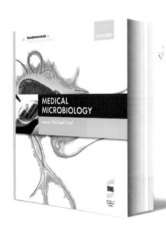

MEDICAL MICROBIOLOGY

EDITED BY Michael Ford

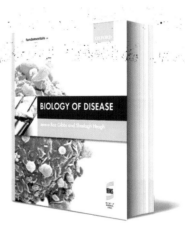

BIOLOGY OF DISEASE

EDITED BY Paul Gibbs and Sheelagh Heugh

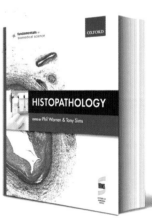

HISTOPATHOLOGY

EDITED BY Phil Warren & Tony Sims

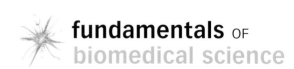

fundamentals OF
biomedical science

Acknowledgement

Mr Nick Davey, Imperial College Healthcare NHS Trust for his help in checking the HLA nomenclature.

An introduction to the Fundamentals of Biomedical Science series

Biomedical Scientists form the foundation of modern healthcare, from cancer screening to diagnosing HIV, from blood transfusion for surgery to food poisoning and infection control. Without Biomedical Scientists, the diagnosis of disease, the evaluation of the effectiveness of treatment, and research into the causes and cures of disease would not be possible.

However, the path to becoming a Biomedical Scientist is a challenging one: trainees must not only assimilate knowledge from a range of disciplines, but must understand—and demonstrate—how to apply this knowledge in a practical, hands-on environment.

The *Fundamentals of Biomedical Science* series is written to reflect the challenges of biomedical science education and training today. It blends essential basic science with insights into laboratory practice to show how an understanding of the biology of disease is coupled to the analytical approaches that lead to diagnosis.

The series provides coverage of the full range of disciplines to which a Biomedical Scientist may be exposed – from microbiology to cytopathology to transfusion science. Alongside volumes exploring specific biomedical themes and related laboratory diagnosis, an overarching *Biomedical Science Practice* volume provides a grounding in the general professional and experimental skills with which every Biomedical Scientist should be equipped.

Produced in collaboration with the Institute of Biomedical Science, the series

- Understands the complex roles of Biomedical Scientists in the modern practice of medicine.

- Understands the development needs of employers and the Profession.

- Places the theoretical aspects of biomedical science in their practical context.

Learning from this series

The *Fundamentals of Biomedical Science* series draws on a range of learning features to help readers master both biomedical science theory, and biomedical science practice.

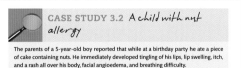

CASE STUDY 3.2 A child with nut allergy

The parents of a 5-year-old boy reported that while at a birthday party he ate a piece of cake containing nuts. He immediately developed tingling of his lips, lip swelling, itch, and a rash all over his body, facial angioedema, and breathing difficulty.

An ambulance was called and he was taken to the local hospital Emergency Department where adrenaline, antihistamines, and oral steroids were administered.

Case studies illustrate how the biomedical science theory and practice presented throughout the series relates to situations and experiences that are likely to be encountered routinely in the biomedical science laboratory.

Method boxes walk through the key protocols that the reader is likely to encounter in the laboratory on a regular basis.

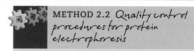

METHOD 2.2 *Quality control procedures for protein electrophoresis*

Electrophoresis requires the running of internal quality control samples, just as other laboratory tests do. It is recommended to run a known paraprotein of known concentration in parallel.

UKNEQAS for immunology runs a scheme for monoclonal protein identification which includes serum and urine protein electrophoresis and also serum and urine monoclone

Clinical correlations bring relevance to the material by placing it in its clinical context.

CLINICAL CORRELATIONS 2.8

Are all monoclonal bands associated with myeloma?

Diseases associated with the presence of monoclonal immunoglobulin include Waldenström's macroglobulinaemia, monoclonal gammopathy of uncertain significance (MGUS), lymphoma, chronic lymphocytic leukaemia, amyloidosis, and heavy chain disease, as well as myeloma. In addition, benign, usually transient, monoclones may be seen in response to infection.

Further features are used to help consolidate and extend students' understanding of the subject

Key points reinforce the key concepts that the reader should master from having read the material presented, while **Summary** points act as end-of-chapter checklists for readers to verify that they have remembered correctly the principal themes and ideas presented within each chapter.

Key Points

Taking an accurate clinical history is the most important tool in allergy diagnosis.

Other techniques such as skin prick and challenge testing, measurement of sIgE antibodies and mast cell tryptase, and basophil activation tests can provide supporting evidence. The decision as to which additional techniques to use is dependent on the complexity of the clinical history.

Key terms provide on-the-page explanations of terms with which the reader may not be familiar; in addition, each title in the series features a **glossary**, in which the key terms featured in that title are collated.

complement

…nt components, mediates many actions, including **opsoniza**-…gen–antibody complexes, inflammation, phagocyte recruit-…brane attack complex which can result in cell lysis.

…ment are triggered in different ways. The alterative and lectin …bial cell surfaces, and the classical pathway is triggered by …uring complement activation, the components are cleaved …lled 'a' for the small fragment and 'b' for the large fragment. …C5a and C5b. C5a binds to the C5a receptor present on a

Opsonization
The binding of complement and antibodies to the surface of a pathogen or foreign substance to aid phagocytosis.

Self-check questions throughout each chapter and extended questions at the end of each chapter provide the reader with a ready means of checking that they have understood the material they have just encountered. Answers to these questions are provided in the book's Online Resource Centre; visit www.oxfordtextbooks.co.uk/orc/hall

| β₂ | C3 |
| γ | Immunoglobulins (γ-globulins) |

SELF-CHECK 2.1

Why it is important to use a protein-selective stain in electrophoresis?

Technical points to note

Cross references help the reader to see biomedical science as a unified discipline, making connections between topics presented within each volume, and across all volumes in the series.

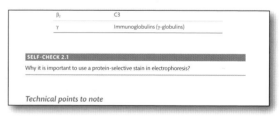

Cross reference
You can read in more detail about nephelometry, turbidimetry, and radial immunodiffusion in the *Biomedical Science Practice* book of this series

− post-streptococcal glomerulonephritis
− C3 nephritic factor.
• C3 is normal and C4 is decreased:
− Type II cryoglobulinaemia associated with hepatitis C infec
− C1 inhibitor deficiency (discussed in more detail in section
− active SLE
− genetic deficiency (C4 null alleles).

Online learning materials

online resource centre

The *Fundamentals of Biomedical Science* series doesn't end with the printed books. Each title in the series is supported by an Online Resource Centre, which features additional materials for students, trainees, and lecturers.

www.oxfordtextbooks.co.uk/orc/fbs

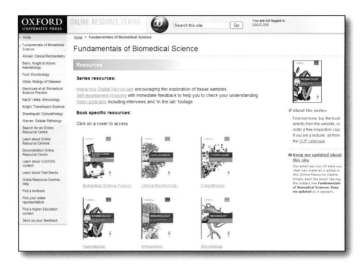

Guides to key experimental skills and methods

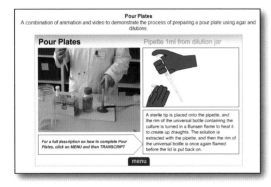

Multimedia walk-throughs of key experimental skills—including both animations and video—to help you master the essential skills that are the foundation of Biomedical Science practice.

Biomedical science in practice

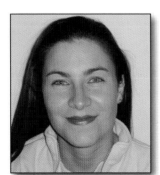

Interviews with practising Biomedical Scientists working in a range of disciplines, to give you valuable insights into the reality of work in a Biomedical Science laboratory.

Digital Microscope

A library of microscopic images for you to investigate using this powerful online microscope, to help you gain a deeper appreciation of cell and tissue morphology.

The Digital Microscope is used under licence from the Open University.

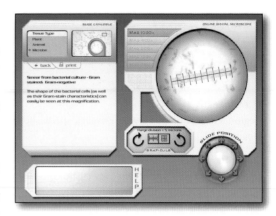

'Check your understanding' learning modules

A mix of interactive tasks and questions, which address a variety of topics explored throughout the series. Complete these modules to help you check that you have fully mastered all the key concepts and key ideas that are central to becoming a proficient Biomedical Scientist.

We extend our grateful thanks to colleagues in the School of Health Science at London Metropolitan University for their invaluable help in developing these online learning materials.

Answers to self-check and end of chapter questions

Answers to questions posed in the book are provided to aid self-assessment.

Lecturer support materials

The Online Resource Centre for each title in the series also features figures from the book in electronic format, for registered adopters to download for use in lecture presentations, and other educational resources.

To register as an adopter visit **www.oxfordtextbooks.co.uk/orc/hall** and follow the on-screen instructions.

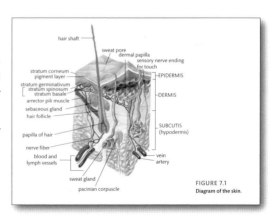

FIGURE 7.1
Diagram of the skin.

Any comments?

We welcome comments and feedback about any aspect of this series.
Just visit **www.oxfordtextbooks.co.uk/orc/feedback** and share your views.

Contributors

I J Ansotegui
Regional Immunology Service, Royal Hospitals, Belfast Health & Social Care Trust

Dawn Barge
Immunology Department, The Newcastle Upon Tyne Hospitals NHS Foundation Trust

Peter J Charles
Translational Research Laboratory, Kennedy Institute of Rheumatology, Imperial College London

Alison Cox
Department of Immunology, Imperial College Healthcare NHS Trust

Alistair Crockard
Regional Immunology Service, Royal Hospitals, Belfast Health & Social Care Trust

Edward Davies
Department of Clinical Allergy and Immunology, King's College Hospital

Tariq El-Shanawany
Department of Immunology, University Hospital of Wales Cardiff

Lynn Follows
Immunology Department, Sheffield Teaching Hospitals NHS Foundation Trust

Angela Hall
Department of Immunology, Imperial College Healthcare NHS Trust

Don Henderson
Imperial College Healthcare NHS Trust

Saiju Jacob
Queen Elizabeth Neurosciences Centre, University Hospital Birmingham NHS Trust

Abid R Karim
Neuroimmunology, Clinical Immunology Service, University of Birmingham

Robert J Lock
Immunology and Immunogenetics, North Bristol NHS Trust

Mo Moody
Department of Immunology, University Hospital of Wales Cardiff

B Paul Morgan
School of Medicine, Cardiff University

Paul Williams
Department of Immunology, University Hospital of Wales Cardiff

Phillip A Whitfield
Immunology Department, Sheffield Teaching Hospitals NHS Foundation Trust

Christine Yates
Immunology Department, Hull and East Yorkshire Hospitals NHS Trust

Online materials developed by

Sheelagh Heugh, Principal Lecturer in Biomedical Science, Faculty of Human Sciences, London Metropolitan University

Dr Ken Hudson, Lecturer in Biomedical Science, Faculty of Human Sciences, London Metropolitan University

Professor Jameel Inal, Professor of Immunology, Faculty of Human Sciences, London Metropolitan University

Contents

Introduction to the clinical immunology laboratory

Learning Objectives

After studying this chapter, you should have some understanding of:

- key aspects of immunology
- the importance of immunology in health
- the role of the biomedical scientist in the immunology laboratory

Introduction

This chapter will introduce you to immunology and its importance in health. Immunology is one of the major pathology disciplines. The others are haematology, transfusion and transplantation science, clinical biochemistry, microbiology, histopathology, and cytopathology. In the clinical setting, results from one discipline should be considered together with those from the other disciplines for meaningful interpretation and diagnosis. Biomedical scientists usually specialize in one discipline but they need, at least, to have a basic understanding and to be aware of the scope of the other disciplines. This book is one in a series which aims to fulfil this need and to provide sufficient detailed information for biomedical specialists in their chosen field to be effective practitioners.

In this opening chapter the topics introduced are the general properties of immunology and the role of immunology as one of the biomedical sciences. It is not within the scope of the book to provide a comprehensive description of the immune system, and readers are directed to more academic textbooks of immunology for this level of detail. Instead, this book provides the new biomedical scientist with an insight into the function of the immune system and the diagnostic techniques used to identify associated malfunctions and disorders. By examining the key immunological principles and scientific basis of laboratory techniques with a focus on the biomedical scientist's role in the diagnostic laboratory, the reader is provided with everything needed to prepare for a specialist qualification in immunology. Current tests, the rationale behind their use, the technologies employed, and the quality measures applied are illustrated by specific case studies showing how the clinician interprets the results to help the patient.

Key Point

The result obtained from one discipline should be considered together with results from other disciplines, in order to provide meaningful interpretation and diagnosis.

1.1 Immunology

Immunology is the branch of biomedicine concerned with the structure and function of the immune system. Immunologists study how the immune system defends the body against attack from micro-organisms and parasites, how it discriminates between self and non-self, how it deals with foreign molecules, and how it recognizes and deals with neoplastic and virally transformed cells, as well as transplanted organs, cells, and proteins. They are also concerned with what happens when the immune system acts against self.

The complexity of immunology can be quite daunting. Traditionally in teaching, immunology is broken down into a description of its **cellular** and **humoral** components, then an explanation of the **innate** and the **adaptive** immune responses, before moving on to more complex subjects including immunoregulation, allergy and hypersensitivity, autoimmunity, malignancy, and immunodeficiency. This facilitates learning, but the scientist must always take a more holistic approach when considering what is being done and how the results affect patients.

Immunology is a rapidly growing field, with many new and exciting discoveries made each year. These enhance our understanding of health and indicate how subtle changes in the immune system have profound effects.

In the diagnostics arena immunological procedures are the basis of many haematological, microbiological, biochemical, and histopathological tests, and there is a lot of cross-over between immunology and the other pathology disciplines. The cells, tissues, and organs of the immune system, as well as the immunologically active substances that they produce are important to all pathologists.

The unique specificity of **antibodies** for their target **antigens** is the basis of many tests. The identification of cell surface proteins and the production of specific antibodies against them have allowed the rapid identification, investigation, and enumeration of **lymphocyte** sub-populations and the derivation of the 'clusters of differentiation' (CD) classification of cells. The CD antigens are used in defining and identifying leukaemias and lymphomas. Antigen capture by antibody is fundamental to diverse techniques, including double diffusion gel-based assays, enzyme and radio immunoassays, nephelometry, Eli-spot assays, immunohistology, flow cytometry, and combined techniques such as Luminex assays. Antibody/antigen technology is branching out also into other fields such as nanoengineering.

Inflammation is a key component of almost all immunological reactions. Interaction of an antibody with its specific antigen activates **complement**, resulting in increased vascular

---

Cell-mediated immunity (cellular immunity)
Immune response mediated by cells such as T lymphocytes.

Humoral immunity
Immune response mediated by antibodies and complement.

Innate immunity
The natural immunity that exists prior to sensitization from an antigen. It is often nonspecific.

Adaptive immunity
The immunity that is acquired following sensitization with antigens.

Antibodies
Antigen-specific proteins that are produced by B lymphocytes in response to exposure to the antigen.

Antigens
Protein molecules recognized by the immune system as foreign and against which the immune system specifically reacts.

Lymphocytes
A type of white blood cell of which there are three subtypes: B cells, which give rise to humoral immunity, and T cells, which give rise to cellular immunity, and Natural killer cells.

Clusters of differentiation (CD)
Cell surface molecules on lymphocytes that are recognized by monoclonal antibodies to allow identification of the cell by flow cytometry.

Inflammation
A characteristic physiological response of tissues to injury. The signs of inflammation are heat, redness, swelling, and pain.

Complement
A group of blood proteins that enhance the immune response.

permeability and mobilization of cells, resulting in an inflammatory infiltrate at the site of reaction. This interplay between complement, antibody, and inflammatory phagocytic cells (**macrophages, neutrophils**) is important for defence against infection. A deficiency in one of these components (**immunodeficiency**) predisposes the individual to repeated infections and disease.

On first exposure to an antigen, the individual becomes immunologically primed and subsequent contact with that antigen leads to secondary boosting of the immune response (**immunological memory**). This immunological priming and secondary boosting leads to the production of antibodies and effector cells. However, in some cases, the memory reaction may be excessive, causing tissue damage (**hypersensitivity**). The most common example is **allergy**.

The immune system has evolved to recognize myriad foreign antigens and inevitably in doing so some lymphocytes are produced that react against the body's own constituents, causing **autoimmunity**.

The **antisera** used in laboratory tests are produced by immunizing animals with the relevant purified antigen. This results in a polyclonal antibody response from different B-cell clones reacting to various determinants (**epitopes**) of the antigen. With the advent of hybridoma technology, **monoclonal antibodies** are increasingly being used. Monoclonal antibodies react with only one epitope on an antigen. They are derived from a single cell hybridized with a nonsecreting myeloma cell to produce an immortalized cell line which can be cultured to produce vast quantities of monoclonal antibodies with precise reactivity. Different reporter molecules are coupled to the antibodies, depending upon the assay technology to be used.

Laboratory tests differ in their **sensitivity** and **specificity**. For optimal results the cut-off points are set such that no diseased patients are test negative (false-negative) and the fewest possible individuals without the disease are test positive (false-positive). The assays described in this book are a mixture of quantitative, semiquantitative, and qualitative. Quantitative assays usually produce precise results, can be standardized against a reference preparation, and can usually be automated. Qualitative assays usually involve considerable technical expertise, and interpretation can be subjective. The endpoint of qualitative assays is of the positive/negative or normal/abnormal type. All immunology laboratories strive to produce a high-quality service reflected in accurate results. This is achieved through internal and external quality assurance schemes and regulation of the laboratory and personnel.

1.2 Immunology in biomedical science

Each immunology laboratory differs in the depth and breadth of service provided according to the needs of the patients it serves and expertise of its staff. Look at Figure 1.1 to see what services can be offered by Immunology.

In the various chapters of this book you will learn more about the role of the immunology service in diagnosis and disease management. The following chapters will describe the importance and relevance of the subject to the immunology service.

In an era of rapidly evolving medical research and development, it is hard to imagine that the original diagnostic laboratories were no more than a corner in a doctor's home, office, or hospital ward, with the doctor himself performing the investigations. Nowadays over 80% of medical interventions rely upon results generated in the pathology service laboratories. The educational and regulatory requirements have grown in parallel with the development

Macrophages

Phagocytic cells found in the tissues that ingest, kill, and digest bacteria, foreign cells, and tissue debris. These cells also play a role in antigen presentation in the immune system.

Neutrophils

Phagocytic white blood cells that ingest and destroy bacteria as part of the innate immune response. These cells rapidly accumulate, in large numbers, at sites of infection and inflammation.

Immunodeficiency

Defects in the immune system resulting in gaps in the body's defence against pathogens.

Immunological memory is the ability of the immune system to 'recall' a previous encounter with an antigen, resulting in a stronger immunological response.

Hypersensitivity

The reaction that causes reproducible signs or symptoms, following exposure to a defined stimulus, in a susceptible individual.

Allergy

A hypersensitivity reaction initiated by immunological mechanisms.

Autoimmune disease (Autoimmunity)

Breakdown of tolerance, resulting in production of antibodies and/or T-cells directed against own cells and tissues.

Antisera

Antibodies that are targeted against a specific antigen. Often used to identify antigens in immunological assays such as ELISA or indirect immunofluorescence (IIF).

Epitope

The region on an antigen that is recognizable by the immune system.

Monoclonal antibodies

Antibodies produced from a single clone of cells, consisting of identical molecules.

Sensitivity

The ability of an assay to correctly identify disease. The number of false negatives.

Specificity

Lack of interference from other elements other than the analyte being measured. The number of false positives.

Cross reference

More precise details on the techniques used within immunology are given in the *Biomedical Science Practice* book of this series.

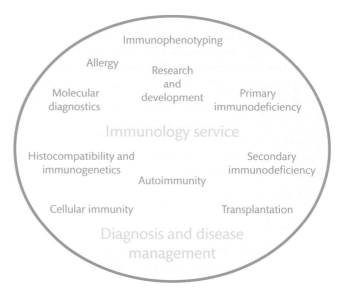

FIGURE 1.1
The breadth and scope of the immunology service.

Cross references

You can look at the virtual immunology laboratory online at http://www.science4u.info/virtuallab/ Here you can find out what tests an immunology laboratory can offer, hear interviews with biomedical scientists, and read about topics such as health and safety and training within an immunology laboratory.

More information on the role of biomedical scientists and the professional development opportunites available can be found on the website of the Institute of Biomedical Science: http://www.IBMS.org

and expansion of the pathology disciplines into independent clinical laboratory professions. Most diagnostic laboratories are found in hospitals and the majority of the professional biomedical scientists are employed in this setting. Those in rural district hospitals tend to be generalists, but in larger institutions such as the teaching hospitals, with their wider scope and increased numbers of tests, many biomedical scientists specialize in specific areas and departments. It is becoming common practice that immunology laboratories will be situated within cross-discipline departments, often linked with either clinical biochemistry or virology departments; however, because of the cross-over between immunology and all the other pathology disciplines, immunology can be found affiliated with any of the other pathology departments. This provides the opportunity for multidisciplinarily trained biomedical scientists, who may be given the opportunity to specialize within more than one discipline.

Within the immunology service laboratory, the specialist areas include immunodeficiency, autoimmunity, allergy and hypersensitivity, cellular and humoral immunity, immunochemistry, transplantation, and malignancy. Biomedical scientists work in all of these areas and, depending upon the laboratory, may be expected to rotate through the various sections. Certainly, trainee biomedical and clinical scientists will have to train and work in each area to gather the knowledge, skills, and competencies to become registered professional scientists. Training and development does not cease at registration, and all scientists are required to keep up to date with advancements in their profession and to demonstrate maintenance of competencies through participation in continuing professional development (CPD). Both the Institute of Biomedical Science and the Royal College of Pathologists run accredited CPD schemes. Biomedical scientists can become Chartered Scientists, which provides international recognition that they are practising science at a fully professional level. Provision of accredited qualifications from the Institute of Biomedical Science gives a framework of qualifications to support advancement in career progression and demonstration of specialized, higher laboratory practice.

Biomedical and clinical scientists should have a presence outside the laboratory. They should participate in **multidisciplinary team** (MDT) meetings and hospital '**grand rounds**', where the results they generate are discussed with clinicians and other health-care professionals in the context of the diagnosis and management of patients. Despite the separate training pathways, there is a lot of overlap in the roles of biomedical and clinical scientists, especially with regard to the timely processing of samples and reporting of results. Depending upon the size and complexity of the laboratory, biomedical scientists predominantly take responsibility for analyses of samples and the assay platforms, while the clinical scientists may take more responsibility for clinical liaison, validation, and research and development, but at the senior levels these boundaries become blurred.

Multidisciplinary team
A group of professionals (i.e. doctors, nurses, scientists) who meet to discuss individual patients, using the knowledge from each discipline to work towards effective diagnosis and treatments.

Grand round
A conference at which clinicians/experts present the case studies of individual patients, or new topics in the field of medicine, and use this as an educational tool for other staff members.

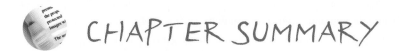

CHAPTER SUMMARY

- Immunology is the branch of biomedicine concerned with the structure and function of the immune system.

- Immunology is a rapidly growing field, with many new and exciting discoveries made each year.

- In the diagnostics arena immunological procedures are the basis of many haematological, microbiological, biochemical, and histopathological tests, and there is a lot of cross-over between immunology and the other pathology disciplines.

- Each immunology laboratory differs in the depth and breadth of service provided, according to the needs of the patients it serves and expertise of its staff.

- Within the immunology service laboratory, the specialist areas range from immunodeficiency, autoimmunity, allergy and hypersensitivity, cellular and humoral immunity, immunochemistry, transplantation, and malignancy.

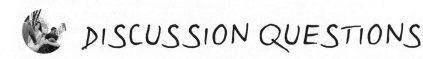

DISCUSSION QUESTIONS

1.1   What are the benefits of cross-disciplinary training?

1.2   What does the title Chartered Scientist mean?

Answers to these questions are provided in the book's Online Resource Centre; visit www.oxfordtextbooks.co.uk/orc/ahmed/

2

Immunoglobulins

Learning Objectives

After studying this chapter you should be able to:

- outline the common features of immunoglobulin structure, function, and pathology
- describe the clinical features of monoclonal gammopathy of undetermined significance (MGUS), myeloma, cryoglobulinaemia, and multiple sclerosis (MS)
- outline the assays and techniques used to test for monoclonal gammopathy of undetermined significance (MGUS), myeloma, cryoglobulinaemia, and multiple sclerosis (MS)
- discuss the limitations of these techniques

Introduction

This chapter describes the investigation of immunoglobulins in the clinical laboratory, both in health and in disease. In the United Kingdom, the investigations are most often performed within clinical chemistry or immunology departments. Often the primary intention is to detect monoclonal gammopathies; however, there is a wealth of information to be seen using serum electrophoresis including inflammatory changes, liver disease, and renal pathology.

It is important to use both quantitative and qualitative measurement of immunoglobulins together when determining a patient's current status. A deficiency in IgA may be missed if only a qualitative screen is performed, as the electrophoretic track may appear normal; conversely, many low-level monoclonal gammopathies will have quantitative levels within the reference range and will be overlooked if the laboratory relies solely on a quantitative screen.

This chapter describes in detail the techniques used in the clinical laboratory for the detection of immunoglobulins, their use, and their interpretation.

2.1 Immunoglobulins

Immunoglobulins are a family of proteins of the humoral immune system that bind to specific targets called antigens. They activate complement, influence effector cells such as natural killer (NK) cells and mast cells through binding to surface receptors, which activate cells or encourage phagocytosis through immune complexes. Each Immunoglobulin molecule consists of two identical heavy chains designated by Greek letters γ (gamma), α (alpha), μ (mu), δ (delta), and ε(epsilon), paired with two identical light chains designated κ (kappa) and λ (lambda). The basic immunoglobulin unit consists of two heavy chains and two light chains. There are five immunoglobulin isotypes or classes named IgG, IgA, IgM, IgD, and IgE, after the corresponding heavy chain (above). The layout of two heavy chains plus two light chains is common to all the immunoglobulin isotypes, with differences in the number and sequence of amino acids dictating differences in size and function. IgG, IgD, and IgE molecules are made up of single four-chain units (monomers). IgA is found predominantly in a two-unit molecule (dimer) and IgM is found as a five-unit molecule (pentamer). In addition, IgG has four subclasses known as IgG1, IgG2, IgG3, and IgG4. IgA has two subclasses; IgA1 and IgA2.

Immunoglobulins are synthesized and secreted by plasma cells in bone marrow and lymph nodes. Plasma cells are the final stage of maturation of B lymphocytes and each plasma cell produces antibody molecules of a single isotype and antigen binding specificity (a clone). The isotype can be switched from M to G, A, or E during B-cell maturation before the plasma cell stage. IgD is a cell surface molecule of unknown function and can be found in low levels in the serum.

Immunoglobulin heavy chains and light chains are produced in different regions of the endoplasmic reticulum and are assembled into a single functional molecule before secretion. However, excess immunoglobulin light chains are produced, which are secreted as independent molecules. The κ free light chains circulate as monomers, whereas the λ free light chains tend to form dimers, or larger polymers. The excess light chains enter the kidneys and because of their low molecular weight they pass through the glomerulus and into the proximal tubule, where they are reabsorbed and degraded into smaller peptides which are then recycled. Normally some 1–10 mg of light chains per day pass into the distal tubule and into the urine but in **monoclonal gammopathies** the capacity of the proximal tubule can be overwhelmed and much higher levels of light chains leak into the urine.

The basic immunoglobulin structure consists of two heavy chains each of about 50 kDa molecular weight and two light chains each of 25 kDa, giving a single unit of at least 150 kDa. The heavy chains have three or four constant regions or domains, depending on the isotype, and one variable domain. The constant domains are named 'constant heavy' (CH) 1, 2, 3, or 4 and are so called because within them the amino acid sequence is highly conserved. They have a substructure of β-pleated sheets of polypeptides cross-linked by disulphide bridges, giving a barrel-like appearance. Look at Figure 2.1 to see the three-CH domain model.

Between CH1 and CH2 is the hinge region which confers flexibility on the molecule allowing antibody binding of antigen in different planes. The hinge region varies in the number of amino acids according to the immunoglobulin isotype.

The CH1 is linked to the variable region domain VH. As the name suggests, the amino acid sequence is more variable, with a small hypervariable region that results from shuffling of the V-region genes. It is the hypervariable region that contributes to the antigen specificity of the antibody molecule.

Linked by disulphide bonds in parallel to each heavy chain (VH and CH1) is the light chain, which may be of κ or λ isotype, but never both. These are similarly divided into a constant light chain domain (CL) and one variable light chain domain (VL).

Monoclonal gammopathy
Disease characterized by the finding of monoclonal immunoglobulin in the serum and/or urine.

Cross reference
See section 2.2 for more information on monoclonal gammopathies.

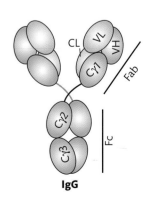

IgG

FIGURE 2.1
Structure of IgG.

Key Point

Immunoglobulin heavy and light chains are organized into barrel-like domains.

Complementarity determining region (CDR)

A short amino acid sequence found in the variable region of an immunoglobulin.

Cross reference

See Chapter 4 for more about complement.

As with the heavy chain VH domain, the VL domain has hypervariable regions, differing in sequence from the VH hypervariable region. The hypervariable regions are also referred to as **complementarity determining regions (CDR)** and on both heavy and light chains they are located in three zones of about five amino acids each in position 25, 50, and 75 approximately. It is the combination of the heavy-chain and light-chain CDRs that give the antibody its specificity, and since the two arms are identical the molecule has two antigen binding sites.

When an immunoglobulin binds to antigen, this causes a conformational change in the hinge region which exposes the C1q binding site in CH2; this then leads to the classical pathway activation of the complement sequence. IgA does not have this function, and is unable to activate complement.

The CH3 domain acts as a ligand for IgG receptors found on cells of the immune system such as neutrophils and NK cells.

The structure of immunoglobulin was elucidated by using enzymes to digest and fragment the molecule. The enzyme papain digests the immunoglobulin molecule at the N-terminus of the inter-chain disulphide bonds, releasing the antigen-binding arms as separate units known as Fab (fragments antigen binding) and the paired CH2 and CH3 domains known as Fc (fragments crystallizable). The enzyme pepsin digests immunoglobulin molecules at the C-terminus of the inter-chain disulphide bonds, leaving both antigen-binding arms linked as a single unit known as F(ab)$_2$ (fragment antigen binding ×2). The remaining CH2 and CH3 domains of the immunoglobulin heavy chain are degraded to small peptides.

Key Point

Immunoglobulin molecules have different effector functions in different domains of the molecule.

Immunoglobulin IgG

IgG follows the three-CH domain model described in section 2.1. The principal differences between the four IgG subclasses are the number of amino acids which constitute the hinge region, and the inter-chain disulphide bonds linking the heavy chains at this point. The key properties of the four IgG subclasses are listed in Table 2.1.

IgG is an immunoglobulin which can be found in the plasma and extracellular spaces. IgG1 and IgG3 antibodies are produced as a result of exposure to T-cell-dependant antigens such as viral protein, while IgG2 antibodies are produced in response to polysaccharide antigen in adults. In children, an IgG1 response is produced following exposure to polysaccharide antigen, as little IgG2 is produced in the first 2 years of life. Children under 2 years of age may present with pneumococcal infections and may not produce a good response to the unconjugated pneumococcal vaccines. The newer protein-conjugated vaccines direct an IgG1 response to the peptide. It is common practice to test for the presence of the IgG subclasses in these circumstances, but a true deficiency of one of the IgG subclasses is rare and it is more clinically relevant to measure antibody responses to pneumococcal antigens.

Cross reference

See Chapter 3.14 on IgG antibodies for more information on immunotherapy.

IgG4 is produced in response to extracellular parasites and multiple exposures to protein antigens. This latter characteristic is exploited clinically to desensitize individuals who have an IgE-mediated hypersensitivity to insect venoms. The IgG4 anti-venom can block the IgE:venom interaction.

TABLE 2.1 **Features of the IgG subclasses**

	IgGl	IgG2	IgG3	IgG4
Serum concentration (adults, g/L)	3.2–10.2	1.2–6.6	0.2–1.9	0–1.3
Hinge region amino acids	16	12	62	12
Interchain bonds	2	4	11	2
Half-life (days)	21	21	7	21
Complement activation	++	+	+++	0
FcRII & III binding	++++	+	+++	+
Antigen	Peptide	Polysaccharide	Peptide	Peptide
Placental transfer	+++	+	++	+

NB: In adults, IgG3 concentrations are higher in females than in males, and IgG4 higher in males than females. Ranges from Protein Reference Unit, Sheffield.

The level of IgG in newborn infants is similar to that of adults due to the active transfer of IgG1 and IgG3 across the placenta. This maternal IgG is catabolized during the first 6 months of life and declines to about 3 g/L or lower as the infant's own synthesis of IgG commences. Adult levels of immunoglobulins (IgG) are not attained until about 15 years of age.

Immunoglobulin IgA

IgA has a CH1–3 heavy chain structure which can be seen in Figure 2.2. It represents about 15% of plasma immunoglobulin, but it is the most abundant immunoglobulin in the tissues. This is because it is the principal immunoglobulin of the gastrointestinal tract, the respiratory tract, and the mucosal surfaces. Its native configuration is that of a dimer linked across CH2 and CH3 by a joining or J chain. In the mucosal compartment, this complex is further enveloped by a molecule called secretory component (SC), which protects the immunoglobulin from proteolytic enzymes. IgA consists of two isotypic subclasses, IgA1 and IgA2, but they are rarely measured as distinct entities.

IgA deficiency is the most common immunoglobulin deficiency, occurring in 1:500–700 white individuals in the United Kingdom, many of whom are asymptomatic. However, some patients are prone to chest infections and a host of associated clinical conditions including coeliac disease, autoimmune endocrinopathies, and pernicious anaemia.

A patient who has an IgA deficiency may go on to develop antibodies against IgA which can be IgG, IgM, or IgE class. This could put the patient at risk of an anaphylactic reaction should they require a blood transfusion, because of the presence of donor IgA.

The patient should be tested periodically for anti-IgA antibodies and carry a card detailing the risk. A few patients may have severe anaphylaxis if exposed to IgA by transfusion. If the patient who has had a reaction has to have further transfusion, it is essential to seek advice from the

Cross reference

Refer to Chapter 10.3 for the clinical correlations associated with low immunoglobulins caused by the absence or loss of function of B cells.

Cross references

See Chapter 7 for more detail about the organ-specific autoimmune diseases such as coeliac disease, autoimmune endocrinopathies, and pernicious anaemia.

Read more about IgA deficiency in the editorial by Lilic and Sewell (2001).

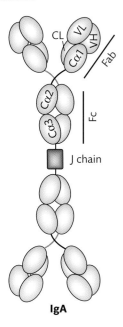

IgA

FIGURE 2.2
Structure of IgA.

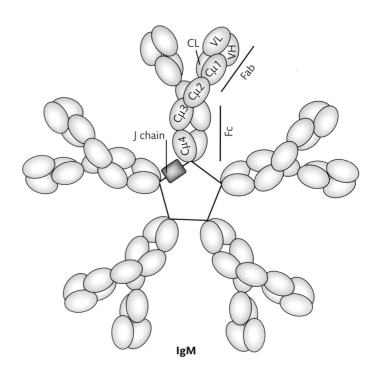

IgM

FIGURE 2.3
Structure of IgM.

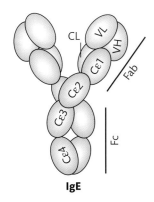

IgE

FIGURE 2.4
Structure of IgE.

Cross reference

See Chapter 3 to read in more detail about the function of IgE and its relationship with allergy.

blood transfusion department as there is a real risk of a repeat reaction unless blood components are specially selected.

Immunoglobulin IgM

IgM has a configuration of four CH domains, with five IgM molecules arranged together linked by J chain, giving a molecular weight of 1×10^6 kDa, which can be seen in Figure 2.3. IgM is predominantly an intravascular immunoglobulin comprising about 10% of the plasma immunoglobulin. Upon binding to antigen, IgM readily activates the classical complement pathway and because it has up to 10 binding sites it will cross-link and form large immune complexes. Isolated IgM deficiency is very rare indeed and is much more likely to be due to suppression by a lymphoproliferative disease or drugs than a primary immunodeficiency.

Immunoglobulin IgE

IgE has a four-CH domain structure and a molecular weight of 195 kDa, shown in Figure 2.4. Its concentration is less than 1% of plasma immunoglobulin and because of this it is measured in the laboratory by different methods from the other immunoglobulins and has different reportable units. The primary function of IgE is to bind to mast cells via high-affinity receptors in response to parasitic worm infestations. Upon binding with the parasite, IgE changes its conformation and triggers the mast cell to discharge its cocktail of proteolytic enzymes, histamine, and tryptase onto the parasite. IgE production is genetically determined, and atopic individuals produce higher levels that correlate with an increased susceptibility to developing allergies in addition to asthma, eczema, and hay fever. Thus, mast cell bound IgE is also responsible for type 1 hypersensitivity allergic responses due to mast cell degranulation. Occasionally, similar reactions can occur due to basophil degranulation due to surface-bound IgE with a similar function.

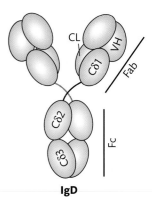

IgD

FIGURE 2.5
Structure of IgD.

CLINICAL CORRELATIONS 2.1

Hyper IgE syndrome

Hyper IgE (Job's) syndrome is a congenital condition characterized by very high plasma IgE, often of more than 50 000 kU/L. Other immunoglobulin levels appear normal. Patients endure frequent abscesses of the skin, respiratory tract, and ears with *S. aureus*, *C. albicans*, and *S. pneumoniae*, among other organisms. The lymphocytes of these patients show diminished responses to mitogen and antigen stimulation. The syndrome has been linked to a defect in the *STAT3* gene on chromosome 4.

Immunoglobulin IgD

IgD is composed of three CH domains and has a molecular weight of 175 kDa, shown in Figure 2.5. Most IgD is integral to the B-cell membranes, with very little detectable in plasma. Indeed, a normal individual may have no detectable plasma IgD.

Many reference ranges have been reported for IgD, commonly in mg/L (Vladutiu 2000), but as there is currently no international mass standard for IgD, the results can be reported as U/mL traceable to British Research standard 67/37 with a reference range of 0–100 U/mL.

CLINICAL CORRELATIONS 2.2

Hyper IgD syndrome (HIDS)

HIDS, one of the periodic fevers, is characterized by sudden onset pyrexia of over 38.5 °C, abdominal pain, vomiting with or without diarrhoea, and skin rashes. About 80% of patients have an IgD level of greater than 100 U/mL, thus 20% of patients have IgD levels within the reference range. The underlying genetic defect is mutations in the *MVK* gene leading to mevalonate kinase deficiency (MKD).

The condition usually commences before the age of 3 and 60% of patients are of Dutch or French heritage.

Table 2.2 shows the immunoglobulin reference ranges for adults. It is important to note that reference ranges for immunoglobulins are age-related. You should look up your local laboratory's reference ranges for children and older people.

TABLE 2.2 Reference ranges for immunoglobulins in adults (18–60 years)

Isotype	Adult reference range
IgG	6.0–16.0 g/L
IgA	0.8–4.0 g/L
IgM	0.5–2.0 g/L
IgD	0–100 kU/L
IgE	0–81 kU/L

2.2 **The monoclonal gammopathies**

Total plasma immunoglobulin is the product of millions of plasma cell clones in bone marrow and lymph nodes. Plasma cell clone reproduction is limited by homeostasis to produce the required amount of immunoglobulin for the required length of time to eliminate an infection. On occasion a plasma cell clone may undergo chromosomal translocations, escape from this control, and reproduce itself millions of times over. Not only does the cell replicate itself but it secretes its programmed immunoglobulin isotype in such large amounts that a discrete band is seen on electrophoresis. Since it is the product of a single cell clone it is referred to as a monoclonal immunoglobulin, the presence of which in a patient is described as a monoclonal gammopathy.

Monoclonal gammopathy can be divided into two groups. The most common presentation is as a coincidental finding during investigation of an unrelated pathology. The patient does not have symptoms attributable to the monoclonal gammopathy, the monoclonal band is less than 30g/L, and the bone marrow has less than 10% plasma cells. This is a condition termed **monoclonal gammopathy of undetermined significance (MGUS)**. The incidence of MGUS increases with age, being 1% in individuals over the age of 50, rising to 10% in those over 80 and with a higher incidence in African-Caribbean patients. The majority of patients will die *with* MGUS rather than *of* MGUS; however, in 1% per year it transforms into the second or malignant form of monoclonal gammopathy known as myeloma. MGUS patients should have a sample analysed at least annually to identify and treat those who progress to myeloma.

Cross reference

Look at section 2.3 for more detail on electrophoresis.

Monoclonal gammopathy of undetermined significance (MGUS)
Monoclonal gammopathy in which the monoclonal quantification and clinical features do not meet the diagnostic criteria for any specific disease.

CLINICAL CORRELATIONS 2.3

What is myeloma?

Myeloma (also multiple myeloma) is a disease associated with a malignant monoclonal proliferation of bone marrow plasma cells, characterized by lytic bone lesions, plasma cell accumulation in the bone marrow, and the presence of monoclonal immunoglobulin in serum and/or urine. Clinical features include bone pain, anaemia, infections, renal failure, and possible hyperviscosity syndrome. Laboratory findings include increased serum calcium, low haemoglobin, raised mean cell volume (MCV), and increased erythrocyte sedimentation rate (ESR). Five per cent of myeloma patients have no identifiable serum monoclone but do have monoclonal free light chains in their urine, whilst in 1% of patients neither a serum nor a urine monoclone can be detected.

Key Point

MGUS must be monitored at least annually as it evolves into myeloma in 1% of patients per year.

The symptoms of myeloma are of insidious onset, and are often due to the organ system most affected by the disease. Thus the patient may present with renal failure, anaemia, severe bone pain, spontaneous fractures of long bones, or collapsed vertebrae. Bone damage is due to the breakdown of the homeostatic control of bone remodelling by osteoclasts and osteoblasts. Osteoclasts dissolve bone and in the myeloma patient their activity is up-regulated in the region of the myeloma cells, as there is an imbalance in the regulatory system. Patients often present with bone pain, which may be severe. As bone is lost the patient is at risk of

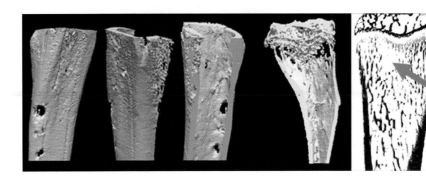

FIGURE 2.6
Osteolytic lesions in multiple myeloma.

spontaneous fractures, particularly in long bones, ribs, or vertebrae and this may lead to admission to orthopaedic wards. Look at Figure 2.6. Loss of bone leads to high plasma calcium levels, leading to renal failure and drowsiness.

The laboratory characteristics of myeloma have common features but are not uniform in all patients and are in part dictated by the type of protein secreted by the abnormal plasma cells. Whole immunoglobulin molecule myeloma (heavy and light chain combined) is the most common, with 60% of cases of IgG and over 20% of IgA isotypes. IgD myeloma represents 1% of patients and IgE myeloma is very rare. IgM myeloma is extremely rare, but has been reported (Dierlamm *et al.* 2002).

CLINICAL CORRELATIONS 2.4

Macroglobulinaemia

The condition Waldenström's macroglobulinaemia is a clonal disease of a preplasma cell called a lymphoplasmacytoid cell, producing monoclonal IgM. These lymphoid cells infiltrate bone marrow suppressing normal plasma cell production, leading to **immune paresis**. Patients often have high levels of monoclonal IgM, leading to hyperviscosity syndrome. Type 1 cryoglobulin may be seen.

Immune paresis
Suppression of normal immunoglobulin production by a malignant bone marrow plasma cell clone.

About 10% of myelomas are of κ or λ light chain only. Large quantities of monoclonal light chain may be produced, but when renal function is good much of this protein overflows into the urine, and it may not readily give rise to a visible band on serum electrophoresis (SEP), or there may be a small band with the same mobility as one of the β or α bands. Upon finding a monoclonal light chain the laboratory must exclude the possible presence of IgD and IgE heavy chains by immunofixation. Light-chain myelomas very often have immune paresis.

Cross references
You can read more about cryoglobulins in section 2.5.

See section 2.3 for more information on how immunoglobulins are quantified and to find out more about serum electrophoresis.

Look at section 2.3 for more information on immunofixation

CLINICAL CORRELATIONS 2.5

What is immune paresis?

Immune paresis is the suppression of normal immunoglobulin production by the malignant cell clone. Low immunoglobulin results may be the only sign of the presence of a small, serum-free light chain or an IgD monoclone. This is why it is important to perform immunofixation on samples from adults with low immunoglobulin results, even if no abnormal electrophoretic band can be seen.

Less than 1% of myelomas apparently do not secrete a monoclonal immunoglobulin. On bone marrow examination there are large numbers of plasma cells (>10% of nucleated bone marrow cells), which by staining with either fluorescein or enzyme-conjugated anti-immunoglobulins demonstrate that their cytoplasm is packed with one immunoglobulin isotype. These abnormal plasma cells lack the mechanism to secrete their immunoglobulin product and are thus called nonsecretory myelomas.

All of the secretory myelomas produce excess free light chains, which may be produced in quantities that overwhelm the tubules and appear in urine as overflow **proteinuria**. These light chains are monoclonal and on urine electrophoresis (UEP) form discrete bands which can be typed as κ or λ by immunofixation. The monoclonal light chains are referred to as **Bence Jones proteins**. As the disease progresses the renal tubules suffer increasing damage and loss, leading to worsening renal function, which may be the presenting clinical feature.

Examples of monoclonal IgG, IgA, and IgM heavy chain only have been described, but these are rare. The monoclone often appears on serum electrophoresis as a smear of protein immunostaining for the heavy chain in question.

The United Kingdom Nordic myeloma forum guidelines suggest concentrations of IgG and IgA isotype monoclones of more than 30 g/L; however, IgD myeloma monoclones are usually of less than 10 g/L. The concentration of the monoclonal immunoglobulin is a reflection of the size of the abnormal plasma cell clone, and it is used as the principal monitor of the success or failure of treatment, which makes it the archetypal tumour marker. Myelomas usually, but not always, have immune paresis, which may lead to repeated infections requiring antibiotic support.

Quantification of patients' monoclonal immunoglobulins is most accurately performed by densitometry or capillary zone electrophoresis (CZE), as described in section 2.3. The immunochemical methods described in section 2.3 for measuring immunoglobulins are not suitable for measuring monoclonal immunoglobulins because they use polyclonal antisera calibrated against polyclonal standards. Monoclonal immunoglobulins often lack some of the epitopes present on normal immunoglobulin and therefore bind differently to the polyclonal anti-immunoglobulin antisera, giving results that are not accurate.

CLINICAL CORRELATIONS 2.6

What is a monoclonal immunoglobulin?

Immunoglobulins are produced by B lymphocytes, with each B lymphocyte producing a specific immunoglobulin. Proliferation of a single (mono) B lymphocyte will produce a 'clone' of those lymphocytes and an associated increase in the serum level of the associated immunoglobulin. All those immunoglobulin molecules will have identical amino acid sequences and identical electrophoretic mobility and so will form a band on electrophoresis pattern. All the molecules in a monoclonal immunoglobulin (MIg, M-protein, paraprotein) will have identical heavy and light chains (see section 2.1 for immunoglobulin structure). Immunofixation identifies the heavy- and light-chain components of the sample and so can determine whether an electrophoretic band is monoclonal or not.

'Biclonal' is the term used for two monoclones present in the same serum.

2.3 Quantification of immunoglobulins

Measurement of serum immunoglobulins

In serum, IgG, IgA, and IgM are amenable to measurement by simple antibody–antigen (Ab:Ag) immune complex formation assays such as nephelometry and turbidimetry. Because there are few IgD assays requested, IgD is usually measured by ELISA. IgE is usually assayed by labelled immunoassays such as ELISA or chemiluminescence. Radial immunodiffusion methods are available for IgG, IgA, and IgM but are rarely used in British laboratories. The most important requirements for either methodology are to maintain **antibody excess** in the reaction mixture and to be aware of when **antigen excess** may occur and how to deal with it. The assays must, therefore, be validated by the manufacturer to use the optimum amount of antibody, dilution of sample, and volume of sample.

In antibody excess the fixed amount of antibody binds antigen, and because of the two binding sites per molecule and the polyclonal nature of antibody, it cross-links to other antigen molecules forming a three-dimensional lattice immune complex in the diluent buffer. With increasing antigen concentration, more of the antibody is consumed in the immune complex. At the equivalence point the amounts of antibody and antigen are equal, the immune complex lattice formation is maximal, and the immune complex forms and redissolves at an equal rate. The addition of more antigen creates an antigen excess condition where the antibody's binding sites become occupied by single antigens and cannot cross-link. Thus the lattice structure begins to break apart and redissolve. With increasing antigen excess the lattice will redissolve completely. The states of antibody and antigen excess were defined by Heidelberger and Kendall in the 1930s and are described by the bell curve named after them (Figure 2.7). It is the amount of immune complex lattice formation that the optical systems in nephelometry and turbidimetry measure, and if the lattice is reduced by antigen excess then a false low result will be produced.

There are various strategies to minimize the interference from antigen excess. All analysers dilute the sample before assaying it, and will redilute samples giving a signal higher than the highest calibrator value. Nephelometers are more sophisticated than turbidimetric systems and they may produce calibration curves with a very broad dynamic range that extends well into the predicted antigen excess zone. A prereaction analysis may also be used, where a small amount of the sample is mixed with the standard volume of antibody and the reaction is monitored for a few seconds. If the lattice formation proceeds rapidly this may be due to very high antigen concentration and the assay is stopped and processed at a higher dilution of the sample.

> **Antibody excess**
> The state in an antibody/antigen mixture where the concentration of antibody exceeds that of antigen.
>
> **Antigen excess**
> The state in an antibody/antigen mixture where the concentration of antigen exceeds that of antibody.

Key Point

You must understand the principle of antigen excess and how the individual analysers deal with this in the routine laboratory setting.

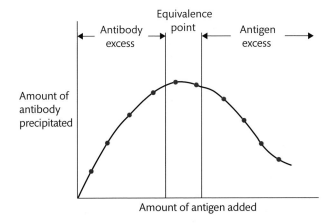

FIGURE 2.7
The Heidelberger–Kendall curve.

Nephelometry is the measurement of light scattered by particles, and has been adapted as immunonephelometry to measure light scattered by immune complexes formed in a small optical cuvette. When the wavelength of the incident light is smaller than the immune complex then forward-angle light scatter predominates. This is known as Rayleigh–Debye scattering and it maximizes the amount of light scattered to the optical detector which is located at an angle from the light path. Increasing scattered light is directly proportional to the antigen concentration.

In turbidimetry, the optical system measures the light transmitted as apparent absorbance, or optical density. The amount of light passed through the reaction mixture is inversely proportional to the antigen concentration.

For optimal performance, both immunonephelometry and immunoturbidimetry include polyethylene glycol (PEG) in the reaction mixture. This high molecular weight polymer is highly hygroscopic and is thought to remove water molecules from around the antibody and antigen, bringing the two closer together and allowing the formation of measurable immune complexes in a few minutes.

All assay systems for immunoglobulin rely on the use of international reference material to standardize instrument calibration. For IgG, IgA, and IgM this is known as CRM 470 and all assays used in clinical laboratories must state that the calibration standard in use is derived from CRM 470. There is no agreed international standard for IgG subclasses and IgD.

Key Point

Use of calibration material traceable to the IRP CRM 470 helps to standardize results between laboratories.

Laboratories must not rely on immunoglobulin quantification to detect the presence of monoclonal bands on the assumption that all significant monoclones will give results higher than the normal range or exhibit immune paresis. There are many examples of clinically significant monoclones—particularly light-chain and IgD isotypes, and most MGUS cases—where the total immunoglobulin assay results are well within the normal range. Only by combining immunoglobulin quantification with serum electrophoresis and immunofixation can the presence of a monoclone be ruled out.

Urine electrophoresis and Bence Jones protein

Excess free light chains produced by plasma cells in myeloma 'overflow' into the urine where they can be detected by urine electrophoresis. This swamping of the reabsorption capacity of renal tubules is called **overflow proteinuria** and it can also be seen with other small, readily filtered proteins such as myoglobin following crush injury.

Overflow proteinuria
Proteinuria caused by glomerular filtration of levels of protein which exceed the reabsorption capacity of the renal tubules.

Monoclonal free light chains in urine were originally known as 'Bence Jones protein', for historical reasons, but the more specific name 'monoclonal free light chains' is to be preferred. Urinary whole monoclonal immunoglobulin (i.e. with both heavy and light chains) is not Bence Jones protein.

Monoclonal free light chains filtering through the kidney may damage nephrons due to the deposition of the proteins in the tubules or tubular damage via tubular toxicity. All patients with suspected myeloma should have both serum and urine electrophoresis performed.

Urine monoclonal free light chains are not necessarily indicative of myeloma or malignant disease (Beetham 2000), but where laboratory data is indicative, information on new serum or urine free light chain monoclones should be telephoned urgently to the requesting source.

Measurement of free light chains

In recent years, The Binding Site Ltd has marketed kits for the assay of serum κ and λ free light chains, known commercially as Freelite™. These assays have been developed for nephelometric and turbidimetric systems. Both assays use polyclonal antibodies to antigenic determinants on light chains which are normally hidden by the partner heavy chain. This allows measurement of the concentration of free light chains in monoclonal gammopathies and it is a particularly suitable method for diseases which express free light chains only, i.e. light-chain myelomas and amyloidosis. The assays also detect free light chain in many samples from patients classified as having nonsecretory myeloma, thus potentially giving the clinicians a diagnostic and monitoring marker for some examples of this disease. Measurement of free light chains also provides a useful marker for the risk of progression to myeloma by MGUS patients. If the MGUS patient has an abnormal κ:λ free light chain ratio, then they are at least 2.6 times more likely to develop myeloma than if the ratio is normal.

The Freelite™ assay requires care and experience in its use and interpretation. Results are expressed in mg/L and patients with light-chain myeloma are sometimes measured with apparently 60 000 mg/L, i.e. 60 g/L, when the electrophoresis strip clearly shows a monoclonal band by densitometry of perhaps 3–4 g/L. The assay is acknowledged to be nonlinear and susceptible to antigen excess, because of the limited number of antigenic epitopes on an abnormal monoclonal light chain. Analytical protocols are provided with the commercial kits for the instruments for which the assay is configured, in an effort to address these issues. However, the controls provided in the kits have target levels of less than 100 mg/L, which is well below the levels seen in myeloma patients. When using these assays, laboratories should consider producing their own high-level controls from pooled patient material.

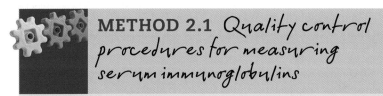

METHOD 2.1 *Quality control procedures for measuring serum immunoglobulins*

Laboratories must establish an internal quality control (IQC) procedure using samples of known concentration and the standard deviation about that known concentration. Using the statistical models and rules developed by James Westgard, the laboratory can apply rules for multiple levels of immunoglobulin concentration and reject runs that exceed these limits. Internal control runs must be performed and recorded before and after each batch of patient samples. Figure 2.8 shows an example of a Levy–Jennings chart.

External quality assessment (EQA) is achieved by the laboratory assaying samples sent from a central body and reporting the results as if they were patient material. In the United Kingdom the National External Quality Assessment Scheme (UKNEQAS) for specific proteins provides this service, dispatching two samples per month to participating laboratories. UKNEQAS provides a report on the participant's performance of the assay compared to other laboratories, performance trends, and differences between assay providers.

Cross reference

Look at http://www.westgard.com/westgard-rules/ for more information on Westgard rules and how to use them in the laboratory.

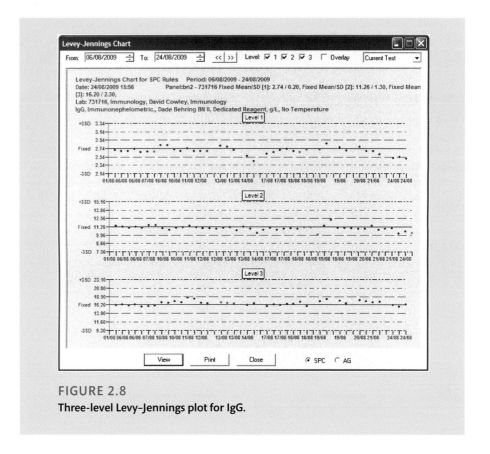

FIGURE 2.8
Three-level Levy–Jennings plot for IgG.

Electrophoresis

Together with serum immunoglobulin measurement, serum and urine electrophoresis form the primary screen for monoclonal gammopathy. Monoclonal immunoglobulin usually produces an abnormal banding pattern on electrophoresis.

Electrophoresis is a technique which uses an electric field to separate molecules according to their electric charge. Most hospital laboratories use automated or semi-automated electrophoresis systems which make analysis faster and simpler. The semi-automated systems use gel electrophoresis techniques, while the fully automated systems are usually capillary zone electrophoresis (CZE). Semi-automated techniques require significant manual input, so it is important to understand how the method works and how to get the best results from it, whereas CZE is more 'press-and-go'. However, both technologies require an understanding of the same two concepts: the isoelectric point and how it relates to the behaviour of proteins in solution, and electroendosmotic flow.

The isoelectric point (pI)

Amino acids are the building blocks of protein and have a general structure as shown in Figure 2.9. When amino acids are placed in solution they form ionic species. Whether an amino acid becomes positively or negatively charged depends upon the nature of the amino acid R group, and the pH of the solution.

When a whole protein is placed in solution, its net charge is the sum of the charges on its component amino acids. The isoelectric point (p*I*) is the pH at which the protein net charge is zero. The p*I* for any given protein is constant and specific for that protein.

When the solution is acidic relative to the p*I* the protein will gain protons from the solution and, if an electric field is applied, the protein will migrate towards the cathode. When the solution is basic relative to the p*I* the protein will donate protons to the solution and will migrate towards the anode.

Most gel systems use an alkaline buffer. At these pH levels all serum proteins have a net negative charge and should move towards the anode.

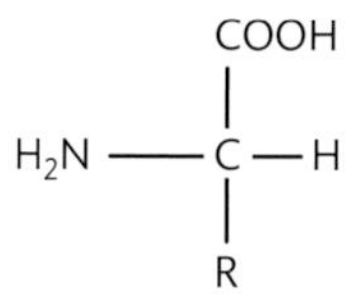

Electroendosmotic flow

Electroendosmosis (sometimes called electro-osmosis or endosmosis) is an effect caused by the use of an immobile support medium which has a negative charge relative to that of a mobile solution. When an electric field is applied to the system the relatively positive ions in the solution begin to flow towards the cathode. The flow strength increases as the charge difference between the two phases (mobile and immobile) increases, and also as the voltage increases.

COOH
|
H_2N —— C — H
|
R

FIGURE 2.9
General structure of an amino acid.

Cross reference
For a more complete explanation of electrophoretic techniques, see Keren (2003).

Gel protein electrophoresis

Method

Separation occurs within a gel (usually agarose on a plastic support) which is loaded with buffer pH 8.6. Sample is applied between the anodal and cathodal ends of the gel. The amount of protein applied to the gel is determined by the concentration of protein in the sample and length of time the sample is allowed to diffuse into the gel.

As the electrophoresis buffer is alkaline relative to the pI of the serum proteins, the proteins become negatively charged. When an electric field is applied the proteins begin to more towards the anode. This may be at different velocities, depending on the net negative charge of the protein.

However, the agarose gel is negatively charged relative to the buffer, and this sets up an electro-endosmotic flow of positive buffer ions towards the cathode. For protein molecules with low net negative charge the pull towards the anode is weaker than the pull of the electroendosmotic flow and, like poor swimmers in a strong current, they are carried towards the cathode.

After electrophoresis the gel is dried and stained with a protein-selective stain. By using a protein-selective stain the molecules of interest, in this case immunoglobulins, can be visualized without excessive interference from other serum components, such as hormones, metabolites, and ions.

A 'normal' serum **protein electrophoresis** pattern shows six major fractions. There are five bands—albumin, α_1, α_2, β_1, and β_2, and a nonbanded γ region. These are shown in Figures 2.10a and 2.10b. Table 2.3 lists some of the proteins that are found in each of the major fractions.

A 'normal' urine protein electrophoresis pattern shows only an albumin band, which can be seen in Figure 2.11.

Protein electrophoresis
The separation of the protein molecules within a solution (usually serum, urine, or cerebrospinal fluid) as a result of their differing mobilities within an electric field.

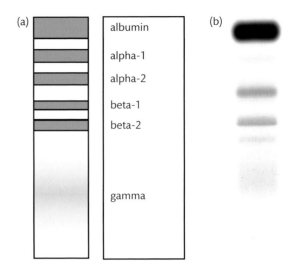

FIGURE 2.10
(a) Diagrammatic representation of serum protein separation in gel electrophoresis (b) Normal serum protein electrophoresis.

TABLE 2.3   Proteins found in the regions of protein electrophoresis

Region	Major proteins present
Albumin	Albumin
α_1	α_1-Antitrypsin, α_1 acid glycoprotein
α_2	α_2-Macroglobulin, haptoglobin
β_1	Transferrin
β_2	C3
γ	Immunoglobulins (γ-globulins)

FIGURE 2.11
Normal urine protein electrophoresis.

SELF-CHECK 2.1

Why it is important to use a protein-selective stain in electrophoresis?

Technical points to note

The gel

- Gels packaged in excess buffer require 'blotting' before use—excess surface buffer can interfere with sample application.
- To prevent distortion of migration, gels need to be uniform. Care should be taken when handling gels and, ideally, gels with obvious defects should not be used.
- Voltage application generates heat. This heat needs to be removed, and one way of achieving this is via a Peltier plate—an electrical device which can provide or remove heat. If the system uses a Peltier plate it is important that the contact between the gel and the plate is uniform so that optimal heat transfer can occur.

Sample preparation

- Serum should be used in preference to plasma, as plasma contains fibrinogen. Haemolysed and lipaemic samples should also be avoided. Early morning urine is preferred as it has a higher protein concentration.

- Urine electrophoresis methods need to be able to detect protein fractions down to approximately 10 mg/L If this cannot be achieved using neat urine, then urine samples should be concentrated before application using an ultrafiltration membrane with a cut-off of <10 kDa, to ensure no free light chains are lost. Sample is loaded onto the membrane and water is either absorbed through the membrane by absorbent pads, or liquid may be pulled through the membrane by centrifugation. Concentration should occur until an albumin band is visible.

- CZE has few advantages to offer over other systems for urine electrophoresis, but if this method is to be used, urine requires concentration and desalting. Desalting improves electrophoretic resolution and is achieved by dialysis.

Sample application

- Sample is applied to the gel surface via an 'application device' which allows consistent application of a number of samples simultaneously. Each sample is loaded into its own reservoir on the applicator from where the sample is 'wicked' down and applied to the gel surface at a steady rate. It is important that the applicator or wick is not overloaded, the result of which can be seen in Figure 2.12.

- Conversely, crystals in urine can impede the flow of sample down the wick and result in under-application, as can cryoglobulin in serum samples.

Staining

- The first step is to fix the proteins within the gel using an acidic solution. Some systems have separate fix and stain solutions, others have a combined fix/stain. If the acid fixative is reused then its pH will increase over time as a result of contamination with pH 8.6 gel buffer. To maintain good staining it is important to replace the fix solution at the recommended intervals.

- Amido Black and Acid Violet are the most frequently used stains. Amido Black is usually used for serum protein electrophoresis staining, and the more sensitive Acid Violet stain is used for urine protein electrophoresis and for immunofixation. An ideal stain binds linearly to protein, meaning that the amount of protein present is directly related to the stain intensity. This allows the quantification of bands within the gel by **densitometry**.

- After staining the gel is 'destained' a number of times to remove background staining, thus enhancing the contrast between the stained proteins and clear gel.

Reading protein electrophoresis gels

A textbook can only give an introduction to reading gels. The only way to learn to read gels is by doing it routinely in a clinical laboratory.

- Before starting to read, prepare your environment:
  - Sit in an area with good lighting and (ideally) no distractions.
  - Find a piece of clean white paper to place behind the gel—this will help show up changes in stain density (some people prefer yellow for reading urine gels).
- Check that any internal quality control samples on the gel have run correctly.

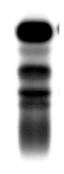

FIGURE 2.12
An example of sample 'overloading' on gel electrophoresis.

Densitometry
The quantitative measurement of optical density.

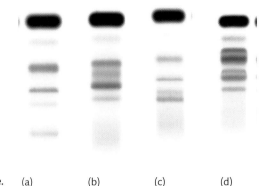

FIGURE 2.13

(a) A strip from a sample containing a monoclonal immunoglobulin;
(b) a sample with haemolysis; (c) a sample with fibrinogen; (d) a sample
with lipaemia. These show patterns which can be mistaken for a monoclone.

(a)   (b)   (c)   (d)

Serum

- Depending which system is being used, there may be five or six regions (in higher–resolution systems the β region can be split). Note whether these five (six) regions are visible.

- Note whether the staining in each region is lower than normal, normal, or greater than normal. (This may not be as easy as it sounds since stain intensity can vary significantly between gels. The usual method is to assess the average intensity for that region over the whole gel and use this as 'normal' for that gel.)

- Note whether there are any extra bands present and where they are in relation to the named regions.

Figure 2.13 shows a strip from a sample containing a monoclonal immunoglobulin and samples with haemolysis, fibrinogen, and lipaemia. These show patterns that can be mistaken for a monoclone.

Table 2.4 details some of the major electrophoresis patterns seen in the laboratory setting.

Using these observations, together with the knowledge of how protein levels alter in disease and information from other blood tests, a final decision can be reached about whether further investigation for monoclonal gammopathy is required. A sample showing an unexplained banding pattern together with immune paresis or with raised IgA or IgM levels should be sent for **immunofixation**.

Immunofixation

Process in which a specific antibody is used to 'fix' antigens within a gel after electrophoresis by means of the formation of antibody–antigen complexes. After removing unfixed molecules by washing and then staining the fixed complexes, the presence or absence of specific molecules in the original sample can be demonstrated.

Cross reference

You can read more about IgM in PBC in Chapter 8.

Key Point

Raised immunoglobulins are seen in many different diseases, e.g. raised IgA in heavy drinkers with renal dysfunction, or raised IgM in primary biliary cirrhosis (PBC). Depending on the clinical reasoning for doing electrophoresis, immunofixation may not be requested.

Urine

- Note whether there is an albumin band present.
- Note whether there are any other bands present.

TABLE 2.4 A breakdown of the major patterns seen on protein gel electrophoresis

A. Single region with altered staining intensity	
Absent α_1 band	Associated with α_1-antitrypsin deficiency, or with an α_1-antitrypsin variant with altered electrophoretic mobility
Absent β_2 band	Usually seen in aged samples. C3 is converted to C3c, which runs in the β_1 region
Reduced γ region	May be associated with reduced immunoglobulins, but may be normal (e.g. in young children) **Need to measure immunoglobulins to assess properly**
Increased γ region	May be associated with increased polyclonal immunoglobulins (e.g. in infection or chronic disease) but may be artefact due to overstaining **Need to measure immunoglobulins to assess properly**
β–γ bridging	Increased staining under the β_2 band is known as β–γ bridging. Seen in liver disease and associated with raised polyclonal IgA and (sometimes) IgM **Need to measure immunoglobulins to assess properly**
B. Altered intensity in several bands	
Acute phase response	Decreased albumin, increased α_1 ($\uparrow\alpha_1$-antitrypsin), increased α_2 ($\uparrow\alpha_2$-macroglobulin and haptoglobin), normal/decreased β_1 ($\downarrow$transferrin), normal/increased β_2 ($\uparrow$C3), normal/increased γ
Chronic inflammatory pattern	As acute phase response but with additional increased γ region
Cirrhotic pattern	Albumin, α_1, α_2, β_1, and β_2 bands all decreased due to reduced protein production by the liver with an increased γ region
Nephrotic pattern	All regions are reduced due to protein loss through the kidney, particularly albumin and the γ regions. The α_2 band is normal or increased as α_2 macroglobulin is too large to be lost in this way. A reduction may be seen in the β band as transferrin is lost, but C3 may be raised
C. Extra bands present[a]	
Bisalbuminaemia	Bisalbuminaemia is an inherited abnormality of albumin in which both normal albumin and an albumin variant are produced. The variant has a different electrophoretic mobility, but may migrate either above or below the normal band. Bisalbuminaemia has no clinical significance
Fibrinogen	If plasma is tested rather than serum, an extra band due to fibrinogen (the protein from which the fibrin clot is formed when blood coagulates) is seen below the β_2 band. A fibrinogen band may obscure a monoclone in this region
Haemoglobin–haptoglobin	Free haemoglobin in blood is scavenged by haptoglobin. The haemoglobin–haptoglobin complex has an electrophoretic mobility different from that of free haptoglobin and this shows as an extra band in the region between the α_2 and β_1 bands. It is most commonly seen in haemolysed samples
Lipoprotein	All samples contain lipoproteins, but they are not usually detectable on gel electrophoresis. In patients with raised lipoprotein levels extra bands with a distinctive shape may be seen in the α and β regions
Monoclonal immunoglobulin	Bands due to monoclonal immunoglobulins can migrate between the α_2 band and the end of the γ region. Their intensity can vary significantly, and small monoclones can easily 'hide' under the normal bands. It is recommended to measure IgG, IgA, and IgM on samples for serum electrophoresis, as abnormal immunoglobulin levels with a normal electrophoresis pattern may suggest a concealed monoclonal band

[a] Extra bands are not necessarily abnormal, but they need to be investigated and accounted for.

The staining patterns seen on urine electrophoresis are much more variable than those seen on serum, and any sample showing either no albumin bands or bands in addition to albumin should be investigated further by immunofixation.

Capillary zone electrophoresis

Method

Separation occurs in a liquid buffer (pH ~10—the exact value depends upon the analyser used) flowing through a fused silica capillary tube. A set volume of sample is then aspirated and introduced into the anodal end of the capillary.

The buffer is alkaline relative to the pI of serum proteins, so the proteins donate protons to the buffer and become negatively charged. When an electric field is applied, the proteins remain at the anode. However, the interior of the capillary has a strong negative charge relative to the buffer, and the application of a high voltage creates a strong electroendosmotic flow of buffer ions to the cathode. The pull of this flow is much stronger than the attraction to the anode and so the proteins begin to move towards the cathode. Proteins with the lowest net negative charge at pH 10 have the weakest attraction to the anode. They travel rapidly in the electro-endosmotic flow and reach the cathode first. Proteins with the highest net negative charge at pH 10 have the strongest attraction to the anode. This retards their movement and they reach the cathode later, as shown in Figure 2.14.

A UV detector at the cathodal end of the capillary detects the proteins as they pass, by using peptide bond UV absorbance at 214 nm. From this, a plot of absorption versus time—an electropherogram—can be constructed. A 'normal' serum protein electropherogram shows the same six major fractions as gel electrophoresis: five bands—albumin α_1, α_2, β_1, and β_2 and a nonbanded γ region (see Figure 2.15a)—whereas urine shows only a trace of albumin, as shown in Figure 2.15b.

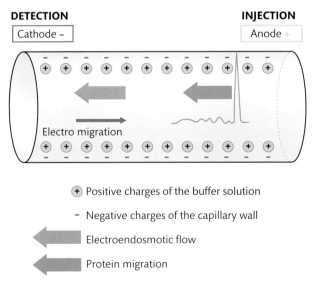

FIGURE 2.14
Protein migration towards the cathode.

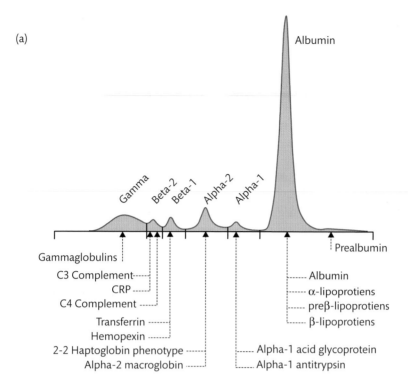

(a)

Albumin

Gamma
Beta-2
Beta-1
Alpha-2
Alpha-1

Prealbumin

Gammaglobulins
C3 Complement
CRP
C4 Complement
Transferrin
Hemopexin
2-2 Haptoglobin phenotype
Alpha-2 macroglobin

Albumin
α-lipoprotiens
preβ-lipoprotiens
β-lipoprotiens

Alpha-1 acid glycoprotein
Alpha-1 antitrypsin

(b)   Urine normale

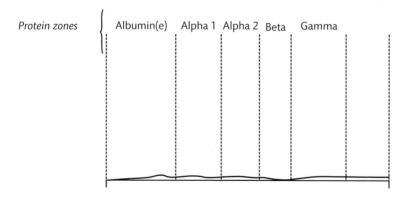

Protein zones

Albumin(e)   Alpha 1   Alpha 2   Beta   Gamma

FIGURE 2.15
(a) Normal serum protein electropherogram; (b) normal urine electropherogram.

Technical points to note

Buffer

- Different buffers are used for different applications. Ensure you are using the correct buffer and that the system has been primed before use.

Sample application and separation

- Urine samples may need special preparation, e.g. desalting, before testing.
- Unlike gel electrophoresis, where each sample has its own individual section of gel, the capillaries in CZE analysers are washed and then prepared for the next sample. It is important

to follow cleaning and maintenance protocols to ensure that the capillaries remain clean and give good performance.

Reading protein electropherograms

As with reading protein electrophoresis gels, the only way to become proficient at reading electropherograms is through practice.

Serum

Although the electropherogram trace for normal serum appears comparable with the pattern seen on gel electrophoresis (i.e. albumin α_1, α_2, β_1, β_2, and a γ region), they are not exactly the same. Some proteins run in different positions, e.g. both the α- and β-lipoproteins run within the albumin peak on CZE.

Some proteins run in the same area but have more visibility on CZE. An example is α_1-acid glycoprotein, which runs in the α_1 region on both gel electrophoresis and CZE. However, whereas it does not stain well on gel electrophoresis because of its heavy glycosylation, it is easily detected by CZE using peptide bond UV absorption. Thus α_1-antitrypsin-deficient samples may be less easily detected using CZE with a six-fraction buffer, as the presence of the acid glycoprotein means that a peak is almost always visible in the α_1 region.

CZE shows extra bands due to haemolysis, fibrinogen, and monoclonal proteins similar to those seen on gel electrophoresis. Unlike gel electrophoresis, CZE also shows extra peaks in the sera of patients given radio-opaque agents (e.g. for coronary angiography). These agents are not proteins, but they absorb UV light at similar frequencies. Peaks can occur in any region of the electropherogram, depending upon the type of contrast media present.

All unusual and/or extra peaks on the electropherogram need investigating further. As with gel electrophoresis, it is possible for small monoclones to hide under normal peaks and so it is recommended to measure IgG, IgA, and IgM on all samples to try and identify those that may contain a concealed monoclonal band.

Urine

All samples with bands other than albumin require further investigation, as do samples without a visible albumin band on electrophoresis.

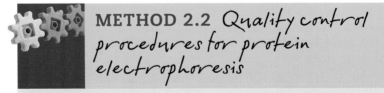

METHOD 2.2 Quality control procedures for protein electrophoresis

Electrophoresis requires the running of internal quality control samples, just as other laboratory tests do. It is recommended to run a known paraprotein of known concentration in parallel.

UKNEQAS for immunology runs a scheme for monoclonal protein identification which includes serum and urine protein electrophoresis and also serum and urine monoclone identification and quantification.

What sample (or samples) would you run as internal quality controls for serum and urine electrophoresis, and why?

Immunofixation

The primary purpose of immunofixation ('fixing') is to identify the presence and determine the isotype (the heavy and light chains present) of a monoclonal immunoglobulin in a sample. The technique uses gel electrophoresis followed by reaction with antisera against heavy and light chains. However, it can also be used to determine the presence or absence of any protein for which a specific antiserum is available. Immunofixation is the only way of determining the presence of a small monoclone under a normal electrophoretic band.

Not all samples showing abnormalities require immunofixation. For example, samples from patients with a known, obvious monoclonal band do not need fixing every time a serum is received in the laboratory unless there is a significant change, such as another band appearing. Similarly, a haemolysis pattern obtained from a haemolysed sample does not need investigation unless other pathology test results suggest that there may also be a monoclone present.

CLINICAL CORRELATIONS 2.7

Why is it important to type the monoclone?

■ Certain diseases are associated with certain monoclone types, e.g. IgM monoclones are associated with Waldenström's macroglobulinaemia.

■ Certain monoclone types such as an IgD monoclone, are associated with a poorer prognosis.

■ The presence of comigrating monoclones with different isotypes can be identified by immunofixation.

■ There are different clinical correlations with free κ and free λ light chains. Free λ light chains are most commonly associated with AL amyloidosis. Free κ light chains are most commonly associated with light chain deposition disease. Prognosis of these two diseases are different, therefore it is important to know the type of free light chain.

Method

Immunofixation has four stages:

1. Electrophoresis: each sample is run in a number of identical lanes (usually six).
2. Antisera application: a general protein fixative (usually acid) is applied to lane 1 to give a reference track and then specific antisera are applied to the other protein lanes. If a corresponding antigen is present in the sample, immune complexes form between it and the antiserum. These complexes lodge ('fix') within the gel matrix. The usual protocol for initial immunofixation is fixative, anti-G, -A and -M heavy chains, anti-κ and anti-λ light chains.
3. Wash: all unfixed proteins are washed from the gel.
4. Stain: all the fixed proteins are stained with a sensitive stain, such as Acid Violet.

By comparing the proteins fixed in each lane, the constituents of an electrophoretic band can be identified and its mono- or polyclonality determined. Undefined bands may be seen

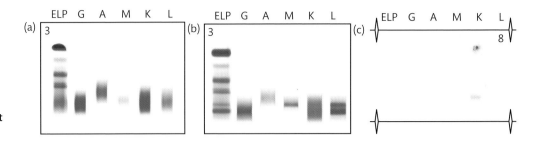

FIGURE 2.16
(a) Normal serum immunofixation;
(b) serum bi-clone IgGλ and IgMλ;
(c) urine κ free light chain.

in the γ region associated with chronic inflammatory states such as infection or autoimmune disease. Look at Figure 2.16 for examples of immunofixation.

Technical points to note

Electrophoresis

- Immunofixation is more sensitive than electrophoresis alone and so serum samples are usually diluted before application. Immunofixation is subject to antibody/antigen excess effects so the dilution factors need to be chosen carefully. Urine samples can be applied neat or concentrated. The concentration factor usually depends upon the urine total protein level.

Antisera application

- Ensure any devices for applying antisera are clean and dry so that there is no carry-over between tracks.
- Immunofixation is capable of giving false-negative results due to antibody or antigen excess. In these situations only small immune complexes are formed. These cannot fix within the gel and are washed out with the other nonfixed proteins. Antigen excess shows as a 'cut-out' hole in the middle of the band. This is shown in Figure 2.17. To confirm this, the serum can be diluted and retested. However, if you have to dilute the sample, either to reduce the likelihood of antigen excess occurring (e.g. if a large monoclone is present or because the immunoglobulin level is raised overall), then there is a possibility of 'diluting out' any small monoclones that might also be present. Complete investigation may sometimes require testing at a number of different sample dilutions.
- Occasionally, there is some difficulty in detecting IgA λ paraproteins, as the λ light chains do not stain. Sometimes changing the anti-λ source to another commercial company resolves this.

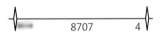

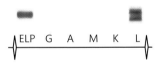

FIGURE 2.17
Antigen excess on immunofixation. See how the band in the λ lane has its centre 'cut out'.

Immunofixation interpretation

Serum

- Bands in the individual antisera lanes must line up with those in the reference lane and must match the pattern seen on electrophoresis. Whole monoclones are most common, free light chain monoclones are not uncommon, and monoclones of heavy chain only are rare but possible.
- IgA paraproteins tend to have a tight band; IgA heavy chain monoclones can appear like a smear due to the fragmented heavy chain.
- Immunofixes showing a possible free light chain monoclone must have IgD and IgE monoclones excluded (usually by further immunofixation with IgD and IgE antisera).

- Where raised polyclonal immunoglobulin is present it may not be possible to identify small monoclones against the deeply stained background, commonly seen in viral infections. Repeat at a higher dilution if necessary.

- Some IgM monoclones may precipitate at the application point and not separate electrophoretically. Pre-treatment with 1 mol/L dithiothreitol (DTT) reduces polymerization by interrupting disulphide linkages between the molecules and can resolve the problem in most cases. (DTT is less hazardous than 2-mercaptoethanol, which was traditionally used for this purpose.)

Urine

Bands in the individual antisera lanes must line up with those in the reference lane and must match the pattern seen on electrophoresis.

Immunotyping by CZE

Immunotyping by CZE is the equivalent of immunofixation, but is currently limited to detection of IgG, IgA, IgM, and free light chain monoclones.

Method

Incubating the serum with specific antiserum (anti-IgG, anti-IgA, anti-IgM, anti-κ light chain or anti-λ light chain), either attached to a bead or in fluid phase, will remove or alter the mobility of the corresponding peak.

The electropherogram obtained for each supernatant is compared with that for nontreated serum. If a monoclone is present, a peak will be seen on the untreated electropherogram. If the monoclone is caused by one of the five isotypes tested, the supernatant from that well will show an electropherogram with the peak missing. The isotype of this well can then be assigned to the monoclone. Monoclonal peaks will show subtraction of the peak in electropherograms corresponding to a single heavy and a single light chain antiserum, while polyclonal peaks will have partial subtractions with both light chain antisera and potentially more than one heavy chain antiserum. This is shown in Figure 2.18.

Technical points to note

- If the monoclonal fraction does not totally disappear on the antisera patterns, then a higher serum dilution may be required.

- Small clones (<5 g) are not easily detectable by immunotyping. It is better to use gel-based methods instead.

Interpretation

- The detected monoclonal peak must be located at the same migration distance as the suspect monoclonal fraction seen in the reference lane.

- Where there is a small monoclone in the presence of raised polyclonal immunoglobulins or under a normal peak, it may not be possible to detect the small subtraction trace produced—if suspicious, confirm with immunofixation.

- Samples which appear to have more than one monoclonal component should be pretreated with a depolymerizing agent and retested to exclude polymerization. This tends to be an issue in hyperviscosity syndrome associated with IgA and IgG3 myelomas.

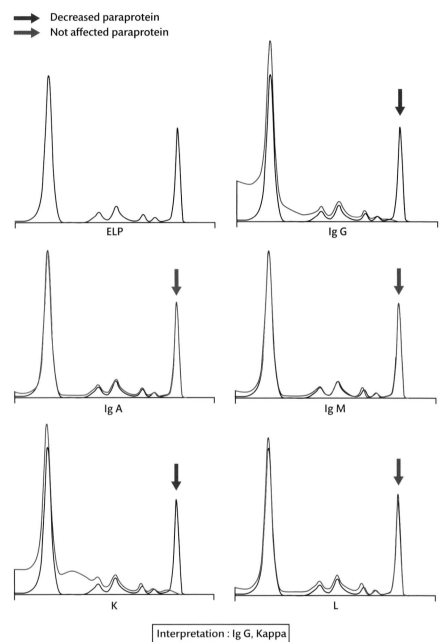

FIGURE 2.18
An example of subtraction showing an IgG κ monoclone.

- Traces showing a possible free light chain monoclone should have IgD and IgE monoclones excluded. This will usually require immunofixation with IgD and IgE antisera, as immuno-subtraction for IgD/IgE is not yet commercially available.

Densitometry

When a monoclonal immunoglobulin is present it requires quantification. Initial quantification can give information about prognosis in some diseases and serial measurements can be used to assess disease progression and therapy effectiveness. Densitometry is used because it allows monoclones to be quantified individually and specifically. This is not the case with immunoglobulin measurements, where monoclonal and polyclonal immunoglobulin cannot be separated and multiple monoclones cannot be quantified separately.

Method

When light is passed through an electrophoresis strip, the amount of light absorbed by the gel at any point is related to the intensity of the stain (the wavelength chosen depends on the stain used). A plot of absorbance over the length of the electrophoresis strip gives the densitometric scan for that sample. Originally this required a densitometer with different light filters for different stains, but it is more usual now to use simple flat-bed scanners with software conversion of the signal into that expected from a densitometer.

If a linear stain has been used, then the stain intensity is directly related to the amount of protein in the strip and the area under the scan is equal to the sample total protein. By dividing the scan using 'gates', the percentage of the total protein in an area can be calculated. If the serum total protein is measured, the monoclone percentage protein can be converted into a monoclone quantification. The plot of UV absorbance against time in the CZE electropherogram is directly comparable with the densitometric plot of light absorbance against gel length and is used to quantify monoclonal peaks in the same way. Look at Figure 2.19 to see a densitometric scan.

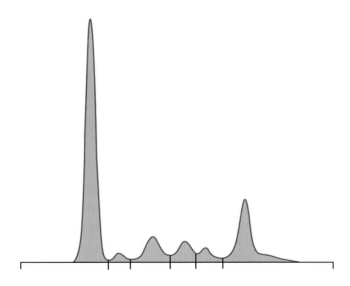

Serum protein electrophoresis

Fractions	%	Ref. %	Conc.	Ref. Conc.
pre-albumi	56.7		21.66	39.00–46.00
alpha-1	2.3		0.88	0.90–1.70
alpha-2	9.7		3.71	5.00–7.00
beta-1	6.5		2.48	4.00–6.00
beta-2	4.3		1.64	1.00–3.00
gamma	20.5		7.83	5.00–11.00

FIGURE 2.19

An example of a densitometric scan.

Technical points to note

- Flat-bed scanners pick up artefacts. Ensure the back of the gel and the scanner plate are free of stain deposits, dust, hairs, etc. before scanning. When analysing the scans, be aware of bands on the scan which are not on the gel. Such artefactual bands are common with urine scans but can also occur with serum.

- There is a nonlinear relationship between dye-binding and protein concentration at high monoclone concentrations.

- Despite the ability of densitometry to gate monoclonal bands individually, the quantification may still not be totally specific for the monoclone. Where a relatively small monoclone overlays a polyclonal background, a significant proportion of the monoclonal quantification will be polyclonal in origin.

- Where a monoclone underlies a normal band (e.g. β_2) it is not possible to quantify the monoclone specifically. Quantification involving subtraction of a nominal value for a normal background band and reporting of the 'corrected' value, or only reporting the area of the peak above the normal band introduces errors. In this case the whole β_2 band should be quantified and then a comment added to the results to say that the quantification includes the normal proteins of the β_2 region.

- Total protein is commonly measured by standard Biuret method; however, different total protein methods can give different results and this can have an effect on monoclone quantification.

- Gating strategies differ between laboratories. It is important that all staff in a given laboratory use the same gating strategy so that results between sequential patient samples are consistent and comparable.

CASE STUDY 2.1 *Myeloma*

A sample was received for serum protein electrophoresis on a 77-year-old man with back pain and anaemia.

- The sample contained a large band which was not present in normal serum.

- Serum immunofixation of the sample identified that the band consisted of a monoclonal immunoglobulin (monoclone) with the isotype IgG κ.

- Using **scanning densitometry** and measurements of serum albumin and total protein, the monoclone was quantified at 30 g/L.

- A 24-hour urine sample from the patient was received for urine protein electrophoresis. This also showed a band that was not present in normal urine.

- Urine immunofixation showed that this band was also monoclonal but, unlike the serum, it consisted of immunoglobulin κ light chains only.

- Following measurement of urine total protein, scanning densitometry was used to quantify the urine monoclone at 0.4 g/24 hours.

The results were telephoned immediately to the requesting clinician as the patient had one of the diagnostic criteria for myeloma: the presence of a monoclonal protein in the serum or urine. A subsequent bone marrow aspirate and trephine showed over 20% plasma cells in the bone marrow and features consistent with myeloma. A skeletal survey showed no lytic bone lesions, but the patient did have renal failure due to AL amyloidosis of κ isotype.

Scanning densitometry (densitometry)

Determination of the density of stain along a protein electrophoresis strip by means of light absorption. If the stain density has a linear relationship to the amount of protein present, the densitometric scan can be used to determine the amount of protein in a given area, e.g. within a monoclonal band.

Monoclone reporting

Once the monoclone has been identified and quantified, a report can be issued to the requesting clinician. All new serum monoclones should have a comment added to the report to suggest that urine electrophoresis be performed if a urine sample has not already been sent. Some results may require clinical staff input or telephoning to the requesting source for urgent attention. This should be protocol-driven within the laboratory but may include results for new large monoclones, new light chain monoclones, and over 50% increases in monoclone quantification.

CLINICAL CORRELATIONS 2.8

Are all monoclonal bands associated with myeloma?

Diseases associated with the presence of monoclonal immunoglobulin include Waldenström's macroglobulinaemia, monoclonal gammopathy of uncertain significance (MGUS), lymphoma, chronic lymphocytic leukaemia, amyloidosis, and heavy chain disease, as well as myeloma. In addition, benign, usually transient, monoclones may be seen in response to infection.

2.4 Cerebrospinal fluid and isoelectric focusing

Cerebrospinal fluid (CSF)

CSF is the fluid that surrounds the brain and spinal cord and protects them from impact. It also bathes the brain in electrolytes and proteins, although its protein content is low (0.15–0.5 g/L) compared with that of plasma. Normally 80% of CSF protein is derived from plasma via ultrafiltration across the blood–CSF barrier, 18% is synthesized within the CSF area, and 2% is released due to cell breakdown. Filtration of protein from the plasma to the CSF is selective, with low molecular weight proteins passing through more readily than those with higher molecular weight. The amount of any individual protein filtered into the CSF is therefore dependent on its molecular mass and relative serum concentration. Thus the concentration of albumin in the CSF is approximately 225 times less than that in plasma (200 mg/L vs 45 000 mg/L), while that of IgG is 500 times less (20 mg/L vs 10 000 mg/L) because of its higher molecular weight.

CLINICAL CORRELATIONS 2.9

Diseases associated with intrathecal IgG synthesis and oligoclonal banding

- Multiple sclerosis (MS)
- Viral infections such as meningitis, encephalitis, subacute sclerosing panencephalitis (SSPE)
- Neurosyphilis
- Bacterial meningitis
- Systemic lupus erythematosus (SLE)
- Sarcoidosis

In healthy individuals all the IgG within the CSF will be plasma-derived. In certain diseases, however, cells migrate across the blood–brain barrier, and where those cells are lymphocytes the CSF may include locally produced (intrathecal) IgG. By comparing the IgG composition of paired serum and CSF, this intrathecal synthesis can be detected by the presence of banding patterns (oligoclonal bands) in the CSF which are not present in serum. Normal electrophoresis is not sufficiently sensitive for this, but a variant of electrophoresis called isoelectric focusing is.

Diffusion ratio

When no intrathecal synthesis is present, the ratio of serum and CSF albumin and IgG should be approximately constant. A diffusion ratio between the proteins can be calculated:

$$(\text{Serum Alb [g/L]}/\text{Serum IgG [g/L]}) \times (\text{CSF IgG [mg/L]}/\text{CSF Alb [mg/L]}) = \text{diffusion ratio}$$

Where intrathecal synthesis is present, the CSF IgG level will be higher than expected from the serum concentration, and the diffusion ratio will increase. A value greater than 0.7 indicates possible intrathecal synthesis.

However, the diffusion ratio can be insensitive and may give a value of 0.7 or less even when isoelectric focusing shows patterns indicating intrathecal synthesis. That is why IgG oligoclonal band detection by isoelectric focusing is the reference method for diagnosis of MS.

Isoelectric focusing (IEF)

IEF is an electrophoretic technique in which the gel is permeated with chemicals (called ampholines) which migrate to set up a pH gradient through the gel when the electric field is applied. The molecules in the sample move through the gel according to their electric charge as before, but that charge alters as the molecules pass through the pH gradient. When the molecules reach their individual isoelectric point (pI)—the pH at which the net molecular charge is zero—they stop migrating. This increases the resolution which can be achieved and means that molecules with similar pI values (which would run together on normal electrophoresis) can be separated.

Technical points to note

- Paired serum and CSF samples should be run side by side. Interpretation is not possible without a concurrent serum sample. If a serum is not taken at the same time as the CSF, then a sample taken within 7 days is acceptable.
- For comparability, serum and CSF samples need similar IgG levels. To achieve this, serum samples should be diluted before application.
- CSF should usually be applied neat, but samples with a raised CSF IgG level may be difficult to interpret. Dilution to ~50 mg/L (with similar for the serum sample) can help.
- IgG in CSF can be unstable and banding patterns can deteriorate over time. Small samples are more prone to this deterioration. Multiple freeze-thawing should be avoided.
- IEF electrophoresis is a high-voltage technique. A large amount of heat is produced during the process and this heat must be removed effectively for good resolution to be achieved.
- After IEF, a staining technique is required which is both sensitive and specific for IgG. One option is immunoblotting: blotting the proteins from the gel onto a nitrocellulose membrane and then using a two-stage immunoenzyme technique for visualization. Another is immunofixation with IgG followed by immunoenzyme staining.

Interpretation

There are five recognized 'patterns' which are shown in Figures 2.20 and 2.21.

- Pattern 1 shows normal diffuse polyclonal IgG in both CSF and serum.
- Pattern 2 shows oligoclonal banding in the CSF but polyclonal IgG in the serum, indicating intrathecal IgG synthesis. This pattern is seen in MS.
- Pattern 3 shows oligoclonal banding in both CSF and serum, but with extra bands in the CSF which are not seen in the serum. This indicates the presence of systemic inflammation, but with additional intrathecal synthesis. This pattern is seen in MS, SLE, sarcoidosis, and CNS infection.
- Pattern 4 shows identical oligoclonal banding in the CSF and serum, indicating systemic disease such as Guillain–Barré syndrome, HIV infection, or another chronic inflammatory state.
- Pattern 5 also shows identical banding in CSF and serum and is associated with the presence of a serum IgG monoclone. The multiple bands are due to isomers of the monoclone which have small charge differences, as glycosylation alters the charge and molecular weight, therefore move differently. These isomers are resolved by IEF but show as a monoclone on normal electrophoresis.
- **Note:** It is impossible to distinguish patterns 2, 3, and 4 without a concurrent serum sample.

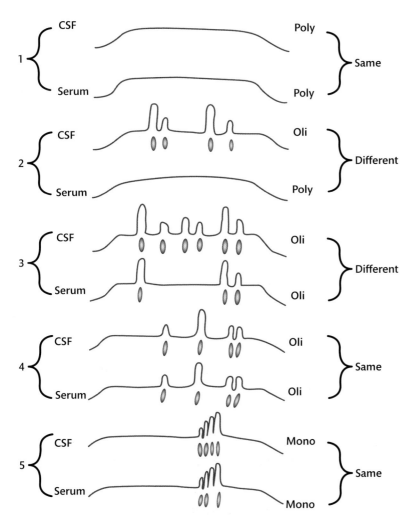

FIGURE 2.20
The five recognized patterns of isoelectric focusing shown diagrammatically.

S   C   S   C   S   C   S   C   S   C

FIGURE 2.21
The five recognized patterns of IEF on a completed nitrocellulose membrane.

Pattern 1   Pattern 2   Pattern 3   Pattern 4   Pattern 5

METHOD 2.3 *Quality control procedures for oligoclonal bands*

■ Because oligoclonal banding patterns 2, 3, and 4 may be unstable, commercial controls are usually monoclonal.

■ UKNEQAS for immunology runs a scheme for CSF oligoclonal bands. There is also a scheme for CSF proteins which includes CSF albumin and IgG (used in the diffusion ratio)

SELF-CHECK 2.3

What are the advantages and disadvantages of monoclonal commercial controls for oligoclonal banding?

Multiple sclerosis (MS)

MS is a chronic inflammatory disease of the CNS. It is the most common disabling neurological disease among young adults—the peak age of onset is between 20 and 40. The cause is unknown, although genetic and environmental factors are thought to influence susceptibility.

In MS there is autoimmune attack on the myelin sheath surrounding the nerve fibres of the CNS. Because the CNS is involved in all nerve activity, symptoms can vary, depending on the site affected. They include fatigue, balance problems, visual disturbances, numbness and tingling, pain, loss of muscle strength, anxiety and depression, cognitive problems, and speech problems. Diagnosis is by patient history, neurological examination, and MRI scan. Demonstration of CSF-specific oligoclonal bands is positive in 80% of patients.

There are four types of MS:

• Relapsing remitting MS: patients have symptomatic episodes (relapse) followed by periods of recovery.

- Secondary progressive MS: as relapsing remitting MS, but the symptoms do not go away after relapse. Approximately 65% of patients with relapsing remitting MS will have developed secondary progressive MS within 15 years of diagnosis.

- Benign MS: as relapsing remitting MS but patients have very few relapses, complete or near-complete recovery after relapse, and minimal disability.

- Primary progressive MS: patients show worsening symptoms and increasing disability from the outset.

2.5 **Cryoglobulins**

Cryoglobulins are immunoglobulins which precipitate at less than 37 °C and then redissolve completely at 37 °C. The propensity to precipitate can occur at any point below 37 °C and varies markedly between individuals. The clinical consequences can also be apparent at any point below 37 °C.

The clinical presentation of cryoglobulin includes purpura, weakness, and arthralgia in over 80% of patients. More than 30% have **Raynaud's phenomenon**, wherein the capillaries of the body's extremities become occluded as the ambient temperature falls, leading to tissue ischaemia and the possible loss of fingers and toes. Renal disease in the form of mesangio-capillary glomerulonephritis is also seen in some 30% of cases of cryoglobulin. Cryoglobulin may be the cause of false results in full blood counts. Haematology analysers often count cryoglobulin complexes as leukocytes or platelets, giving abnormally high results.

> **Raynaud's phenomenon**
> Spasm of the tiny artery vessels supplying blood to the extremities during periods of low ambient temperature.

Wintrobe and Buell first reported cryoglobulin in 1933. The classification discussed here is that of Brouet *et al.* (1974), which divides cryoglobulins into three types:

- **Type 1 cryoglobulins:** These consist solely of monoclonal immunoglobulin and are invariably associated with a monoclonal gammopathy such as myeloma or Waldenstrom's macroglobulinaemia. Most are IgM, some IgG, and rarely IgA. The cryoprecipitation occurs within a few hours of storing the patient's plasma at 4 °C and is due to the abnormal structure of the pathological monoclone, which cannot maintain the colloid state in the cold. They account for some 10% of cryoglobulins.

- **Type 2 cryoglobulins:** These consist of a mixture of immunoglobulins of different isotypes. There is usually one monoclonal immunoglobulin directed against the Fc portion of IgG, usually IgM κ. They are seen in hepatitis C virus (HCV) infections and Sjögren's syndrome and account for approximately 60% of cryoglobulins.

- **Type 3 cryoglobulins:** These are a mixture of polyclonal immunoglobulins, usually polyclonal or oligoclonal IgM and IgG. The IgM acts as a rheumatoid factor (RF) and binds to the Fc portion of IgG. They are seen in viral and bacterial infections and some autoimmune disorders. They account for approximately 30% of cryoglobulins.

Types 2 and 3 cryoglobulins can take up to a week to form fully when a plasma sample is stored at 4 °C, but the clinical significance of a cryoglobulin that takes up to a week to form at 4 °C is debatable.

Using the most sensitive serological assays, as many as 80% of mixed cryoglobulins are positive for antibody to HCV, although this varies with the population under study and the methods employed. Furthermore, polymerase chain reaction (PCR) studies reveal HCV RNA in the purified cryoprecipitate. HCV infection has been associated with autoimmune disease such as autoimmune hepatitis. Anti-immunoglobulin RF is produced as part of the antiviral immune response to enhance the clearance of virus:antivirus complexes, thus explaining the coexistence of HCV in the immunoglobulin precipitate and RF. HCV infects lymphocytes and has been associated with non-Hodgkin's lymphoma, a B-cell dyscrasia. Lymphoma may develop in the mixed cryoglobulinaemia patients who are followed up long-term, and it is possible that the monoclonal IgM type 2 variant is a precursor of lymphoma. When viewed from the perspective of HCV infection, depending on the population in question, as many as half of the HCV patients have detectable cryoglobulin without the associated clinical symptoms. However, only a minority of HCV-infected patients will develop clinical cryoglobulinaemia (Ferri *et al.* 2002).

Cryofibrinogen is the result of abnormal fibrinogen molecules native to plasma, which precipitate at less than 37 °C. Ferri *et al.* (2002) regard these as false positive but there are examples that cause clinical symptoms indistinguishable from cryoprecipitable imunoglobulins. Cryofibrinogen may also be seen in the plasma of normal individuals.

Cryoglobulin analysis

Sample collection for cryoglobulin analysis, referred to as the preanalytical phase, is of crucial importance to obtain a valid result. The precipitation occurs at less than 37 °C and at ambient temperature, in a non-anticoagulated sample tube, some of the cryoglobulin will be bound up in the fibrin clot and lost to analysis. Lack of control of the temperature in the preanalytical phase is the most important factor in failing to detect a cryoglobulin. The following protocol for the collection of cryoglobulin samples is recommended.

Sample collection

The venepuncture is performed in a warm room. Place about 250 mL of water at 37 °C into a vacuum flask or a Dewar flask. A sample without anticoagulant and an EDTA blood tube are labelled with the patient's details, using a ballpoint pen, and these are then prewarmed by placing them in a plastic bag in the 37 °C flask. Similarly, the syringe or vacuum phlebotomy system must be prewarmed, again by placing them in a plastic bag in the 37 °C flask. Alternatively, the clinic could have a stock of tubes and blood-drawing equipment in a 37 °C incubator ready for use.

Once the blood is obtained it must be placed in the 37 °C flask at once and forwarded to the laboratory without delay. On receipt, the laboratory must check the temperature of the water, which must be not less than 37 °C and not more than 41 °C. If these limits are exceeded the samples must be rejected.

The laboratory must then transfer the samples to a 37 °C waterbath/incubator and leave to clot for a minimum of 1 hour. Centrifuge the samples at 37 °C to separate the serum and EDTA plasma. Very few laboratories have a centrifuge with a controlled 37 °C option, so the samples should be left in a 37 °C incubator or water bath and the red cells allowed to sediment by gravity over several hours. Samples received in the afternoon of the working day can be safely left overnight at 37 °C but it should be acknowledged that they will not be suitable for certain tests that may be requested subsequently. Two labelled secondary tubes for each of the serum and plasma samples are prepared, one set of which is transferred to a refrigerator at 4–6 °C and the other pair kept at 37 °C. These are then left for not less than 3 days and up to 7 days.

Sample analysis

The analytical phase of cryoglobulin analysis begins with the visual examination of the samples. The samples incubated at 37 °C should be reviewed first in order to establish the background turbidity, if any. The samples at 4 °C are then examined. If there is no precipitate, or turbidity then the test is negative and no further action is required. If precipitate or turbidity is seen or suspected then further analysis is required.

Type 1 monoclonal immunoglobulin cryoglobulins can precipitate within a few hours. As well as precipitating, they may occasionally form a solid gel with little or no free fluid. These may completely liquefy when put back in the incubator at 37 °C for a few minutes. The gel formation makes further analysis difficult, as it is not possible to wash the cryoglobulin and remove uninvolved protein. Since these are due to pathological monoclones they can be investigated by the usual serum electrophoresis and immunofixation procedures maintained at 37 °C.

Cryoprecipitate can appear as flocculates or a fine precipitate covering the bottom of the tubes.

Any type of cryoglobulin seen requires further investigation. A refrigerated centrifuge must be pre-chilled to 4 °C. Centrifuge the samples to form a pellet and mark the tube to indicate the fluid level. Transfer the supernatant fluid to a labelled, clean tube for possible use later. The cryoglobulin pellet is re-suspended in 0.15 mol/L saline solution pre-chilled to 4 °C and centrifuged again. The saline supernatant is discarded and the wash cycle repeated at least three times. Maintaining the cryoprotein at 4 °C throughout this phase of the analysis is essential. This includes taking care not to handle the bottom of the tube containing the cryoprecipitate with one's fingers, as heat can be transferred. The recommended number of washes varies between laboratories, but it should be pointed out that each wash cycle will lose a little of the cryoprotein.

The hallmark of cryoglobulin is to precipitate at less than 37 °C and redissolve at 37 °C. At the end of the wash cycle the cryoglobulin is re-suspended in 0.15 mol/L saline to its original volume and placed overnight at 37 °C. Precipitate that has not redissolved is not cryoglobulin but is likely to be lipid or fibrin in nature and therefore the test for cryoglobulin is negative. If incubation at 37 °C has dissolved the cryoglobulin, then it must be characterized further by immunofixation. The total protein content of the dissolved cryoglobulin is typically small (e.g. <1 g/L), thus it is advisable to use the same highly sensitive immunofixation protocol as used for urine Bence Jones protein analysis. Type 2 cryoglobulin presents most frequently as an IgM κ monoclone with polyclonal IgG κ and IgG λ staining. Type 3 cryoglobulin on immunofixation typically reveals polyclonal IgM and IgG staining. Cryofibrinogen can be detected with anti-fibrinogen on immunofixation.

Quantification of cryoglobulin can be attempted, but there is no standardization. The total protein content of the washed cryoglobulin can be determined by using the same assay as that for urine total protein. Alternatively, the IgG, IgA, and IgM content of the washed cryoglobulin can be determined, although the variables in the washing process and the lack of references ranges make this difficult to interpret.

CASE STUDY 2.2 *Cryoglobulin*

A 32-year-old man presented with vasculitis, purpura of the lower limbs, and arthralgia.

The clinical history revealed a 7-year period of intravenous drug abuse. Routine bloods were obtained for urea and electrolytes (U&E), liver function test (LFT), and full blood count (FBC). The total protein was 66 g/L (reference range 63–79 g/L), albumin was 28 g/L (reference range 35–48 g/L) and globulin was slightly elevated at 38 g/L (range 18–36 g/L).

The haematology analyser had revealed abnormally high figures for the red and white cell counts. On examination of the blood film the cell counts were estimated to be low. The presence of cryoglobulin was postulated to be the cause of the high analyser cell counts, as cryoprecipitates are known to pass through the cell count apertures and trigger a signal to the analyser.

The clinical team obtained the samples required for the investigation of cryoglobulin and, in view of the history of drug abuse, the patient was tested for antibodies to hepatitis B, (HBV), HCV, and HIV.

The cryoglobulin analysis demonstrated a large cryoglobulin which was cold washed and typed as an IgM κ monoclone in a background of polyclonal IgG. This complex had a total protein content of 15 g/L and was reported to be consistent with type 2 cryoglobulinaemia. The patient was positive for rheumatoid factor 1200 IU/mL (range 0–15 IU/mL). There was antibody to HCV and detectable HCV RNA.

The HCV infection was treated with pegylated interferon-α over 6 months. During this time the FBC, U&E, and LFT were analysed at monthly intervals. The FBC was tested following warming of the sample to 37 °C on all occasions. The clinical chemistry results were always reported from samples at ambient temperature and the results were consistently similar to the original sample. The presence of the large monoclonal IgM suggests that the serum total protein and globulin levels were grossly underestimated due to the cryoprecipitation at ambient temperature which was removed by centrifugation in the clot. Unfortunately, this was not pointed out to the clinicians or the clinical chemistry laboratory.

After 6 months' treatment the patients' symptoms had significantly resolved. The HCV RNA was no longer detectable and the cryoglobulin analysis showed a markedly reduced IgM κ monoclone in a background of polyclonal IgG.

In summary, cryoglobulins may be classified as one of three types, the first and least common of which is solely monoclonal immunoglobulin, which is associated with a B-cell dyscrasia. The mixed cryoglobulins, types 2 and 3, can be distinguished on immunofixation by the presence or absence of monoclonal IgM with polyclonal immunoglobulin. Types 2 and 3 are associated with HCV infection; around half of these patients will have a cryoglobulin but only a minority will have symptoms associated with cryoglobulinaemia.

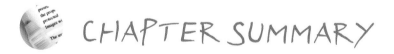 CHAPTER SUMMARY

- Immunoglobulins are key effector molecules in adaptive immunity with template structures of two identical heavy chains and two identical light chains.

- Clonal expansion of plasma cells produces monoclonal gammopathies which may be benign or malignant.

- Monoclonal gammopathies present a measureable band on electrophoresis which can be used to monitor the size and progress of the tumour.

- Monoclonal free light chains can overflow into the urine, where they are known as Bence Jones protein.

- Recently, assays have been developed to measure monoclonal free light chains directly in serum.

- Immunoglobulins and fibrinogen may spontaneously precipitate at temperatures below 37 °C, leading to the formation of cryoprecipitates.

- Although standardization of the assay is poor, cryoprecipitates have been classified into four subtypes: cryoglobulin types 1, 2, or 3, and cryofibrinogen.

- Intrathecal synthesis of IgG is an important diagnostic feature of MS.

- Because of the low level of protein in CSF the analysis requires the use of IEF enhanced by immunoblotting or immunofixation.

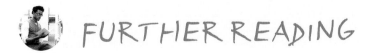 FURTHER READING

- Andersson M *et al.* (1994) Cerebrospinal fluid in the diagnosis of multiple sclerosis: a consensus report. *J Neurol Neurosurg Psychiatry*, **57**, 897–902.

- Dispenzieri A *et al.* (2009) International Myeloma Working Group guidelines for serum-free light chain analysis in multiple myeloma and related disorders. *Leukaemia*, **23**, 215–224.

- Johnson S *et al.* (2006) Guidelines on the management of Waldenström's macroglobulinaemia. *Br J Haematol*, **132**, 683–697.

- Keren D (2003) *Protein Electrophoresis in Clinical Diagnosis. Arnold*, London.

- Lilic D, Sewell WAC (2001) IgA deficiency: what we should—or should not—be doing. *J Clin Pathol*, **54**, 337–338.

- Miller D *et al.* (2008) Differential diagnosis of suspected multiple sclerosis: a consensus approach. *Mult Scler*, **14**, 1157–1174.

- Smith A, Wisloff F, Samson D. (2005) Guidelines on the diagnosis and management of multiple myeloma. *Br J Haematol*, **132**, 410–451.

- UK Myeloma Forum (2004) Guidelines on the diagnosis and management of AL amyloidosis. *Br J Haematol*, **125**, 681–700.

- UK Myeloma Forum and Nordic Myeloma Study Group (2009). Guidelines for the investigation of newly detected M-proteins and the management of monoclonal gammopathy of undetermined significance (MGUS). *Br J Haematol*, **147**, 22–42.

- Ward AM, Sheldon J, Rowbottom A, Wild GD (2007) Protein Reference Unit Handbook of Clinical Immunochemistry. 9th edition, PR Publications, Sheffield.

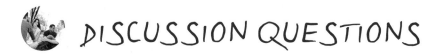

DISCUSSION QUESTIONS

2.1 Immunoglobulin molecules are composed of highly conserved subunits. Name the subunits and describe their structure.

2.2 Which of the heavy chain domains is concerned with: (a) complement activation; (b) opsonization; (c) antigen binding?

2.3 What are the effector roles of each of the IgG subclasses?

2.4 How does antigen excess lead to falsely low results in nephelometry and turbidimetry?

Answers to these questions are provided in the book's Online Resource Centre; visit www.oxfordtextbooks.co.uk/orc/ahmed/

3

Allergy

Learning Objectives

After studying this chapter you should be able to:

- outline the immunological basis of allergy
- describe the major clinical features of allergic disease
- describe the clinical and laboratory techniques used to diagnose allergy
- discuss the advantages and limitations of these techniques
- outline the role of flow cytometry in determining basophil activation

Introduction

The incidence of allergy in developed countries is increasing. In the United Kingdom the incidence of common allergic diseases has trebled over the past 20 years to become one of the highest in the world. It is estimated that approximately one-third of the population will develop allergic symptoms at some point in their lives. This, along with diagnostic and therapeutic developments, is impacting significantly on clinical and laboratory practice. This chapter provides an overview of how clinical and laboratory investigations come together to provide accurate diagnoses leading to effective management and enhanced quality of life.

The terms which are used in allergy are different to those that you will have come across in previous chapters describing other immunological diseases. To help you understand the content of this chapter, a brief description of the terms that are most commonly used is provided in section 3.1.

3.1 Allergy terminology

Allergy is defined as a hypersensitivity reaction initiated by immunological mechanisms. This relatively simple, all-encompassing definition was proposed by expert panels of the European Academy of Allergology and Clinical Immunology (EAACI) and the World Allergy

Allergy
A hypersensitivity reaction initiated by immunological mechanisms.

TABLE 3.1 Gell and Coombs (1963) classification of hypersensitivity

Type		Mechanism
I	Immediate hypersensitivity	IgE-mediated mast cell degranulation leading to release of vasoactive mediators
II	Cytotoxic antibody	IgG and IgM mediation of cell destruction by ADCC or complement
III	Immune complex	Antibody–antigen complex deposition leading to complement activation and inflammation
IV	Delayed-type hypersensitivity	Th1 mediated cytokine release leading to macrophage recruitment and activation

ADCC, antibody-dependent cell-mediated cytotoxicity.

Hypersensitivity

The reaction that causes reproducible signs or symptoms, following exposure to a defined stimulus, in a susceptible individual.

Atopy

A genetic predisposition to produce prolonged IgE antibody responses to commonly occurring allergens.

Cross reference

You can read more about atopy in sections 3.5 and 3.6.

Organization (WAO) as a means of unifying nomenclature and improving communication between health-care professionals. However, the term is more frequently restricted to the description of type 1 (IgE-mediated) immediate **hypersensitivity** reactions. A hypersensitivity reaction can be mediated by cells or antibodies. In the majority of cases the antibody responsible for an allergic reaction belongs to the IgE isotype class and the reaction is described as IgE-mediated allergy. All other hypersensitivity reactions, mediated by antibodies of other immunoglobulin classes and/or cells, are known as non-IgE-mediated allergy. There are four types of hypersensitivity as defined by Gell and Coombs (1963); these are briefly listed in Table 3.1.

The reason why some individuals develop persistent allergic symptoms is that they have a genetic predisposition to produce prolonged IgE antibody responses to commonly occurring allergens. This condition is known as **atopy**. It may be an individual or familial tendency, and usually develops in childhood or adolescence. Nonatopic individuals who have similar exposure to allergens do not produce a prolonged IgE antibody response.

Atopy is a clinical definition and cannot be used until IgE sensitization has been documented by detection of IgE antibodies in serum or by a positive skin prick test.

3.2 Allergens

Allergens

Antigens that induce immune responses which cause allergy.

Hapten

A complex of a small molecule with a carrier, usually protein.

Cross reference

Comprehensive lists of recognized allergens can be found at http://www.allergome.com/ and http://www.allergen.org/Allergen.aspx.

Antigens that induce immune responses which cause allergy are known as **allergens**. Most allergens are of biological origin, e.g. plant pollens, animal hair and dander, mites, moulds, plant- and animal-derived foods. Allergens are predominantly proteins and display considerable heterogeneity in molecular size, composition (glycosylation), and conformational structure. Low molecular weight chemicals can act as **haptens**, which can behave as allergens and bind to IgE antibodies.

Many hundreds of allergens have been described and an internationally agreed form of nomenclature has been developed as a means of standardization and classification. The nomenclature system, established by the International Union of Immunological Societies (IUIS) Allergen Nomenclature Subcommittee, assigns allergens according to a standardized scheme. For example, the major pollen allergen of the white birch *Betula verrucosa* is named Bet v 1. The first three letters are from the plant's genus, followed by the letter of the specific family, and a number indicating the order of discovery of the allergen.

3.3 **Allergy mechanisms**

An allergic response can be broadly divided into two phases, which can be seen in Figure 3.1:

- An induction phase, in which the immune system forms IgE antibodies in response to initial exposure to the allergen.
- A reactive phase, in which an allergen binds to IgE molecules, present on Fc receptors on mast cells and basophils, causing the cells to release preformed or rapidly synthesized mediators.

Induction phase: sensitization

When an allergen comes in contact with the immune system for the first time it is captured and processed by antigen-presenting cells (APC). Presentation of the allergenic epitope, in association with MHC class II and costimulatory molecules, to T cells then occurs. Depending upon the nature of the APC, characteristics of the allergen, levels of allergen exposure, activation of toll-like receptors and cytokine microenvironment, T cells can differentiate into distinctive sub-populations. These sub-populations are distinguished on the basis of their predominant cytokine profile. In allergy, Th2 lymphocytes (producers of IL-4, IL-5, and IL-13) are pivotal in signalling B lymphocytes to produce IgE antibodies. These specific IgE antibodies are released

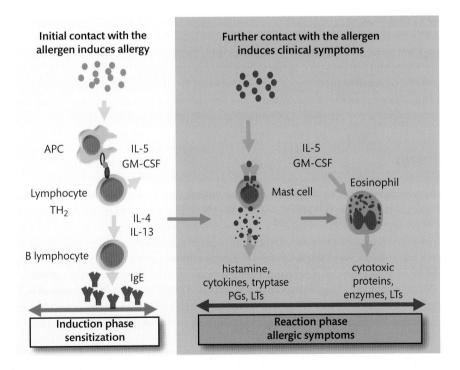

FIGURE 3.1
Diagrammatic representation of the induction and reaction phases of an allergic reaction, showing the interaction between cellular and soluble components. APC, antigen presenting cell; IL, interleukin; GM-CSF, granulocyte macrophage stimulating factor; PGs, prostaglandins; LTs, leukotrienes.

into the circulation but they are rapidly removed by binding to high-affinity Fc receptors on the surface membranes of basophils and mast cells. The binding and concentration of specific IgE antibodies on the surface membranes 'sensitizes' the cells.

Reactive phase: allergic response

In the reactive phase, subsequent exposure to allergen results in cross-linking of the cell-bound IgE molecules on the surface of the sensitized cells. This results in release of potent preformed mediators (histamine, heparin, proteases) from mast cells and basophils. In addition, synthesis of a second set of chemical mediators (leukotrienes, prostaglandins, thromboxanes, chemotactic factors) occurs. These mediators are released into the tissues several hours after the reaction. The actions of both sets of mediators result in the characteristic features of allergic reactions: vasodilatation, swelling, and itch. How these features present in different forms of allergic disease is described in section 3.4.

SELF-CHECK 3.1

Can you describe the immunological mechanisms which give rise to allergic symptoms?

3.4 Clinical features of allergic diseases

An important concept to understand is that allergy is a systemic disease and not an organ-specific disease. Allergy can present with different clinical features and patients can present with single or multiple clinical manifestations. Indeed, it is not unusual for changing patterns to emerge over time. To illustrate the variety of presentations and symptoms that are associated with allergy, the major clinical features of the most common allergic conditions are described below.

Asthma

Asthma is a chronic inflammatory disorder of the airways with variable airflow limitation that causes recurrent episodes of wheezing, breathlessness, chest tightness, and cough, particularly at night. According to the Global Initiative for Asthma (GINA) guidelines, asthma is classified according to severity into four stages: intermittent; mild, moderate, and severe persistent. The inhalant allergens are, in most cases, the main triggers of allergic asthma. Among these, house dust mites, storage mites, grass pollen, and pet dander are the most frequent, either alone or in combination. Occasionally, foods, drugs, hymenoptera venoms, and chemical allergens can cause allergic asthma. Interestingly, the major allergen of house dust mites is the faeces and most people with suspected bird allergy turn out to be allergic to house dust mites that thrive in the birdcages.

Rhinitis

Rhinitis is the most prevalent respiratory disease, affecting more than 15% of the population. Most cases are IgE-mediated. Nasal itching, blockage, watery rhinorrhoea, loss of sense of smell, and frequent sneezing are the major symptoms of rhinitis. Allergic rhinitis induced by pollen during the spring and summer seasons is known as hay fever. The major allergens in rhinitis are the same as mentioned previously for asthma. Any patient affected by allergic rhinitis should be studied for asthma and vice versa.

Rhinoconjunctivitis

Allergic rhinitis accompanied by watery and itchy eyes is referred to as allergic rhinoconjunctivitis. In most cases, treatment of the nasal symptoms also improves the allergic conjunctivitis.

Urticaria

In urticaria the hypersensitivity reaction that occurs in the skin is characterized by erythematous areas which may be variable in size, extension, and degree of itchiness. Urticaria, which has an allergic basis, is usually triggered by food and drug allergens.

Angioedema

Angioedema is frequently associated with urticaria. Whereas urticaria affects the epidermis, producing a superficial erythema, angioedema impacts the deeper dermal level, inducing skin swelling. Drugs, foods, and insect stings are the most common allergens inducing angioedema. Nonsteroidal anti-inflammatory drugs (NSAIDs) and angiotensin-converting enzyme (ACE) inhibitors are groups of drugs that may induce episodes of urticaria/angioedema.

Cross reference
There are different causes of angiodema. Another common type seen in the clinical immunology laboratory is hereditary angioedema (HAE) caused by a problem with the complement cascade. You can read in more detail about this in Chapter 4.

Eczema

Eczema describes a local erythematous inflammation of the skin. When related to other allergic clinical manifestations, it is known as atopic eczema. Special attention should be paid to atopic eczema that appears in early childhood and is induced by foods such as cow's milk and egg. This is because most of the affected children will develop respiratory allergy in later years. Close contact with various metals and chemicals may result in a delayed local eczema that appears 48–72 hours after the contact. This is known as contact dermatitis.

Anaphylaxis

Anaphylaxis is the most severe allergic reaction and involves more than one bodily system: skin, respiratory system, blood, cardiovascular system, gastrointestinal tract. It can be life-threatening, and fatalities occur if adrenaline is not promptly administered. Almost universally, patients experiencing an anaphylactic attack report a 'feeling of impending doom'. Many allergens can induce anaphylaxis, but the most frequent are:

- foods: peanuts, tree nuts, and shellfish
- drugs: antibiotics, muscle relaxants, and painkillers
- venoms: Hymenoptera (bees and wasps)
- latex.

Establishing an accurate diagnosis is crucial for patient management and treatment. This is achieved through both clinical and laboratory investigations. The various elements of the investigative strategy are shown in Figure 3.2 and described in detail in sections 3.5 and 3.6.

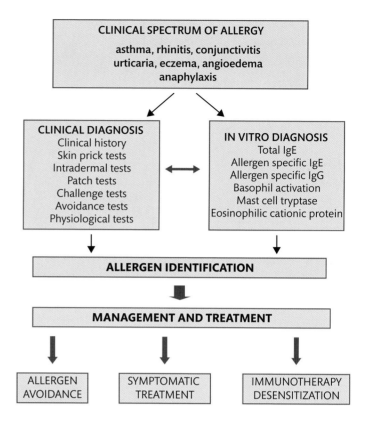

FIGURE 3.2
Investigative strategy for allergy diagnosis and management.

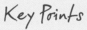

Allergy is a systemic disease.

Allergy patients can present with single or multiple manifestations.

Clinical symptoms can change over time.

3.5 Clinical diagnosis

Clinical history

Taking an accurate clinical history is the most important tool for diagnosis of allergic diseases. This includes collecting information about time of onset of disease; frequency and duration of symptoms; day–night variation; shape, size, and distribution of skin lesions; occurrence in relation to different triggers and conditions; exercise; food and drug intake; personal and familial history; type of work and hobbies; relationship to the menstrual cycle; quality of life; and concurrent therapy.

Depending on the type of allergy under investigation, a number of specific points should be queried.

- For respiratory allergy, it is important to know whether symptoms are seasonal or persistent and whether the patient identifies any triggers (animals, dust, workplace).

- In food allergy, it should be established whether the reaction is different depending on whether the food is raw or cooked.
- In suspected drug allergy, the lapsed time between drug intake and the onset of symptoms should be noted and whether the patient has taken the same drug before and after the allergic episode.

A number of *in vitro* tests can also be used to aid diagnosis, and these are described below.

Skin prick test

Skin prick testing is the 'gold standard' diagnostic method in the allergy clinic. It is useful for the diagnosis of most IgE-mediated allergies. The selection of allergens to test is determined according to the clinical history. Most allergens can be obtained from commercial sources. Sometimes the suspected allergen is not available and testing is performed directly using the suspected product which is applied to the skin, removed, and the skin pricked with a lancet. It is important to check that the patient is not taking antihistamines as this will diminish the sensitivity of the test.

METHOD 3.1 *Skin prick testing*

Liquid allergen drops are placed on the volar aspect of the forearm and pricked with a 1-mm lancet. A positive reaction is identified by a weal and flare around the site of the skin prick (Figure 3.3a). Weal size is measured after 15 minutes. A reaction is considered positive when the weal is at least 3 mm in diameter and equal to or greater than the weal formed by a histamine-positive control solution. Physiological saline is used as the negative control.

Patch test

Patch tests are used for the diagnosis of contact dermatitis. The test is performed on the patient's back by applying adhesive patches containing the different suspected chemicals. After 48 hours the patch is removed and the eczematous reactions are identified. This can be seen in Figure 3.3b.

Challenge test

Challenge tests can take a number of forms—oral, inhaled, injected, or direct contact—depending on the nature of the allergy. The procedure exposes the patient to progressively increasing concentrations of the allergen, to a point where a normal level of exposure is reached. This is compared with the reaction observed with placebo. Careful monitoring of signs and symptoms is undertaken throughout the procedure by trained health-care personnel and, as the procedure carries some risk, emergency treatment is available.

Double-blind placebo controlled challenge (DBPCC) is the preferred method for both diagnostic purposes and scientific studies. However, the process is time-consuming and requires specialist expertise. Consequently, open challenge (investigator and patient aware of the

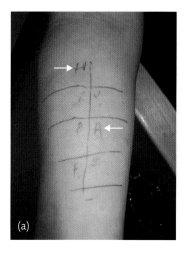

Histamine	
Rocuronium	Vecuronium
Propofol	Atracurium
Fentanyl	Saline

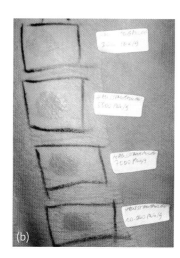

(a)

(b)

FIGURE 3.3

(a) Skin prick testing in a patient who experienced a perioperative anaphylactic reaction. Weal and flare reactions (arrowed) were observed for histamine (positive control) and atracurium (a muscle relaxant drug). Negative reactions were observed for saline (negative control) and other anaesthetic drugs; (b) demarcated areas of eczematous rash following patch testing.

Figure 3.3a courtesy of Dr M Shields.

test substances) is more commonly undertaken. For practical reasons open tests are the first approach, particularly when the probability of a positive outcome is estimated to be low.

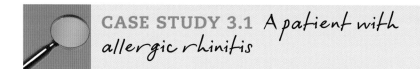

CASE STUDY 3.1 A patient with allergic rhinitis

A 19-year-old man reported a history of sneezing, nasal blockage, itchy nose, and watery eyes occuring each year during the spring and summer months. He also develops a wheeze after exercise but at no other times. He reported a tingling feeling in his lips when eating melon.

The patient had a history of eczema and was allergic to eggs as an infant. He had experienced no other allergic symptoms until 3 years ago. He is not on any medication.

His mother has a history of wasp allergy and his father has a history of hay fever. The family do not have any pets.

Skin prick tests were carried out to house dust mite, cat dander, dog dander, horse dander, storage mites, grass pollen mix, tree mix, timothy grass and cocksfoot, apple, banana, avocado, peach, melon, strawberry, and raspberry. Results were positive to timothy grass, cocksfoot, and melon and negative to all other skin prick tests. Blood was also taken for measurement of total serum IgE and specific-IgE to the above allergens. Specific IgE positivity to timothy grass (57.2 kU/L), cocksfoot (79.5 kU/L), and melon (1.44 kU/L) was observed.

A diagnosis of allergic rhinitis and oral allergy syndrome induced by melon was made.

The patient was advised not to eat melon and to avoid grassy areas during the summer months. Additional measures to reduce exposure to grass pollen such as wearing wrap-around sunglasses and staying indoors with the windows closed when the pollen count is high were recommended. He was also advised to take antihistamine tablets on a regular basis over the spring and summer months. A nasal corticosteroid was also prescribed to be taken daily during this time.

He is an ideal candidate for desensitization with grass pollen. Commencement of immunotherapy at the end of the grass pollen season was proposed.

Key Points

Taking an accurate clinical history is the most important tool in allergy diagnosis.

Other techniques such as skin prick and challenge testing, measurement of sIgE antibodies and mast cell tryptase, and basophil activation tests can provide supporting evidence. The decision as to which additional techniques to use is dependent on the complexity of the clinical history.

3.6 Laboratory diagnosis

Allergen-specific IgE antibody tests

Allergen-specific IgE antibody (sIgE) testing is the commonest laboratory procedure employed in the diagnosis of allergic disease. The assays have developed significantly over the past 40 years and continue to evolve in the areas of allergen characterization, antibody detection, and instrumentation.

Originally described in the late 1960s, the radioallergosorbent test (RAST) was the first routine technique used for determining sIgE in serum. This 'first generation' assay employed cyanogen bromide-activated paper discs as the solid phase (allegrosorbent) and used a birch pollen-specific IgE calibration curve from which the levels of sIgE could be interpolated. Results were semi-quantitative and organized into classes of reactivity related to skin prick test positivity. These are described in Table 3.2.

'Second generation' methods, introduced in the early 1990s, offered marked improvements in assay convenience and performance. These included:

- developments in solid phase allergosorbent materials or use of a liquid-allergen matrix resulting in enhanced antigen–antibody kinetics and assay sensitivity
- the use of nonisotopic detection methods (spectrophotometry, fluorimetry, enzyme-enhanced chemiluminescence)
- reporting of quantitative sIgE results (kU/L) standardized to a WHO International Reference preparation for IgE.

In addition, systems became semiautomated, resulting in faster turn-around times for results.

Further refinements have been introduced with 'third generation' assays, most notably in the extension of the lower limit of detection to 0.1 kU/L, and in the availability of random access automated analytical platforms.

TABLE 3.2 Classification of allergen-specific IgE reactivities

Class	kU/L	Interpretation
0	<0.35	Negative
1	0.35–0.7	Weak positive
2	0.7–3.5	Positive
3	3.5–17.5	Positive
4	17.5–52.5	Strong positive
5	52.5–100	Strong positive
6	>100	Strong positive

Adapted from *PRU Handbook of Clinical Immunochemistry*, 9th edition, 2007; reproduced with permission.

Test performance characteristics

The performance characteristics (diagnostic sensitivity/specificity, positive and negative predictive values) for sIgE tests have been widely studied. For most common food and inhalant allergens correlation of sIgE positivity with clinical features and/or skin testing reactivity is generally good.

In the investigation of food allergy the tests may be particularly useful in defining a patient's clinical sensitivity. This is based on the construction of probability curves, from which sIgE threshold limits for the respective foods are defined. This information can be used by clinicians when considering challenge testing: a sIgE below the threshold limit has 95% probability of a negative test result, and a sIgE result above the threshold limit indicates a 95% probability of a positive challenge test.

Specific IgE antibody levels measured with different commercial assays cannot be considered as equivalent. This is largely due to variability in the composition and immunogenicity of the allergen preparations used in the assays. Therefore, when considering performance characteristics of respective assays the analytical platform on which results are obtained should be borne in mind, as the results obtained from different systems may not be interchangeable. This caveat also applies in the general sense that complete concordance between *in vitro* sIgE testing and skin testing cannot be expected, the former measuring circulating IgE antibodies, the latter, cutaneous mast cell reactivity.

Cross reference

You can read more about allergen standardization in section 3.7.

SELF-CHECK 3.2

Can you describe the investigative strategies used in allergy diagnosis?

3.7 Allergen standardization

Identification of specific IgE reactivity, leading to an accurate diagnosis, is dependent on the quality of the allergen extract employed. Most allergen extracts used in commercial assays are prepared by chemical extraction from raw material. Ensuring standardization of allergen preparations poses significant challenges for manufacturers because of:

- the heterogeneous mixture of allergenic and nonallergenic components in the biological material
- the requirement to be able to extract all relevant allergens at biologically (and diagnostically) appropriate concentrations
- variability in source material, e.g. climate/pollution affecting the nature of pollens; species variability in food allergens; contamination of source material by moulds or insect proteins.

In addition, many biological sources contain allergens with strong potential for cross-reactivity, i.e. IgE antibodies binding to structurally similar epitopes from different species. The use of heterogeneous extracts containing such structures may potentially result in false-positive and clinically erroneous results. Although significant progress has been made towards standardizing allergen preparations, the potential for variability remains. This can be seen, for example, when quality control returns for specific IgE testing from different assay manufacturers are compared. As a means of addressing some of these issues, recombinant allergens are being produced and introduced into diagnostic practice.

Cross references

You can read in more detail about quality assurance in section 3.11.

You can read more about recombinant allergens in section 3.9.

3.8 **Cross-reactivity**

Allergen cross-reactivity is a phenomenon that always needs to be considered in allergy testing. It can occur due to:

- biochemical similarity between antigenic determinants
- cross-reactive carbohydrate determinants (CCD).

Biochemical similarity

This form of cross-reactivity occurs because sIgE antibody recognizes the same or similar antigenic determinants from a variety of allergen sources. Generally, cross-reactivity can occur when a sequence homology of over 70% is present between the respective antigenic determinants. It is usually associated with allergens that are common to organisms across various taxonomic groups, e.g. tropomyosin, profilin, lipid transfer proteins, chitinases.

Clinically, oral allergy syndrome is a common feature of cross-reactivity of pollen with fruit and vegetable allergens. Similarly, multiple allergies to fish and shellfish can occur.

Cross reference

Several databases are available which can be used to determine or predict allergen cross-reactivity, e.g. http://www.allergome.com/, http://www.allergen.org/

Cross-reactive carbohydrate determinants (CCDs)

Many plant glycoproteins are composed of complex carbohydrate structures covalently bound to proteins. These carbohydrate entities share significant similarities in structure and this can result in nonspecific binding to CCDs. This phenomenon can result in false-positive results in sIgE assays. Suspicion of a false-positive result may arise when discrepant results are obtained from sIgE assays and skin testing and/or sIgE results are not consistent with the clinical history.

As a means of establishing the likelihood of CCD false positivity, patient sera can be tested with sIgE reagents to a number of allergens, e.g. bromelain or horseradish peroxidase, that contain CCD but rarely cause allergy. If the serum under test is positive to bromelain, this would suggest that CCD is responsible for the false results.

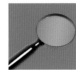

CASE STUDY 3.2 *A child with nut allergy*

The parents of a 5-year-old boy reported that while at a birthday party he ate a piece of cake containing nuts. He immediately developed tingling of his lips, lip swelling, itch, and a rash all over his body, facial angioedema, and breathing difficulty.

An ambulance was called and he was taken to the local hospital Emergency Department where adrenaline, antihistamines, and oral steroids were administered.

The boy had no previous history of allergy and has a healthy diet. He was not on any medication. The family do not have any pets. His mother has a history of asthma and hay fever.

Skin prick tests were carried out to the following nuts: almond, brazil nut, cashew nut, peanut, hazelnut, pine nut, pistachio, and walnut. Results were positive for peanut and negative for all other nuts. Blood was sent for total serum IgE and specific IgE to all of the above nuts as well as common inhalant allergens. Peanut-specific IgE was positive (>100 kU/l). Negative results were obtained for all other allergens tested.

A diagnosis of food allergy to peanut was made.

The parents were advised that their son should avoid all nuts and food containing nuts in his diet. Although the patient tested positively only to peanut, contamination of other nuts and nut products is common. Therefore the advice is to avoid all nuts.

His parents should carry antihistamine medication at all times as well as adrenaline autoinjectors. Training was given on when and how to use the autoinjectors. His school was informed that he has a peanut allergy and his parents were advised that he should wear a medical alert bracelet.

3.9 Recombinant allergens

Using recombinant DNA techniques the molecular characterization of many allergens can be defined. This has important implications for allergy diagnosis and treatment. First, the actual disease-eliciting components of a given allergen can be identified: e.g. for birch pollen seven allergenic components are described in Table 3.3. Secondly, panels of recombinant allergens with consistent quality and without genetic or biological variation can be produced and used as diagnostic tools. This can be applied in a number of ways, as shown in Figure 3.4:

- **as an extract replacement:** combining a number of recombinant allergens which represent the sum of the relevant epitopes
- **as an additive to extracts:** spiking natural extracts with recombinant allergens that are not optimally represented in the extracted material
- **as a single component:** using individual recombinant allergens for quantitation of specific IgE antibodies that have diagnostic value, particularly for therapeutic decision-making.

With these enhanced diagnostic reagents it becomes possible to resolve a patient's reactivity at the level of individual disease-eliciting components. The term 'component resolved diagnosis' (CRD) is used to describe this diagnostic approach.

TABLE 3.3 Allergen components of *Betula verrucosa* (birch) pollen

Protein	Common name	Biological function
Bet v 1	PR-10 protein	Pathogen response protein
Bet v 2	Profilin	Actin-binding protein
Bet v 3	4 EF-hand calcium-binding protein	Calcium-binding protein
Bet v 4	Procalcin	Calcium-binding protein
Bet v 6	Isoflavone reductase	Isoflavone reductases
Bet v 7	Cyclophilin	Petidylprolyl isomerase

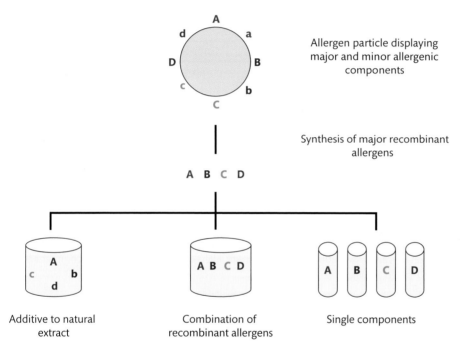

Allergen particle displaying major and minor allergenic components

Synthesis of major recombinant allergens

A B C D

Additive to natural extract

Combination of recombinant allergens

Single components

FIGURE 3.4

Diagrammatic representation showing three ways in which recombinant allergens can be used as *in vitro* diagnostic reagents.

Look at Figure 3.5. Using the example of birch pollen allergy, CRD could be undertaken as follows:

1. The patient's serum is tested for specific-IgE reactivity to birch pollen extract.

2. If positive, the serum is then analysed using recombinant reagents for reactivity to individual components.

3. The CRD is defined as positivity to the major component (Bet v 1); minor components (Bet v 2/4); both major and minor components.

This information may help to inform the clinician as to whether a patient may benefit from specific immunotherapy (SIT). Immunotherapeutic reagents for birch pollen are usually standardized against Bet v 1, which is the major allergenic component to which 90% of patients

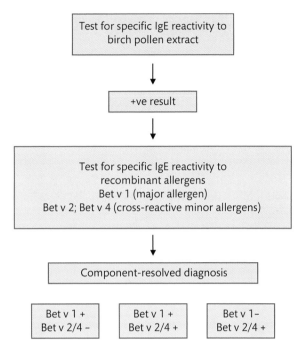

FIGURE 3.5

Component-resolved diagnosis (CRD) for birch pollen allergy. Schematic representation showing how the combination of testing with natural extract reagent and recombinant allergens leads to a CRD.

react. Therefore, patients who are monosensitized to Bet v 1 are potentially suitable for SIT. Conversely, patients for whom Bet v 2 or Bet v 4 are the predominant allergenic components are unlikely to benefit from Bet v 1-based SIT.

Although SIT has significant potential for management of allergic patients, it is currently not in widespread clinical practice because:

- there is limited availability of recombinant allergen panels to facilitate comprehensive CRD-based testing
- relatively small numbers of SIT agents are available.

Key Points

Most allergens are proteins. They are heterogeneous in size, degree of glycosylation, and conformation.

Cross-reactivity between different allergens is common and due to biochemical similarity or sharing of cross-reactive carbohydrate determinants.

Recombinant allergens can be used to determine the disease-eliciting components of a given allergen.

Component-resolved diagnosis (CRD) can be established using recombinant allergens.

SELF-CHECK 3.3

What do you understand by the term 'component-resolved diagnosis'?

3.10 **Microarray-based allergy testing**

Based on the development of DNA microarray technology in the 1990s, the application of protein microarrays to diagnostic testing in autoimmunity, infectious diseases, and allergy is now emerging. For allergy, this advancement has coincided with developments in recombinant technology leading to novel forms of multiple allergen testing, by microarray/biochips, becoming available.

The assays are based on immobilization of allergen proteins (purified or recombinant) on to glass slides or silicon chips. The surfaces of these supports are treated to ensure stability and appropriate orientation of the proteins. The allergens are 'spotted' robotically in a distinctive pattern or array. When serum is applied to the slide/chip, each micron-sized spot becomes a reaction site for an antigen–antibody reaction. Bound IgE is then detected by a fluorescently labelled anti-human IgE antibody and fluorescence measured using a microarray scanner. Fluorescence images are analysed by customized software which relates fluorescence intensity of the respective spots to values derived from a calibrator serum which is incorporated in the assay. Results are reported semiquantitatively (kU antigen/L) or in classes.

Using allergen microarrays, simultaneous determination of sIgE reactivities to a large number of allergens, using very small volumes (microlitre amounts) of serum, is feasible. This may have a role in screening but the development of 'symptom-based' chips or dedicated microarrays to common groups of allergens, such as foods or pollens is likely to be more beneficial. There is also the potential to develop specific recombinant allergen microarrays for component-derived diagnosis.

Microarray-based assays have the potential to revolutionize laboratory allergy diagnostic testing. However, at present, significant work is required to establish the diagnostic characteristics of these assays in relation to third-generation immunoassays and to demonstrate economic benefits.

3.11 **Quality assurance**

The principles that apply to quality-assuring allergy test results are similar to those described for other immunological assays. Good laboratory practice will incorporate both internal quality control and external quality assurance schemes.

Internal quality control

Internal quality control for sIgE assays relies on the inclusion of sera and/or commercial preparations of known sIgE concentrations in the assay. These reagents are selected to have sIgE levels across the dose–response curve and are incorporated at a variety of positions within the assay set up. Assay verification is undertaken by monitoring results of Levy–Jennings plots and by applying Westgard rules.

The extensive range of allergens for which tests are available presents a particular difficulty for internal quality control of sIgE assays. There is a limited repertoire of standardized sIgE commercial preparations, and laboratories have difficulty in obtaining sufficient quantities of patient sera covering a complete range of specificities. Thus, it is common practice for laboratories to incorporate a limited number of sera with sIgE positivity to the most clinically appropriate allergens. Inconsistency in allergen extract preparations may result in batch-to-batch variability and so results for internal quality control should be monitored carefully.

External quality assessment

External quality assessment refers to a programme of interlaboratory proficiency testing. Such programmes are available from commercial companies or independent providers. Proficiency testing provides a benchmark of accuracy of results reported by clinical laboratories. The schemes also enable laboratories to assess their performance with other laboratories using similar or different analytical systems.

In the United Kingdom the principal scheme is organized by the United Kingdom National External Quality Assessment Service (UKNEQAS). For allergy, two programmes are offered:

- **UKNEQAS for IgE:** This programme distributes serum samples for total IgE quantitiation. Results are displayed as an all-laboratories trimmed mean (ALTM) with accompanying method-specific statistics. Individual laboratory performances are expressed in terms of mean running bias index score (MRBIS), standard deviation of the bias index score (SDBIS), and mean running variance index score (MRVIS), and assessed over a running analytical window of 10 samples.

- **EUROEQAS for allergen-specific IgE:** This programme distributes serum samples for the assessment of sIgE antibody reactivity. Distributions are drawn from a panel of 15 common or clinically relevant sIgE specificities. Results are reported to the scheme in kU/L and in classes or grades. Individual laboratory performances are expressed in terms of MRBIS, SDBIS, MRVIS and assessed over a running analytical window of 12 samples. The overall quantitative performance is expressed as the overall mean running variance index score (OMRVIS), which is the mean of all the individual allergen-specific MRVISs. Semi-quantitative classes/grades are assessed by a misclassification index (MI) and scored in relation to a consensus-designated response value (class 0–1, negative; class 2–6, positive).

An example of the cumulative results from approximately 250 laboratories (reporting 10 different methods) for specific IgE reactivity to four allergens from a single serum sample is shown in Figure 3.6. Clear columns indicate the distribution of values for all methods; solid columns represent the cumulative results reported by approximately 50 laboratories using the same assay. You can see from the distribution of results that for house dust mite there is general consensus across the range of methods. However, for cat, grass, and tree pollen there is a clear distinction between the high values obtained using the assay represented by the solid columns and the other methods.

Whether these higher results reflect enhanced analytical sensitivity or false positivity is unknown. Undoubtedly the composition of the allergen extract is a significant factor and characterization of the epitopes in each allergen preparation may help in understanding these differences. However, interpatient variability in sIgE reactivity to standardized allergen preparations does occur and, as quality control samples are drawn from a patient population, a degree of variability is always likely. The use of recombinant allergen preparations may reduce variation, but will not eliminate it entirely.

Although the scheme can highlight discrepancies between methods, it cannot identify the cause(s). Therefore, laboratories should, as a minimum requirement, confirm that their analytical performances are in keeping with results for their peer group. From Figure 3.6 you can see that there is generally good agreement between the laboratories using the method identified by the solid columns. In situations such as this, laboratory personnel should advise the clinicians who use the service of the patterns of reactivity determined by the analytical platform used.

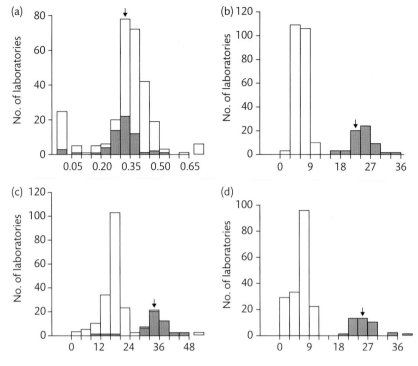

FIGURE 3.6

Cumulative results from an EUROEQAS specific IgE distribution which tested for reactivity to four allergens: (a) house dust mite; (b) cat; (c) grass pollen; (d) birch pollen. Solid columns indicate values reported by laboratories using the same assay, clear columns represent the distribution of values reported using different analytical platforms. *x*-axis, kU/L; *y*-axis, number of participating laboratories.

Reproduced with permission from UKNEQAS.

As part of the UKNEQAS quality assessment programme, a web-based educational tool (http://www.immqas.co.uk) is available. In the allergy section, individuals select their level of expertise then navigate through a series of virtual patient results, answering questions and suggesting additional tests and potential diagnoses. Completed assessments are compared with respective peer group responses and can be logged on a personal achievement folder.

3.12 **Total IgE measurements**

Although detection of allergen-specific IgE antibodies has an important role in allergy diagnosis, measurement of total serum IgE is of very limited value. Total IgE levels are age-dependent (the values are shown in Table 3.4) and vary widely in allergic and nonallergic individuals. There is no clear cut-off level to indicate allergic disease. High levels of sIgE may occur when the total IgE concentration is within the normal range. Alternatively, high levels of total IgE (>1000 kU/L) may give rise to false-positive sIgE results, so measuring total IgE may be helpful if nonspecific positivity is suspected.

Total IgE measurements can be useful in a number of nonallergic conditions such as parasitic infections; immunodeficiency (hyper IgE syndrome, Wiskott–Aldrich syndrome, Omenn's syndrome); vasculitis (Churg–Strauss syndrome), and IgE myeloma.

TABLE 3.4 Age-related serum IgE levels (kU/L)

Age	Median	95th centile
Newborn	0.5	5
3 months	3	11
1 year	8	29
5 years	15	52
10 years	18	63
15 years	22	75
Adult	26	81

Adapted from *PRU Handbook of Clinical Immunochemistry*, 9th edition, 2007; reproduced with permission.

SELF-CHECK 3.4

In what circumstances are total IgE measurements useful?

3.13 IgG antibodies

Allergen-specific IgG antibodies may be detected in patients with allergic disease. The clinical value of measuring allergen-specific IgG antibodies (often termed precipitating antibodies) is limited to a relatively small number of conditions in which chronic exposure to inhaled allergens gives rise to elevated levels of these antibodies.

Precipitating IgG antibodies (precipitins)

Chronic exposure to organic dusts containing, for example, moulds or bird droppings can result in hypersensitivity reactions involving lung interstitium and terminal bronchioles. Specific IgG antibodies can be detected in serum from patients with pulmonary diseases such as:

- **farmer's lung:** IgG antibodies to *Saccharopolyspora rectivirgula* (formerly *Micropolyspora faeni*) or *Thermoactinomyces vulgaris*
- **allergic alveolitis and allergic bronchopulmonary alveolitis**: IgG antibodies to *Aspergillus fumigatus*
- **bird fancier's lung:** IgG antibodies to avian serum/faecal extracts.

Traditionally, these antibodies are detected by the Ouchterlony plate double diffusion technique whereby the antigen/antibody reaction is visualized as a precipitin line. Hence the terminology: precipitating IgG antibodies or precipitins. Specific IgG immunoassays, similar to IgE immunoassays, are now more commonly employed.

The presence of specific IgG in the serum indicates exposure to the antigen and hence the antibodies can be detected in both symptomatic and asymptomatic subjects. However, a high level of antigen-specific IgG in a symptomatic individual would be supportive of the diagnosis.

Immunotherapy

The proposal that desensitization may work, in part, by stimulating the production of blocking IgG antibodies has led to the suggestion that specific IgG and/or IgG subclasses (predominantly IgG4) could be used to monitor immunotherapy. Successful aeroallergen immunotherapy may be accompanied by increased levels of allergen-specific IgG, but this is not a universal finding. Consequently, because specific IgG/subclass levels do not necessarily correlate with control of clinical symptoms, monitoring of specific antibodies has not entered mainstream clinical practice. An exception appears to be wasp and bee venom desensitization, where quantifying venom-specific antibodies can be used to guide dosing schedules.

Food allergy

Determination of food-specific IgG has no clinical relevance in the investigation of food allergy. IgG antibodies to dietary antigens can be detected in healthy individuals, and food-specific IgG antibody levels do not correlate with the results of oral food challenges.

SELF-CHECK 3.5

Can you identify the conditions in which allergen-specific IgG antibody testing provides useful diagnostic information?

3.14 Flow cytometric analyses

A novel approach to the laboratory diagnosis of allergy is offered by the analysis of allergen-induced basophil activation by flow cytometry. The basis of the test is the demonstration of an altered membrane phenotype on activated peripheral blood basophils. In practice, the methodology is similar to that used for immunophenotypic analysis of lymphocyte subpopulations involving immunofluorescence labelling of membrane antigens with monoclonal antibodies and detection and quantitation by flow cytometry.

Flow cytometric basophil activation test

Interaction of allergen with membrane-bound IgE results in cross-linking of the IgE molecules and subsequent basophil stimulation. As well as secretion of bioactive mediators, up-regulation of several activation markers occurs, most notably CD63 and CD203c. The general characteristics of these molecules are summarized in Table 3.5 and Figure 3.7.

The attraction of this method is that it may more accurately mimic the *in vivo* situation of allergen challenge rather than, as with specific IgE testing, indicate previous exposure to

TABLE 3.5 Surface membrane characteristics of CD63 and CD203c on unstimulated and stimulated basophils

	CD63	CD203c
Unstimulated	Barely detectable	Constitutively present
Stimulated	Up-regulation within 10 min. Expressed at high density	Up-regulation within 5 min. Expressed at lower density than CD63

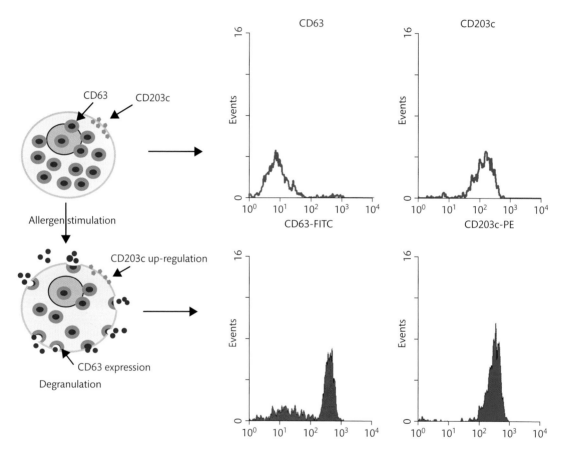

FIGURE 3.7

In resting basophils CD63 is located in intracellular granules. On activation the granules fuse with the surface membrane and CD63 is expressed on the cell surface. This can be detected by flow cytometry. Upper left quadrant: background immunofluorescence signal; lower left quadrant: positive signal. CD203c is constitutively expressed on the surface membrane of resting basophils and up-regulated following activation. This can be detected by flow cytometry. Upper right quadrant: low-level immunofluorescence signal; lower right quadrant: positive signal. x-axis, fluorescence intensity; y-axis, number of events.

Adapted, with permission, from Ebo *et al*. (2006) *Allergy*, **61**, 1028.

the allergen. The technique may be particularly applicable in situations where specific IgE tests are unavailable or have poor diagnostic sensitivity or specificity, for example, in drug allergy. The assays are labour-intensive, however, and unlikely to replace specific IgE testing in most cases.

METHOD 3.2 Basophil activation test

Basophils, either in whole blood or from buffy coat or gradient sedimentation preparations, are incubated with allergen extract. Positive (IgE) and negative (saline) controls are included.

Cell suspensions are labelled with fluorochrome-conjugated monoclonal antibodies:

■ anti-IgE (to facilitate identification of basophils on flow cytometry plots)

■ anti-CD63 and/or CD203c (activation markers).

Flow cytometric analyses are performed. Basophils are identified on the basis of side-scatter laser light and fluorescence signals. The percentage of CD63-or CD203c-positive basophils is determined (see Figure 3.8).

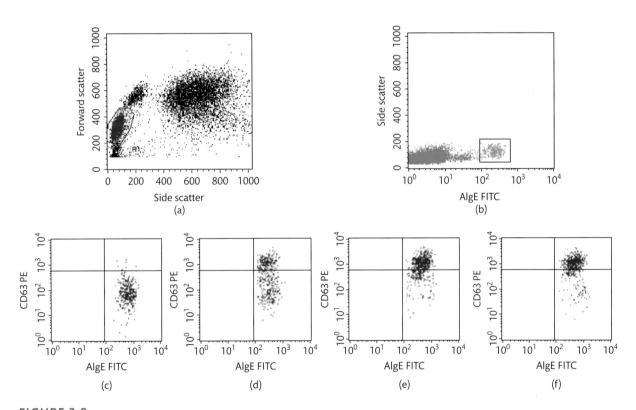

FIGURE 3.8

Flow cytometric dot plots demonstrating basophil activation and CD63 positivity in a patient with latex allergy. (a) Peripheral blood leukocytes distinguished on the basis of forward and side-scatter laser light signals. A gate is drawn electronically around the lymphocyte population (red); (b) basophils (green) are identified from within the gated lymphocyte population on the basis of side-scatter laser light and green fluorescence signals; CD63 reactivity in: (c) unstimulated basophils, negative control (<3%; upper right quadrant); (d) basophils stimulated with IgE, positive control (50%); (e) basophils stimulated with latex allergen, 0.12 µg/mL (72%); (f) basophils stimulated with latex allergen, 0.03 µg/mL (78%).

Figure courtesy of Dr ML Sanz.

Evaluative studies have reported good correlation with clinical diagnoses for inhalant allergy (pollens, house dust mite), Hymenoptera venom allergy, and latex allergy. A representative series of flow cytometric plots following the basophil activation test conducted on a blood sample from a patient with latex allergy is shown in Figure 3.8. The diagnostic sensitivity of the test is lower for drugs, probably reflecting the weaker allergenicity of these molecules. Nonetheless, the technique has potential diagnostic utility in the investigation of reactions caused by neuromuscular blocking agents and β-lactam antibiotics.

Internal quality control for the basophil activation test relies on concurrent analysis of a blood sample from a healthy individual.

Key Points

Basophil activation tests can provide useful *in vitro* diagnostic information, particularly when specific IgE tests are unavailable or have poor diagnostic sensitivity or specificity, e.g. drug allergy.

Allergen-induced basophil activation is assessed by flow cytometric analysis of CD63 or CD203c expression.

3.15 Measurement of mediators released during allergic reactions

Cross reference

Two mediators which have a role in allergy diagnosis are described in sections 3.16 and 3.17.

As we have seen in section 3.3, a number of preformed or newly synthesized mediators are released during an allergic reaction. However, very few of these molecules are measured in the routine diagnostic laboratory. This is because of difficulties of detection, either because the molecules have short half-lives or standardized assays are unavailable.

3.16 Mast cell tryptase

Mast cell tryptase exists in two major forms: α-tryptase and β-tryptase. Both forms of the enzyme are synthesized and secreted as precursors: pro-α-tryptase and pro-β-tryptase, respectively. Together, pro-α-tryptase and pro-β-tryptase make up the baseline levels of mast cell tryptase detected in the circulation. As these enzymes are virtually unique to mast cells, blood levels typically reflect the body's mast cell content; i.e. the higher the tryptase level, the greater the number of mast cells present.

As well as being directly secreted, β-tryptase is stored, in a tetrameric form, in secretory granules in mast cells, where it is the principal preformed mediator within these structures. Activation of mast cells (by IgE- and non-IgE-mediated mechanisms) results in degranulation and release of β-tryptase and other preformed mediators (e.g. histamine; heparin). Thus, detection of elevated levels of β-tryptase in the circulation is an indication of mast cell activation.

Following degranulation, mast cell tryptase levels in the blood peak within 1 hour, with a return to normal levels within 12 hours. This contrasts with histamine, also released during mast cell activation, where maximal blood levels are observed within 5 minutes of degranulation, with a return to baseline within 30 minutes. Given this short time frame, collection of blood samples for histamine analyses can pose problems. Hence, measurement of mast cell tryptase is the preferred assay for clinical laboratories assessing mast cell activation, e.g. in anaphylaxis.

Measurement

Serum or plasma mast cell tryptase may be measured by fluorescence immunoassay. The capture antibody employed in the assay identifies both α- and β-tryptase and so detects total tryptase. The normal range in serum/plasma is 2–14 ng/ml, most of which is α-tryptase. Following mast cell degranulation the predominant form that is measured is β-tryptase.

Clinical utility

Mast cell tryptase measurements are useful in the laboratory investigation of mastocytosis or suspected anaphylaxis.

Mastocytosis

Mastocytosis is a disease characterized by proliferation of mast cells in various tissues (bone marrow, skin, liver, spleen, gastrointestinal mucosa). Cutaneous (generally indolent) and systemic (generally aggressive) forms of the disease are described. Clinical manifestations are caused by mast cell infiltration into tissues and release of bioactive mediators acting locally or at distant sites. Microscopic analysis of tissue biopsy, in which increased numbers of mast cells are detected, is a key laboratory test. However, measurement of mast cell tryptase is also helpful in that increased levels, usually over 20 ng/ml (rarely >100 ng/ml) are found. Monitoring mast cell tryptase levels during cytoreductive therapy may be helpful, as decreasing levels will reflect a reduction in mast cell burden.

Anaphylaxis

Mast cell tryptase levels are elevated in most cases of anaphylaxis. However, the timing of sample collection is critical for detection of anaphylaxis-induced tryptase release. A series of samples taken within 1 hour of the reaction and at 3 and 24 hours post-reaction is recommended. This allows for detection of mast cell tryptase within the period of maximal release (1–3 hours) and determination of the patient's baseline level (24 hours). Time of venepuncture in relation to the reaction should be clearly indicated on the samples and a clinical history including information about drugs or foods taken before the reaction, or insect stings should be provided. This allows for a proper interpretation of results to be made.

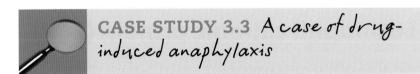

CASE STUDY 3.3 A case of drug-induced anaphylaxis

A 44-year-old woman was scheduled for an emergency appendicectomy. Anaesthesia for this procedure was induced using fentanyl (an opioid) and propofol. In order to pass an endotracheal tube a muscle relaxant, suxamethonium, was also administered. All these medicines were given over 30 seconds in a rapid manner. Within minutes a red urticarial rash developed over her arms and chest. At the same time her heart rate became fast, 140 beats/min (normal 60–90) and when checked her blood pressure had fallen dangerously to 52/40 mmHg (normal 120/80). She also developed a wheeze.

Allergic anaphylaxis was immediately suspected and the patient was given 100% oxygen and intravenous fluids. 0.5 mg of adrenaline, 10 mg chlorphenamine, and 200 mg hydrocortisone were administered intravenously.

Within 10 minutes the blood pressure had returned to normal and the wheeze settled.

Blood samples were taken for mast cell tryptase at 15 minutes and 6 and 24 hours following the reaction. These revealed levels of 81.2, 22.0, and 4.1 ng/ml, respectively. Suxamethonium-specific IgE measured on the 24-hour sample was also elevated, at 2.4 kU/L.

The patient had skin testing performed 6 weeks following the reaction to determine which of the drugs used had caused the reaction. Skin prick testing was positive for suxamethonium. As there is cross-reactivity between the suxamethonium and other anaesthetic muscle relaxants, she had skin testing to the muscle relaxants commonly used in anaesthesia. This showed that the patient was also allergic to rocuronium and vecuronium but not the others.

The patient was advised to wear a medical alert bracelet and warn doctors and nurses of her allergy if she needed any further surgery.

Other allergic conditions

Mast cell tryptase measurements may be useful in investigating reactions to insect venom, as basal serum levels may predict the severity of reaction. Furthermore, the test may help to exclude mastocytosis, which is an important consideration if immunotherapy is being considered.

Unlike drug or venom-induced anaphylaxis, the levels of mast cell tryptase determined in food-related reactions are rarely significantly elevated.

Measurement of mast cell tryptase in post-mortem blood (up to 24 hours after death) may provide supportive evidence for anaphylactic shock.

SELF-CHECK 3.6

Why is it important to know the time of blood sampling in relation to an anaphylactic reaction when interpreting mast cell tryptase levels?

3.17 Eosinophil cationic protein (ECP)

ECP is a single-chain, zinc-containing protein which is stored in the secretory granules of eosinophils. Activation of the cells results in release of ECP. The secreted protein exhibits a number of properties:

- cytolytic actions against bacteria, viruses, parasites
- stimulation of mucus production in the airways
- histamine release from basophils and mast cells.

Within the airways release of ECP may contribute to epithelia damage, increased hypersensitivity leading to chronic inflammatory airways disease. Consequently, ECP has been investigated as a potential biomarker of airway inflammation, particularly in asthmatic patients.

Measurement

ECP can be measured by fluorescence immunoassay. The assay is straightforward, but standardization of sample collection and handling is critical for assay reproducibility. This is because of *in vitro* release of ECP which occurs during the clotting process. Consequently, serum ECP measurement combines the physiological level with that released by *in vitro* activation. The latter element reflects the propensity of activated eosinophils to release granule proteins. As 'primed' eosinophils are a feature of airway inflammation, ECP is more readily released from these cells than from 'unprimed' eosinophils. Thus, discrimination between the levels observed as a consequence of airway inflammation compared with those detected in health is enhanced. Serum measurements are regarded, therefore, as being superior when assessing and monitoring airway inflammation.

A number of practical controls should be set in place if ECP assays are undertaken:

- use of blood collection tubes with gel barriers to decrease cell transfer to the serum phase
- standardization of clotting times (60–120 minutes) and temperature (20–24 °C)
- transfer of serum into a fresh tube within 1 hour of separation.

Values of more than 15 µg/mL are considered to be elevated for both adults and children (>2 years).

Clinical utility

In asthmatic patients, ECP levels in blood (and bronchoalveolar lavage and sputum) reflect airway inflammatory status. Monitoring ECP during anti-inflammatory therapy (e.g. with corticosteroids) may be helpful in assessing compliance and/or efficacy of treatment.

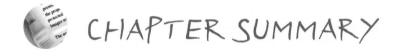 CHAPTER SUMMARY

- The incidence of allergic disease is increasing.

- Allergy is a hypersensitivity reaction. IgE antibodies initiate a two-stage reaction: induction/sensitization and reactive phases.

- Allergy is a systemic disease. Patients can present with single or multiple symptoms.

- Allergy diagnosis is based on clinical assessment supplemented by laboratory investigations. Taking an accurate clinical history, skin testing and appropriate selection of allergen-specific IgE tests are the primary diagnostic tools used to diagnose allergic disease.

- Allergens are heterogeneous, and IgE antibody cross-reactivity can occur.

- Recombinant allergens can be used to define disease-eliciting components and allow component-resolved diagnoses (CRD) to be made.

- Quality assurance for allergy testing can be problematic. No reference standards are available for any allergen preparation. Consequently, assessment of results should be made with a peer group using a comparable assay platform.

- Allergen-specific IgG antibody testing can aid in the diagnosis of respiratory conditions caused by chronic exposure to inhaled allergens. Food-specific IgG antibody testing is not useful in the investigation of food allergy.

- Determination of *in vitro*-induced basophil activation by flow cytometry has a role in the investigation of certain allergic reactions, e.g. in suspected drug allergy.

- Circulating levels of mast cell tryptase are raised during anaphylaxis. Detection of elevated levels in serum would support a diagnosis of anaphylaxis provided the blood sample has been taken within 3 hours of a suspected reaction.

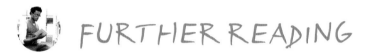

FURTHER READING

- Ahlstedt S, Murray CS (2006) **In vitro diagnosis of allergy; how to interpret IgE antibody results in clinical practice.** *Primary Care Resp J*, **15**, 228–236.

- Crameri R (2006) **Allergy diagnosis, allergen repertoires and their implications for allergen specific immunotherapy.** *Immunol Allergy Clin North Am*, **26**, 179–189.

- Ebo DG, Sainte-Laudy J, Bridts CH, *et al.* (2006) **Flow-assisted allergy diagnosis: current applications and future perspectives.** *Allergy*, **61**, 1028–1039. A comprehensive review explaining how flow cytometry can be used in allergy diagnosis.

- Gell PGH, Coombs RRA (eds.) (1963) *Clinical Aspects of Immunology*, 1st edition. Blackwell, Oxford. The original definition of the four types of hypersensitivity.

- Hamilton RG, Adkinson NF (2004) **In vitro assays for the diagnosis of IgE-mediated disorders.** *J Allergy Clin Immunol*, **114**, 213–225.

- Kay AB, Kaplan AP, Bousquet J, Holt PG (2008) *Allergy and Allergic Diseases*, 2nd edition. Wiley-Blackwell, Oxford. A major reference source which describes the scientific basis of allergy and the aetiology, diagnosis, and treatment of allergic diseases.

- Schwartz LB (2006) **Diagnostic value of tryptase in anaphylaxis and mastocytosis.** *Immunol Allergy Clin North Am*, **26**, 451–463.

- Simons FER *et al.* (2007) **Risk assessment in anaphylaxis; current and future approaches.** *J Allergy Clin Immunol*, **120**, S2–24.

- Vrtala S (2008) **From allergen genes to new forms of allergy diagnosis and treatment.** *Allergy*, **63**, 299–309.

- Williams P, Sewell WA, Bunn C, Pumphrey R, Read G, Jolles S (2008) **Clinical immunology review series: an approach to the use of the immunology laboratory in the diagnosis of clinical allergy.** *Clin Exp Immunol*, **153**, 10–18. A paper that explains the role of the diagnostic laboratory in the assessment of patients with allergic disease.

- Wohrl S *et al.* (2006) **The performance of a component based allergen microarray in clinical practice.** *Allergy*, **61**, 633–639.

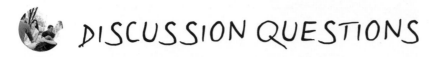

DISCUSSION QUESTIONS

3.1 What are the relative advantages and disadvantages of natural extracts and recombinant allergens as diagnostic tools?

3.2 How should quality assessment be undertaken in a laboratory performing allergy tests?

3.3 What is the role of flow cytometry in allergy diagnosis?

Answers to these questions are provided in the book's Online Resource Centre; visit www.oxfordtextbooks.co.uk/orc/ahmed/

4

Complement

Introduction

The complement (C) system consists of a group of soluble plasma proteins which interact with one another in three distinct enzymatic activation cascades:

- the classical pathway (CP)
- the alternative pathway (AP)
- the lectin pathway.

The naming of the classical and alternative pathways is historical, as the classical pathway was described first. However, in evolutionary terms the alternative pathway is likely to have arisen first. The names are potentially confusing; it should be remembered that the alternative pathway is not an alternative to the other pathways, but a pathway in its own right with its own role in immune defence. Complement plays a central role in innate immune defence, providing a system for the rapid destruction of a wide range of invading microorganisms. The control of complement activation is essential to prevent rapid consumption of complement *in vivo*. The control is provided by ten or more plasma- and membrane-bound inhibitory proteins acting at multiple stages of the system. The major source of most of the complement components and soluble control proteins is the liver. Other tissues and cells may synthesize specific proteins and local synthesis by macrophages and other cells at sites of inflammation may be of importance in maintaining local concentrations in the tissues during activation. Figure 4.1 shows an overview of the complement system.

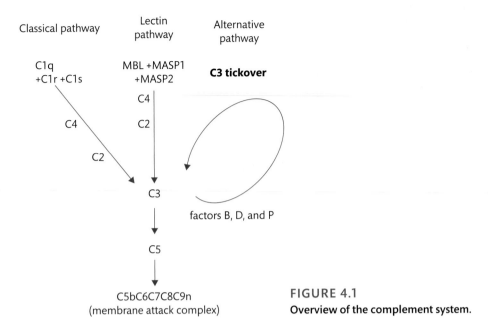

FIGURE 4.1
Overview of the complement system.

Key Point

The classical and alternative pathways are so named for historical reasons. Each is an important pathway in its own right.

4.1 **Actions of complement**

Complement, through its different components, mediates many actions, including **opsonization** of targets, clearance of antigen–antibody complexes, inflammation, phagocyte recruitment, and formation of the membrane attack complex which can result in cell lysis.

The different pathways of complement are triggered in different ways. The alterative and lectin pathways are triggered by microbial cell surfaces, and the classical pathway is triggered by antibody-antigen complexes. During complement activation, the components are cleaved into active forms. These are labelled 'a' for the small fragment and 'b' for the large fragment. For example, C5 is cleaved into C5a and C5b. C5a binds to the C5a receptor present on a number of cell types, including endothelial cells and phagocytes, and mediates an inflammatory response. C5b binds to C6 and C7 and initiates assembly of the membrane attack complex which punches holes in cell membranes. Look at Table 4.1 for a list of complement components and their actions.

Classical pathway

The first step in the **classical pathway** involves binding of C1q to aggregated or immune complex-bound IgG or IgM antibody. C1 is a large multicomponent complex with a molecular weight of approximately 800 kDa. It consists of a single molecule of C1q and two molecules each of C1r and C1s. Binding of multiple heads of the C1q molecule by aggregated IgG or

Opsonization
The binding of complement and antibodies to the surface of a pathogen or foreign substance to aid phagocytosis.

Classical pathway
The complement pathway that is triggered by antibody bound to particulate antigen. Many other substances, including components of damaged cells, bacterial lipopolysaccharide, and nucleic acids can also trigger the classical pathway in an antibody-independent manner.

TABLE 4.1 Complement components and their functions

Pathway	Component	Action
Classical	C1q	Binds to Fc portion of antibodies (IgM and IgG in particular) leading to activation of C1r
	C1r	Cleaves and activates C1s
	C1s	Cleaves C4 and C2
	C4	C4b binds to C2, which is then cleaved by C1s (C4a is a weak inflammatory mediator)
	C2	As part of C4b2a cleaves C3 and forms C4b2aC3b, which cleaves C5
Lectin	MBL	Binds to sugars present on bacterial cell walls and activates MASP2
	MASP1 and 2	Cleaves C4 and C2, leading to the formation of C4b2a3b as above
Alternative	C3	Spontaneously hydrolyses (tickover) forming C3a and C3b
	Factor B	Binds to C3b on bacterial cell wall and is then cleaved by factor D. The resultant C3bBb cleaves C5
	Factor D	Cleaves factor B into Ba and Bb
	Properdin	Stabilizes the C3bBb complex
Common	C3	Activated as above C3a mediates inflammation C3b cleaves and activates C5 by the classical and lectin pathways
MAC	C5	C5a is a potent inflammatory mediator C5b initiates formation of the MAC
	C6 and C7	Bind to C5b forming C5b67 C5b67 insert into the target cell membrane
	C8	Binds to C5b67 and anchors the complex more tightly to the cell membrane
	C9	Multiple C9 molecules bind to C5b-8 and polymerize, forming an open pore in the cell membrane

MAC, membrane attack complex.

IgM triggers activation of the other components of the C1 complex. C1r and C1s are homologous single-chain molecules with a molecular weight of 80 kDa, which associate with one another and with C1q in a calcium-dependent complex (Reid 1986, Reid and Day 1989). Conformational changes in C1q trigger the autoactivation of the proenzyme C1r, and activated C1r in turn activates C1s in the complex. C1s in the activated C1 complex will cleave and activate the next component of the classical pathway, C4.

C4 is a large (200kDa) plasma protein containing three disulphide-bonded chains (α, β, and γ) (Schreiber and Muller-Eberhard 1974, Janatova and Tack 1981). C1s cleaves plasma C4 at a single site near the N-terminus of the α chain, releasing a small fragment, C4a (Mw ~9 kDa) and exposing a labile, reactive thioester group in the α chain of the large fragment, C4b. Once exposed in C4b the thioester forms covalent amide or ester bonds with exposed amino or hydroxyl groups respectively on the activating surface, locking the molecule to the activating surface. Membrane-bound C4b provides a receptor for the next component of the classical pathway, C2.

C2 is a single-chain plasma protein of molecular weight 102 kDa. In the presence of Mg^{2+} ions, C2 binds membrane-bound C4b and is cleaved by C1s in an adjacent C1 complex. The C-terminal fragment, C2a, remains attached to C4b to form the C4b2a complex, the next enzyme in the classical pathway.

C3, a 185-kDa heterodimeric molecule, is the most abundant of the complement components (1–2 mg/mL in serum) and is essential for activity of both the classical and alternative pathways (Lambris 1988). C3 binds the C4b2a complex and is cleaved by the C2a enzyme, releasing a small fragment, C3a (9 kDa), from the N-terminus of the α chain and exposing in the large fragment, C3b, a labile thioester group. C3b binds via the thioester either to the activating C4b2a complex or to the adjacent membrane (Kozono et al. 1990, Ebanks et al. 1992). C3b bound to the activating C4b2a complex constitutes a new enzyme, C4b2a3b, the C5-cleaving enzyme (convertase) of the classical pathway.

C5 is a heterodimeric protein of 190 kDa molecular weight that is structurally related to C3 and C4 but lacks a thioester. C5 binds to C3b in the C4b2a3b convertase and is cleaved by C2a in the complex. A small fragment, C5a (~10 kDa), is released from the N-terminus of the α chain, whilst the large fragment, C5b, remains attached to the convertase.

Alternative pathway

The key component of the **alternative pathway** is C3, but three other proteins, factor B (fB), factor D (fD), and properdin are also required. Factor B, a single-chain protein closely related to C2, binds C3b in a Mg^{2+}-dependent manner. This renders factor B susceptible to cleavage by factor D, a 26-kDa serine protease present in plasma in its active form. Cleavage exposes a serine protease domain in the large (60-kDa) fragment, Bb (Gotze 1986). The C3bBb complex can then cleave more C3 to generate C3b. Properdin binds and stabilizes the C3bBb complex.

Initiation of the alternative pathway occurs spontaneously, a phenomenon known as 'tick-over'. C3 in plasma is hydrolysed to form a metastable $C3(H_2O)$ molecule which binds factor B in solution and renders it susceptible to cleavage by factor D to form a fluid phase C3 convertase (Lachmann and Hughes-Jones 1984, Law and Dodds 1990). The surface features of many microorganisms and foreign cells favour amplification of the alternative pathway and rapidly become coated with C3b molecules.

Binding of a second C3b molecule to the C3bBb complex generates the C5-cleaving enzyme of the alternative pathway, C3bBbC3b. C5 is cleaved by Bb in a manner identical to that described above for cleavage in the classical pathway, in which the large fragment C5b remains attached to the convertase.

Lectin pathway

The more recently described **lectin pathway** provides a second antibody-independent means of activation of complement on the surfaces of bacteria and other microorganisms. Mannan-binding lectin (MBL) is a high molecular weight serum lectin made up of multiple copies of a single 32-kDa chain that binds mannose and N-acetylglucosamine residues in bacterial cell walls (Reid and Turner 1994, Turner 1991, Holmskov et al. 1994). The structure of MBL resembles that of C1q and it too is associated with a serine protease, MBL-associated serine protease (MASP). The MBL–MASP complex activates C4 in a manner identical to that described above for the activated C1 complex.

Alternative pathway
The complement pathway that provides a rapid, antibody-independent route for activation and amplification of complement on foreign surfaces.

Lectin pathway
A means of activation of complement on bacterial and other microorganism surfaces. It is antibody-independent and shares C2, C3, and C4 with the classical pathway, to which it is highly analogous.

Membrane attack pathway

The membrane attack pathway involves the noncovalent association of C5b with the four terminal complement components to form an amphipathic membrane-inserted complex, the **membrane attack complex (MAC)**. C5b, while attached to the C5 convertase, binds C6, a large single-chain plasma protein. The C5b6 complex then binds C7, a single-chain protein homologous to C6, which triggers the release of the complex from the convertase. The C5b67 complex binds tightly to the surface membrane of the microorganism through its labile hydrophobic binding site. C8 is a heterotrimeric protein and binds C7 in C5b67, causing the complex to insert deeper in the membrane. Finally, multiple copies of C9 bind the C5b-8 complex to form a large transmembrane pore, the MAC, which can cause lysis of the target cell by allowing free diffusion of molecules in and out of the cell.

Membrane attack complex (MAC)

A large transmembrane pore formed from the terminal complement components which can cause lysis of the target cell by allowing free diffusion of molecules in and out of the cell.

Key Point

All three complement pathways result in the formation of C5 convertase, leading to the formation of the membrane attack complex (MAC), which can result in the lysis of target cells.

SELF-CHECK 4.1

Can you name the three complement pathways and what triggers them?

4.2 Regulation of complement

The complement system is tightly controlled at multiple stages in the pathway by regulatory proteins present in plasma and on cell membranes (Morgan and Harris 1999).

The first step of the classical pathway is regulated by C1 inhibitor (C1inh), a serine protease inhibitor which binds activated C1 and removes C1r and C1s from the complex (Davis 1988, Davis 1989). C1inh is the only plasma inhibitor of activated C1 and even partial deficiency can result in uncontrolled activation of complement in peripheral sites, with resultant inflammation—the syndrome known as **hereditary angioedema (HAE)**.

Hereditary angioedema (HAE)

Genetic mutations resulting in the decreased levels of C1 esterase inhibitor in serum are found in approximately 85% of patients (type I). The remaining 15% of patients have normal or elevated serum concentrations, but the protein produced by one allele is dysfunctional (type II). This results in episodes of angioedema.

Control of the C3 and C5 convertases is provided by factor I (fI), a serine protease which, in the presence of essential cofactors, cleaves C3b and C4b to inactivate the convertases. In plasma, two proteins act as cofactors for fI; factor H (fH) in the alternative pathway and C4bp in the classical pathway. Both fH and C4bp also inhibit the pathways by accelerating the decay of the convertases. On the membrane, decay-accelerating factor (DAF) acts to accelerate the decay of convertases, whereas membrane cofactor protein (MCP) acts as cofactor for the cleavage of C4b and C3b by fI, irreversibly inactivating the enzyme. Complement receptor 1 (CR1) is a large transmembrane protein which has both decay-accelerating and cofactor activities.

The membrane attack pathway is also regulated by inhibitors present in the fluid phase and on membranes. The fluid-phase C5b-7 complex is the target of S-protein (vitronectin) and clusterin, abundant serum proteins which, among their many roles, help regulate complement activation by binding the hydrophobic site in C5b-7. On the membrane, CD59 binds

TABLE 4.2 Complement control proteins

Control protein	Mechanism of action
Liquid phase	
C1 esterase inhibitor (C1inh)	Binds and deactivates C1qrs complex
Factor I (fI)	Cleaves C3b and C4b
C4-binding protein (C4bp)	Accelerates decay of C4b2a and acts as a cofactor for fI cleavage of C4b
Factor H (fH)	Accelerates decay of C3bBb and acts as a cofactor for fI cleavage of C3b
Membrane bound	
Complement receptor 1(CR1)	Accelerates decay of both C4b2a and C3bBb. Acts as a cofactor for fI cleavage of C3b and C4b
Decay-accelerating factor (DAF)	Accelerates decay of C4b2a and C3bBb
Membrane cofactor protein (MCP)	Cofactor for fI cleavage of C3b and C4b
CD59	Prevents formation of the membrane attack complex (blocks incorporation of C9)

to C8 in the C5b-8 complex and blocks incorporation of C9 and assembly of the MAC (Lachmann 1991).

Table 4.2 summarizes the complement control proteins.

SELF-CHECK 4.2

Name five proteins involved in the regulation of complement. For each protein, describe its method of action.

4.3 **Complement deficiencies**

Deficiencies of almost every complement protein and regulator have been described and more detailed accounts of the various complement deficiencies can be found in several reviews (Morgan and Walport 1991, Colten and Rosen 1992, Figueroa *et al.* 1993). Several of the assays to be described in this chapter are useful in screening for complement deficiency, but an understanding of the symptoms associated with deficiencies of different components is essential for selecting the right tests.

Deficiencies of components of the classical pathway (C1, C4, or C2) are associated with an increased susceptibility to immune complex disease, a consequence of the failure of immune complex solubilization. The frequency and severity of disease is greatest with deficiencies of one of the subunits of C1 (C1q, C1r, C1s), closely followed by total C4 deficiency, each giving rise to a severe immune complex disease which closely resembles systemic lupus erythematosus (SLE). Deficiency of C2 is the most common homozygous complement deficiency in white people, but causes much less severe disease. Inherited or acquired deficiency of C1 esterase inhibitor can lead to episodes of swelling.

C3 is an essential component of all activation pathways and is vital for efficient opsonization of bacteria. C3 deficiency is associated with a marked susceptibility to bacterial infections.

Cross references

Two recent reviews focusing on complement in disease are Pettigrew *et al.* (2009) and Botto *et al.* (2009).

Look at section 4.5 for more information on C1 inhibitor deficiency.

You can read in more detail about SLE in Chapter 5.

Haemolytic uraemic syndrome (HUS)

A deficiency or mutation in factor H or factor I can lead to a susceptibility to HUS, which consists of the triad of thrombocytopenia, Coombs negative microangiopathic haemolytic anaemia, and acute renal failure.

Deficiencies of the regulators factor I and factor H cause a secondary deficiency of C3 and also present with recurrent bacterial infections. Furthermore, a deficiency or mutation in either factor H or I can lead to susceptibility to atypical **haemolytic uraemic syndrome (HUS)**, which is the most common cause of renal failure in children.

Deficiencies of the alternative pathway components are rare. A few individuals deficient in factor D or factor H have been described, all of whom have presented with recurrent *Neisseria* infections, usually meningococcal meningitis. Deficiency of the positive regulator properdin is the most common disorder of the alternative pathway and is also associated with meningococcal infection.

Deficiencies of terminal pathway components (C5, C6, C7, C8, or C9) also cause susceptibility to *Neisseria* infection—often presenting as meningococcal meningitis or systemic meningococcal infection.

Use of deficient and depleted sera to characterize complement deficiencies

Sera deficient in or depleted of individual components can be used to identify the specific component that is missing in complement-deficient individuals. Table 4.3 lists the complement

TABLE 4.3 The component proteins of the complement system. The proteins that constitute the classical, alternative, and membrane attack pathways are listed

Component	Structure	Plasma conc. (mg/L)
Classical pathway		
C1	Complicated molecule, composed of 3 subunits, C1q (460 kDa), C1r (80 kDa), C1s (80 kDa) in a complex (C1qr$_2$s$_2$)	180
C4	3 chains from a single precursor: α, 97 kDa; β, 75 kDa, γ, 33 kDa	600
C2	Single chain: 102 kDa	20
Alternative pathway		
fB	Single chain: 93 kDa	210
fD	Single chain: 24 kDa	2
Properdin	Oligomers of identical 53-kDa chains	5
Common		
C3	2 chains: α,110 kDa; β,75 kDa	1300
Terminal pathway		
C5	2 chains: 115 kDa, 75 kDa	70
C6	Single chain: 120 kDa	65
C7	Single chain: 110 kDa	55
C8	3 chains: α, 65 kDa; β, 65 kDa; γ, 22 kDa	55
C9	Single chain, 69 kDa	60

Modified from Morgan BP, Harris CL (1999) *Complement Regulatory Proteins*. Academic Press, London.

METHOD 4.1 *Depletion of sera of individual complement components*

Complement C1

C1 is a euglobulin and can be removed from serum by dialysis against low ionic strength buffer. Dialyse fresh serum (5 mL) overnight at 4 °C against 2 L of 10 mmol/L barbitone buffer pH 7.4 containing $CaCl_2$ (5 mmol/L) and NPGB [nitrophenylguanidinobenzoate] (0.1 mmol/L). Centrifuge at 5000 g for 15 min at 4 °C. Store C1-depleted serum (R1) in aliquots at −70 °C.

Complement C4

The thioester group in C4 (and C3) is inactivated by treatment of serum with ammonia. To 8.5 mL of serum (guinea pig serum is most commonly used) add 1.5 mL NH_4OH diluted to 150 mmol/L in H_2O. Incubate for 45 min at 37 °C; adjust pH to 7.4 with dilute HCl. Store C4-depleted serum (R4) in aliquots at −70 °C.

Complement C2

C2 and factor B are the most heat labile of the complement components. Place fresh serum (1 mL) in a glass tube preheated in a 56 °C water bath and incubate at 56 °C for precisely 6 min with constant shaking. C2-depleted serum (R2) generated in this manner should be stored on ice and used immediately.

Complement C3

Incubation of serum with zymosan efficiently depletes C3 and partially depletes C5 and the terminal components. Zymosan depletion of C3 works better in guinea pig serum than in human serum. Incubate 1 mg boiled zymosan (Sigma) in 10 mL serum at 37 °C for 60 min; centrifuge (1000 g, 5 min) to pellet zymosan. Store supernatant (R3) in aliquots at −70 °C.

Complement factor B

Place fresh serum (1–2 mL) in a glass tube preheated to 50 °C in a water bath. Incubate for 20 min with continuous shaking. Factor B-depleted serum generated in this manner should be stored on ice and used immediately.

Complement factor D

Factor D can be selectively depleted from serum by virtue of its small size. Apply fresh serum (1 ml) to a Sephadex G-75 gel filtration column (0.5 × 30 cm) equilibrated in veronal buffered saline (VBS). Factor D is significantly retarded on this column. Develop the column in VBS and pool the void volume fractions, containing the bulk of the serum proteins minus factor D. Store in aliquots at −70 °C.

Mannose-binding lectin (MBL)

MBL can be depleted from serum by utilizing its affinity for specific carbohydrates.

---

components, their structure, and normal plasma concentration. If a particular patient serum fails to restore haemolysis when mixed with a particular deficient or depleted test serum, then the patient and test sera must be missing the same component. Human and animal sera deficient in many individual components are now widely available from many suppliers, but they are expensive and of variable quality. It may be easier to generate depleted sera in-house for use in these assays. Sera may be depleted of individual complement components by 'classical' or immunochemical methods. 'Classical' methods for depletion are summarized in Method 4.1 above.

With the increasing availability of monoclonal antibodies against the complement components, immunoaffinity methods are now widely used to generate depleted sera. The general principle involves immobilizing the appropriate monoclonal antibody on Sepharose and applying fresh serum to the column at 4 °C. The completeness of the depletion can be easily assessed in haemolytic assays. Orren and colleagues have described a simple and sensitive haemolysis-in-gel assay utilizing known complement-deficient sera to simultaneously screen patient serum for deficiencies of each of the terminal complement components (Egan *et al.* 1994). Although, with the increasing availability of the essential reagents, assays of this sort could easily be established in most clinical immunology laboratories, we do not advise this course of action. Artefacts induced in sample handling and the influence of *in vivo* complement activation can make interpretation of results difficult. Laboratories experienced in complement assays will be better equipped to recognize and correct these problems.

Key Point

Sera deficient in or depleted of individual components can be used to identify the specific component that is missing in complement-deficient individuals.

Complement in pathology

Cross reference

Section 4.4 provides more detail about the assays available for measuring complement activity.

Activation of complement occurs in a large number of inflammatory diseases and is likely to be an important contributor to tissue damage in these diseases. Complement deposition can be detected in the tissues and products of complement activation are found in the plasma. Assays for individual complement components may be of help in identifying complement activation, but measurement of complement activation products is a far more sensitive and specific approach.

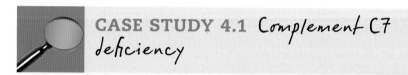

CASE STUDY 4.1 Complement C7 deficiency

A woman aged 37 was admitted to hospital with group C meningococcal septicaemia, having previously had meningococcal meningitis twice aged 35 and 16. She recovered fully after treatment, a CT scan showed no cranial bony abnormality, and upon discharge she was started on lifelong penicillin V 250 mg once daily.

She was found to have a serum C3 concentration of 1.31 g/L (normal 0.97–2.0), C4 0.18 g/L (normal 0.14–0.45), classical pathway CH_{50} activity 174 (normal 1000–1200 units) and alternative pathway CH_{50} 0 (normal 80–200 units). Immunochemical assays of individual serum complement components revealed a complete deficiency of C7.

Her daughter and three siblings had CH_{50} values within the normal range, but one brother had a low classical pathway CH_{50} activity (430 units) with a normal alternative pathway CH_{50} (176 units).

She was immunized with the tetravalent meningococcal vaccine that contains relevant immunogens of the A, C, Y, and W135 meningococcal groups, as patients with terminal pathway complement deficiencies are at risk of infection with all of these strains (Morgan and Orren 1998). This vaccine is different from the usual commercially available bivalent meningococcal vaccine which contains immunogens from groups A and C only. Neither contains immunogens from the remaining group B, as effective vaccines for group B organisms do not yet exist.

4.4 Measurement of complement activity

Sample handling for measurement of complement components

Most of the complement proteins are heat-labile and so correct handling of samples is essential if reliable, meaningful results of complement assays are to be obtained. Improper handling of samples may result in incorrect or uninterpretable results. This applies especially to assays of complement haemolytic activity and complement breakdown products. Serum is used for measurement of C3 and C4 and for measuring the haemolytic activity of the classical and alternative pathways (CH_{50} and AP_{50} assays). Clotted blood taken for these assays (2–4 mL) should reach the laboratory on the day of venesection, where sera should be assayed directly or separated, aliquotted and frozen (at $-20\,°C$ for up to one month, $-70\,°C$ for longer periods). Repeated freezing and thawing of specimens should be avoided as it can lead to loss of activity. For assays of complement activation products, EDTA plasma is used. By chelating Ca^{2+} and Mg^{2+}, EDTA inhibits *in vitro* activation through the classical, alternative, and lectin pathways. Again, plasma should be obtained fresh and either assayed immediately or stored frozen as described above. Some commercial additives have been developed specifically to inhibit *in vitro* activation of complement. The advantages of these agents over EDTA are minor.

Key Point

The handling of samples for complement analysis is critical to ensure that reliable results are achieved in the laboratory.

Assays of complement haemolytic activity

Assay of the serum complement haemolytic activity (CH_{50}) involves measuring the ability of all the complement protein molecules involved to lyse target cells. This measures the functional activity of the whole system from initiation through to endpoint. The only compelling indication for measuring CH_{50} is when a deficiency of a complement component protein is suspected. There is rarely any reason to assay CH_{50} in any fluid other than serum. Patients who have complement deficiencies typically present clinically in one of three ways:

- a second infection with *Neisseria meningitides*, the causal organism of meningococcal meningitis and meningococcal septicaemia (which can occasionally coexist). Any patient who has two or more infections with this organism should have the CH_{50} assayed (whether this should be assayed after the first episode of meningococcal infection is debatable)

- failure to clear immune complexes, giving a clinical picture resembling systemic lupus erythematosus (SLE)

- recurrent infections, usually bacterial.

Classical pathway activity CH_{50}

The classical pathway CH_{50} measures the amount of a serum sample required to lyse 50% of a standardized suspension of sheep erythrocytes (Esh) coated with optimal amounts of rabbit anti-Esh antibody (EshA; made by preincubation with antibody and subsequent washing). The assay assesses activity from C1q activation through to cell lysis by the membrane attack pathway. Different dilutions of a standard and the test sera are incubated with EshA in different wells of a 96-well microtitre plate and the degree of haemolysis in each well is measured. This enables calculation of the amount of classical pathway haemolytic activity per mL of test serum. The measured CH_{50} will be dependent on the concentration of EshA in the system, the relative concentrations of reactants, ionic strength, and many other variables, and so it is important to standardize the assay conditions.

Alternative pathway activity CH_{50}

The alternative pathway CH_{50} measures the activity of the alternative pathway from initiation of C3 activation through to lysis. Washed rabbit erythrocytes (Erb) without any antibody bound to their surface are used as the target cells because Erb are extremely susceptible to non-antibody-dependent haemolysis by human complement (i.e. haemolysis via the alternative pathway). The reagents and conditions used are similarly standardized. Selectivity for the alternative pathway is improved by using the chelating agent ethylene glycol tetra-acetic acid (EGTA) with excess magnesium, the former eliminating the calcium-dependent function of C1 and in the presence of the latter permitting the assembly of the magnesium-dependent C3bBb complex.

Cross reference

Other technologies in use for measuring CH_{50} activity are detailed later in this section.

Key Point

You must find our which technology is used by your local laboratory and what considerations are taken into account for the quality control, technical aspects, and interpretation of the results provided by the test system in place.

Standardization and quality control

The classical pathway assay is standardized against a commercially available freeze-dried standard material. Each lot of material has an ascribed value for the classical pathway CH_{50}. This material is also included in every alternative pathway assay, although no value for the alternative pathway CH_{50} has been ascribed to it by the manufacturers.

Internal quality control is achieved by running an aliquot of a standard normal human serum in every assay run. This material is obtained from a single normal donor, aliquotted, and frozen at −70 °C and a fresh aliquot used for each assay. There is currently no external quality assurance scheme available for complement haemolytic activity assays.

Expression of results in CH_{50} units/mL from activity in X_{50} µL

The classical pathway CH_{50} results are expressed in arbitrary units using the following calculation, on the basis that the amount of complement haemolytic activity is inversely proportional to the amount of serum required to produce 50% haemolysis of the erythrocyte (X_{50}):

$$CH_{50} = (1/X_{50}) \times 2000$$

The alternative pathway CH_{50} results are expressed similarly. A different multiplication factor is used to generate a different range of values for results:

$$CH_{50} = (1/X_{50}) \times 200$$

Normal ranges for these assays should be calculated locally. The normal ranges for the classical pathway and alternative pathway CH_{50} were calculated in our laboratory by measuring a number of normal sera. This provided a range of 1000–2000 units/mL for the classical pathway and 80–200 units/mL for the alternative pathway. Some laboratories report the haemolytic activity as a percentage of normal; more than 50% activity when compared with a normal serum is considered to be normal activity.

Inter-run correction factor

As this is a bioassay, a significant amount of variation may occur from one assay run to another. This has the potential of producing results that may be significantly influenced by variables such as the laboratory temperature or extraneous influences upon the susceptibility of the erythrocytes to haemolysis. In order to compensate for these variables it is recommended to modify the calculated CH_{50} values obtained.

The necessary modification is made by multiplying every measured test CH_{50} value by a correction factor, as follows:

$$\text{Corrected serum } CH_{50} = \text{Measured serum } CH_{50}$$
$$\times (\text{Standard material mean } CH_{50}/\text{Standard material measured } CH_{50})$$

(The standard material mean CH_{50} is the running mean of many serial measurements of the standard material CH_{50}.)

Acceptability of results

In order to measure the CH_{50} values of the test sera accurately, the absorbance of the samples and the standard are measured at 3-minute intervals. This provides multiple calculations of the CH_{50} at different incubation times. As the standard material has an expected value (from experience ±15% from its target value), the incubation time that gives a CH_{50} standard value nearest to the target value is chosen, and it is at this time that the patient's CH_{50} values are reported.

When a patient's serum gives a low CH_{50} result, it is recommended to perform a repeat assay without a prior dilution step. This will attempt to quantify low levels of haemolytic complement.

Interpretation of results

Values of CH_{50} activity that are high or in the low normal range do not have any clinical significance. Low values of CH_{50} most often result from complement consumption. The serum concentrations of C3 and C4 may or may not be low, and so clinical details are required to clarify such situations. Low values of alternative pathway CH_{50} activity are frequently seen in infants;

these values usually rise into the normal range after a few months. In such cases, repeat assays after a suitable interval are recommended, with prophylactic antibiotics being recommended in the interim if clinically indicated.

Key Points

When interpreting functional complement assay results, the levels of complement C3 and C4 must be taken into account.

Clinical details are required to interpret the results of complement assays.

Alternative assays for measuring CH_{50}

Several assays have been described which have sought to establish a simplified system for measurement of CH_{50} levels, removing the requirement for erythrocytes as indicator cells.

Numerous liposome-based assays have been reported (Bowden *et al.* 1986, Canova-Davis *et al.* 1986, Yamamoto *et al.* 1995). A commercially available kit (Autokit CH50; Wako Ltd, Osaka, Japan) utilizes liposomes loaded with the enzyme glucose-6-phosphate dehydrogenase (G6PD). The antibody-sensitized liposomes are incubated with the test and control sera and released enzyme is quantified in the supernatant by monitoring the conversion of NAD in the substrate buffer to NADH (increased absorbance at 340 nm). The kit is simple, sensitive, and correlates well with assays utilizing EshA as an indicator.

Recently, several protocols have been described for measurement of CH_{50} which eliminate altogether the need for an indicator cell or liposome. Enzyme immunoassay (ELISA) methods measure the appearance of complement activation products and generate results which can be expressed in CH_{50} equivalent units (Goldberg *et al.* 1997, Zwirner *et al.* 1998). A commercially available kit measures the generation of the terminal complement complex (TCC). These assays have also been shown to correlate well with 'classical' CH_{50} techniques.

The Binding Site total haemolytic complement assay is an adaptation of a traditional radial immunodiffusion assay. It uses the principle that sheep erythrocytes coated with anti-sheep erythrocyte antibody (haemolysin) will activate the classical pathway in the presence of normal serum. Erythrocytes coated with haemolysin are incorporated into an agarose gel. Serum is added to wells in the plate and incubated to allow diffusion of complement components. Activation of the classical pathway results in a clear zone of haemolysis around the well and the diameter of this zone will be proportional to the haemolytic activity of the sample (see Figure 4.2). A similar assay is available for the alternative pathway. This uses the principle that chicken erythrocytes will bind C3b. The formation of C3 convertase activates the alternative pathway, resulting in haemolysis of the erythrocytes.

SELF-CHECK 4.3

Why is sample handling for CH50 important?

Immunochemical measurement of individual components

The complement proteins C3, C4, and C1 inhibitor (C1inh) are present in serum at sufficient concentrations and antisera of uniformly good quality are commercially available so as to

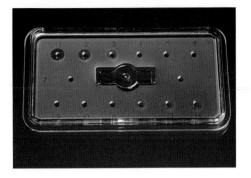

FIGURE 4.2

Haemolysis of sheep erythrocytes coated with anti-sheep erythrocyte antibody by complement.

Courtesy of The Binding Site.

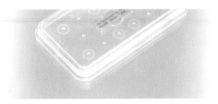

FIGURE 4.3

Measurement of complement component protein by RID.

Courtesy of The Binding Site.

allow them to be reliably assayed by nephelometry or turbidimetry. Other complement proteins (C1, C2, C5–C9) may be assayed immunochemically by radial immunodiffusion (see Figure 4.3). They have alternatively been assayed by rocket electrophoresis, but this is a cumbersome method that is now infrequently used.

Standardization and quality control

Most of the immunochemical assays have been standardized using an international reference preparation for plasma proteins provided by the International Federation of Clinical Chemistry (IFCC).

Internal quality control is achieved by running an aliquot of a standard normal human serum in every assay run. This material is obtained from a single normal donor, aliquotted and frozen at −70 °C and a fresh aliquot used for each assay. UK NEQAS offer external quality control schemes for complement C3, C4, and C1 inhibitor (both antigenic and functional activity).

Interpretation of results

You need to understand the complement pathways and the relationship of the different components in order to interpret the immunochemical results.

- An increase in the plasma concentrations of C3 and C4:
  - commonly seen during inflammation. C3 and C4 are acute phase proteins and can be seen together with an increase in CRP and ESR (erythrocyte sedimentation rate). As C3 and C4 increase as acute phase proteins, levels can sometimes appear normal even when the proteins are being rapidly consumed.
- A decrease in both C3 and C4:
  - commonly seen when the classical pathway is activated
  - immune complex-mediated diseases such as SLE
  - consumption of the complement components (sepsis).
- C3 is decreased and C4 is normal:
  - commonly seen when the alternative pathway is activated (Gram-negative sepsis)

Cross reference

You can read in more detail about nephelometry, turbidimetry, and radial immunodiffusion in the *Biomedical Science Practice* book of this series

— post-streptococcal glomerulonephritis

— C3 nephritic factor.

- C3 is normal and C4 is decreased:

    — Type II cryoglobulinaemia associated with hepatitis C infection

    — C1 inhibitor deficiency (discussed in more detail in section 4.6)

    — active SLE

    — genetic deficiency (C4 null alleles).

CASE STUDY 4.2 *Complement values in neonates*

An only child, aged 11 weeks, of nonconsanguineous parents, presented with a group B meningococcal meningitis. He was born by vaginal delivery at 36 weeks gestation after spontaneous rupture of the membranes and developed pneumonia soon after birth (with no organism isolated), again aged 5 weeks, and RSV bronchiolitis at 7 weeks.

While he was ill 5 weeks after birth his serum C3 concentration was 0.66 g/L (normal 0.97–2.0), C4 0.14 g/L (normal 0.14–0.45), classical pathway CH_{50} activity 1106 (1000–1200 units) and alternative pathway CH_{50} 0 (80–200 units).

Primary complement deficiency or alternatively a combination of complement consumption due to pneumonia and delayed acquisition of adult serum levels were considered as possibilities. He was thus started on regular prophylactic broad-spectrum antibiotic treatment.

When well, aged 12 weeks, the serum C3 concentration was 0.90 g/L, C4 0.14 g/L, classical pathway CH_{50} activity 2139 (1000–1200 units) and alternative pathway CH_{50} 70 (80–200 units).

This case illustrates firstly that age-specific ranges for relevant complement values still require definition, particularly for neonates (despite there being a higher incidence of meningitis in childhood than adulthood) and secondly that prophylactic antibiotic treatment may need to be started empirically and later withdrawn when complement values normalize.

Measurement of activation fragments and complexes

Assay of fragments and/or complexes generated during complement activation provides an accurate and dynamic picture of the complement activation status at the time of sampling. The small fragments C4a, C3a, C5a, and Bb; the large fragments iC3b and C4d; and the complexes C1r, C1s/C1inh, C3bBbP, and SC5b-9 (TCC) all represent potential targets for assay (Wurzner *et al.* 1997). Judicious choice of assays can yield information on the pathway by which complement is activated, as well as the degree of activation. Of the fragments, C3a has been most used as an index of complement activation. C3a is rapidly inactivated in serum by removal of a single Arg residue from its C-terminus and all available assays measure both C3a and its metabolite C3adesArg. Radioimmunoassays for C3a(desArg) are commercially available and have been widely used in research and diagnosis. ELISA assays for C3a(desArg) have more recently become available. A comprehensive panel of ELISA assays for complement activation products is commercially available. The best of the ELISA assays depend upon the generation of neoantigens in complement fragments or complexes not expressed by the native components. ELISA assays utilizing antibodies against neoepitopes in the SC5b-9 complex have proved particularly useful.

4.5 C1 inhibitor deficiency

Hereditary and acquired angioedema

C1 inhibitor functions as an essential regulator of the complement, coagulation, and contact (kinin-forming) systems. It is a serine protease inhibitor and acts as a suicide protein in that it becomes consumed during its inhibition of complement C1r and C1s, the contact system factor XII and kallikrein and the coagulation factor XI (Davis *et al.* 1993a). Lack of inhibition of these systems by C1 inhibitor leads to the formation of vasoactive peptides, whose precise identity remains uncertain. The molecule is encoded at a single locus, and expression of adequately functioning paternal and maternal alleles is necessary to provide sufficient serum enzymatic activity for health. When one copy encodes a dysfunctional or nonexpressed protein, clinical angioedema results (homozygous deficiency is not compatible with life). Subcutaneous swellings lasting 1–5 days are important to control, as they are embarrassing and frequently misconstrued by others as indicating violence. Abdominal swellings can mimic an acute abdomen and upper airways swelling can cause life-threatening laryngeal oedema. Some patients report relatives who have died of unexplained asphyxia.

Hereditary angioedema (HAE) has an autosomal-dominant inheritance, but symptoms may sometimes first appear only in adulthood. Heterozygotes manifest the condition and thus it is not too uncommon, affecting about 1 in 50 000 people (Davis 1988). In more than 20% of patients with HAE the mutations are spontaneous and therefore there is no family history of disease (Agostoni and Cicardi 1992). Many types of mutation result in the absence of a protein product of that allele in serum, and reduced immunochemical concentrations of C1 inhibitor are found in approximately 85% of patients (type I HAE). The remaining 15% of patients have normal or elevated serum concentrations, but the protein produced by one allele is dysfunctional, usually due to point mutations causing amino acid substitutions at or near the enzyme's active site (type II HAE) (Davis *et al.* 1993b).

Acquired angioedema (AAE) is rare and due to increased consumption rather than deficient production of C1 inhibitor. Autoantibodies to C1 inhibitor bind to the molecule in such a way as to allow it to become cleaved by other plasma proteases, or consumed and cleaved during its interaction with the C1r–C1s complex while preventing its inhibition of the complex's activity (Mandle *et al.* 1994). Serum assays thus show reduced C1 inhibitor function (due to consumption) but immunochemical levels as measured by nephelometry may be normal due to the presence of cleaved C1 inhibitor. The latter may be detected by staining a western blot of the patient's serum with an anti-C1 inhibitor antibody, when two bands are seen that represent the normal and cleaved molecules, respectively. In addition, the serum concentrations of C1, C4, and C2 are reduced as they are consumed. These autoantibodies may occur in association with leukaemia, lymphoma, and rarely other tumours (type 1 AAE) (Cicardi *et al.* 1996). They may alternatively occur in isolation or in relation to nonorgan-specific autoimmune diseases such as rheumatoid arthritis and SLE (type II AAE).

Differential diagnosis of angioedema

A thorough drug history should be taken, as some drugs such as angiotensin converting enzyme (ACE) inhibitors can cause angioedema. Patients with C1 inhibitor deficiency usually have low plasma levels of C4 (which is the substrate of the C1r–C1s complex) in between attacks, and these fall significantly further during attacks. When assessing new patients it is expedient to assay serum immunochemical concentrations of C3, C4, and C1 inhibitor at the same venesection. Low serum C4 can be present in C1 inhibitor deficiency. If this is not confirmed by immunochemical assay, then C1 inhibitor function should be assayed. If this is normal, then assay of C1 and investigations for causes of types I and II AAE should be undertaken. Usually, all laboratory results are normal and no cause is found.

Laboratory diagnosis—C1 inhibitor functional assay

C1 inhibitor function may be measured in assays that have haemolytic or esterolytic endpoints. The latter involves incubating appropriate dilutions of normal and test sera and a standard reference material with a substrate which yields a coloured product following hydrolysis by C1 inhibitor. Such assays should always be performed in specialist or reference laboratories. Many laboratories have used a commercially available chromogenic assay for C1-inhibitor activity, which contains chromogenic substrate for C1s, substrate buffer, and freeze-dried purified C1s. ELISA-based assays for C1 inhibitor functional activity are also commercially available.

Treatment of C1 inhibitor deficiency

HAE

Treatment varies according to the patient's clinical phenotype. Tranexamic acid (which inhibits some of the proteases which cleave C1 inhibitor) taken prophylactically or as required often controls symptoms adequately. In more clinically resistant cases the anabolic, androgenic steroids danazol or stanozolol (which increase transcription of many genes, including the normally functioning copy of C1 inhibitor) are required (Frank et al. 1976, Waytes et al. 1996). They may have unacceptable androgenic adverse effects in women (especially if pregnancy is desired) and they are contraindicated in prepubertal children as they limit growth. Acute upper airway obstruction requires emergency treatment. In the United Kingdom, C1 esterase inhibitor concentrate (a blood product) is used. Fresh frozen plasma is a poor substitute for C1 esterase inhibitor, and, in cases where significant complement consumption has occurred, may even worsen the situation by providing a fresh supply of complement components. Adrenaline, while life-saving in allergic reactions, provides no benefit in the treatment of HAE. Bradykinin inhibitors, which have recently become available, provide another treatment option for HAE.

AAE

The treatment of AAE is different from that of HAE, in that attempts at increasing C1 inhibitor synthesis are less likely to be helpful. Treatment is aimed at the underlying disorders—anti-tumour treatment in type I AAE and appropriate immunosuppression in type II AAE.

CASE STUDY 4.3 Hereditary angioedema

One month after starting the oral contraceptive pill, an 18-year-old woman was admitted with abdominal pain that was observed for 3 days and resolved spontaneously, allowing her discharge from hospital.

She had previously been entirely well, but then began to have deep cutaneous swellings affecting her arms and hands. Elective dental treatment had once caused facial swelling requiring hospital admission for 3 days. Over the following year she continued to have occasional swellings and, while well, was found to have serum concentrations of C3 1.31 g/L (0.97–2.0), C4 0.07 g/L (0.14–0.45), and C1 inhibitor 0.09 g/L (0.15–0.35).

The oral contraceptive pill was stopped and daily danazol treatment started, but extreme aggression necessitated its withdrawal. Tranexamic acid 1–1.5g tds for 7 days as required (additionally prophylactically for any dental treatment) resulted in satisfactory management, with only four minor swellings in the following 2 years.

SELF-CHECK 4.4

Which laboratory tests should be performed in the investigation of HAE?

4.6 Autoantibodies against complement components and complexes

Numerous autoantibodies directed against complement components have been described; so far all are directed against neoepitopes on activated or conformationally altered molecules. The reasons why some individuals develop an antibody response against these neoepitopes is not known.

Autoantibodies to the collagen-like region (CLR) of C1q (anti-C1qCLR) have been detected in numerous individuals (Strife *et al.* 1989, Wener *et al.* 1989). These antibodies only bind solid-phase C1q.

ELISA systems in which C1q or its CLR are immobilized on the plate have been developed and have demonstrated the presence of anti-C1qCLR antibodies in SLE, membranous glomerulonephritis, rheumatoid vasculitis, hypocomplementaemic urticarial vasculitis (HUVS), and other diseases. The presence of anti-C1q CLR antibodies correlates strongly with the severity of renal disease in SLE. Virtually all patients with HUVS have anti-C1q CLR antibodies; the presence of these antibodies has been used as a diagnostic aid for this syndrome (Wisnieski and Naff 1989, Wisnieski *et al.* 1995).

Autoantibodies against C1 inhibitor have been demonstrated by ELISA in some patients with AAE. It has been suggested that the autoantibody binds at a site close to the reactive centre of C1-Inh and thus blocks function (Mandle *et al.* 1994). The frequency of such antibodies in AAE is still not certain.

Autoantibodies to the C3 convertase complexes are termed nephritic factors. C3 nephritic factor (C3 NeF) is an IgG autoantibody that stabilizes the C3bBb convertase, promoting the continued activation of C3 and profound hypocomplementaemia. C3NeF has been found in association with membranoproliferative **glomerulonephritis (MPGN)** and partial **lipo-dystrophy**. Published assays for C3NeF measure the capacity of the test serum to enhance complement activation through the alternative pathway in a fluid-phase activation assay. The products of complement activation (usually C3 breakdown products) are measured after a defined incubation by two-dimensional electrophoresis, ELISA, or other appropriate method. Testing for C3NeF should be considered in patients with a low C3 and the presence of glomer-ulonephritis and/or partial lipodystrophy.

C4 nephritic factor (C4NeF) an IgG autoantibody which stabilizes the C3 convertase of the classical pathway C4b2a, has been reported in patients with SLE and glomerulonephritis (Daha *et al.* 1976). The measurement of C4NeF is not performed routinely.

SELF-CHECK 4.5

What is C3 nephritic factor? When would you measure it?

4.7 **Complement allotyping**

It is apparent that most complement components, receptors, and regulators are **polymor-phic**, some with several tens of different **allotypes**. Analysis of polymorphisms in comple-ment proteins can provide information of relevance for genetic studies and insights into function of the different allotypes. Analysis can be undertaken at the phenotypic and geno-typic levels. Most of the complement polymorphic variants can now be easily **genotyped**. Phenotypic analyses involve methods such as SDS-PAGE analysis and isoelectric focusing, separating different allotypes on the basis of altered size or charge of the protein. In recent years, allotype-specific monoclonal antibodies have been developed for several of the com-plement components, including C4, C6, and C7. These provide a very easy and rapid way of assessing the relative frequencies of different complement component allotypes (Wurzner *et al.* 1997).

ELISAs specific for the two isotypes of C7 have been used in numerous research studies but have not found a place in clinical practice. Indeed, although of considerable academic interest, it is debatable whether allotyping of complement components has any place in the clinical laboratory. Where allotyping might be of use is in the determination of null **alleles** in a patient with chronically low C4 level—could this be due to consumption (e.g. immune complexes in SLE) or reflection of a genetic deficiency? The problem here is that C4 null alleles are very complex to analyse, at both protein and genetic level. With the exception of the null allelles responsible for complete or subtotal complement deficiencies, no comple-ment allotype has yet been directly implicated in any disease process. However, most recent genome-wide association studies have not yet excluded the C4 gene as a susceptibility gene for SLE.

Glomerulonephritis (MPGN)
Inflammation of the glomeruli of the kidney.

Lipodystophy
The progressive loss of fat. Lipodystrophy may be congenital or acquired, and may affect all of the body (generalized lipodystrophy) or just parts of the body (partial lipodystrophy).

Polymorphism
Variations in a gene locus at a frequency greater than 1% (adj. **polymorphic**).

Allotypes
Allelic polymorphisms in a gene that can be determined using specific antibodies for the gene product.

Genotyping
The process of defining the genotype of an individual using laboratory techniques such as DNA sequencing and PCR. This is useful in determining if an individual has disease-associated genes.

Alleles
Variations of a single genetic locus.

Cross references

For more information on polygenic variations of C4, you can read Yang *et al.* (1993).

For more information on the involvement of C4 allotypes in the pathogenesis of human diseases, you can read Samano *et al.* (2004).

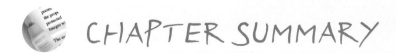

CHAPTER SUMMARY

- Complement is an important part of the immune system. There are three pathways which initiate complement activation, the classical, lectin, and alternative pathways. All the pathways result in the cleavage of C3 forming C3a and C3b, the cleavage of C5 forming C5a and C5b, and the formation of the membrane attack complex (MAC).

- Complement activation results in opsonization of targets, clearance of antigen–antibody complexes, inflammation, phagocyte recruitment, and formation of the MAC, which can result in cell lysis.

- Deficiency of complement components leads to susceptibility to infection. Deficiency of the classical pathway can increase the risk of SLE due to a lack of clearance of immune complexes.

- There are many regulatory proteins which normally hold the activation of complement under tight control. Deficiency of these can lead to disease, hereditary angioedema (HAE) being one example.

- The assessment of complement in the laboratory requires samples which have been handled appropriately. Laboratory tests can assess both the concentration of complement components, and their function.

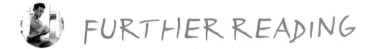

FURTHER READING

- Botto M, Kirschfink M, Macor P, *et al*. (2009) Complement in human diseases: lessons from complement deficiencies. *Mol Immunol*, **46**, 2774–2783.

- Pettigrew HD, Teuber SS, Gershwin ME (2009) Clinical significance of complement deficiencies. *Ann N Y Acad Sci*, **1173**, 108–123.

- Samano EST, *et al*. (2004) Involvement of C4 allotypes in the pathogenesis of human diseases. *Rev Hosp Clin Fac Med Sao Paolo*, **59**, 1381–1344.

- Yang Y, Chung EK, Zhou B, *et al*. (2003) Diversity in intrinsic strengths of the human complement system: serum C4 protein concentrations correlate with C4 gene size and polygenic variations, hemolytic activities and body mass index. *J Immunol*, **171**, 2734–2745.

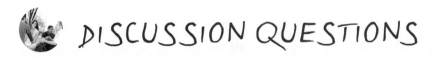

DISCUSSION QUESTIONS

4.1 Name the ways in which the complement system protects against infection.

4.2 HAE results from a deficiency of which complement regulator and what is the inheritance? What symptoms might a patient with HAE suffer from? What treatments are available?

4.3 Compare and contrast the classical and lectin pathways.

Answers to these questions are provided in the book's Online Resource Centre; visit www.oxfordtextbooks.co.uk/orc/ahmed/

5

Autoimmune rheumatological disease

Learning Objectives

After studying this chapter you should be able to:

- outline the clinical presentation of the autoimmune rheumatological diseases seen in the immunology laboratory
- outline the assays and techniques used to test for autoantibodies seen in autoimmune rheumatological diseases
- understand the performance characteristics of these tests
- describe the autoantibodies tested in the clinical immunology laboratory to aid diagnosis of autoimmune rheumatological diseases
- describe common patterns of immunofluorescence routinely seen on HEp-2 slides

Introduction

The laboratory plays an increasing role in the diagnosis and clinical management of patients with rheumatic diseases. It is therefore essential that the results of laboratory tests are both accurate and reliable, and give clinicians correct information. It is also important to keep clinicians informed of the changes occurring in the rapidly evolving field of investigation of autoantibodies.

In rheumatology the detection of autoantibodies is useful in diagnosis, prognosis, and monitoring disease activity. The first two are firmly established, while with certain exceptions, such as the quantitation of anti-double-stranded DNA, the value of the third is still not fully assessed.

This chapter focuses on the rheumatic diseases seen in the clinical laboratory and the tests used to aid their clinical diagnosis.

5.1 Systemic lupus erythematosus (SLE)

SLE is a disease that most commonly affects women of the age group 20–45. Cases do occur in men but it is approximately nine times as common in women. It can occur in children and there is no sex bias before the onset of puberty. SLE is a multisystem disease capable of affecting many different organs in the body. In reality it is probably not one disease but a group of closely related diseases which share common features. As a result of this, the symptoms of SLE vary greatly from person to person. For some patients with SLE it represents little more than a mild nuisance condition, but for some the disease is very troublesome, even life-threatening as a result of major organ failure. This heterogeneity is reflected in the 11 criteria laid out for the diagnosis of the disease, from which each patient only requires 4 to fulfil the diagnosis, thus giving many possible combinations. Thus there is no typical clinical presentation and diagnosis can often be delayed whilst other diseases are excluded.

From the American College of Rheumatology 1997 update of the 1983 revised criteria for classification, the 11 diagnostic criteria are:

- malar rash
- discoid rash
- photosensitivity
- oral ulcers
- nonerosive arthritis involving >2 peripheral joints
- pleuritis **or** pericarditis
- renal disorder: persistent proteinuria **or** cellular casts
- neurological disorder: seizures **or** psychosis in the absence of drugs or known metabolic disorders
- haemotological disorder: haemolytic anaemia **or** leucopenia **or** lyphopenia **or** thrombocytopenia
- immunological disorder: antibodies to dsDNA **or** Sm **or** positive finding of antiphospholipid antibodies (anti-cardiolipin, lupus anticoagulant or a false-positive syphilis test)
- positive anti-nuclear antibodies.

There is a strong genetic background to SLE. It is associated with null alleles within the complement region of chromosome 6 and with genes within the HLA region (DR2 in African Caribbeans and DR3 in whites).

The **aetiology** of this disease remains unclear. There are strong indications from human and mouse studies that deficiencies in **apoptosis**, the clearance of apoptotic material, and the removal from the circulation of **immune complexes** may all play a role in the induction of antibodies to self-antigens which are the characteristic hallmark of this disease. These defects probably result in a failure of the body to clear potentially antigenic material from the circulation, thus allowing it to be processed by the immune system. However, it remains debatable what role, if any, autoantibodies play in the **pathogenesis** of this disease. Complement levels (C3 or C4) may be decreased as a result of increased breakdown and may be used to monitor disease activity.

Cross reference

More information on the criteria for diagnosing SLE and other rheumatological diseases can be found at http://www.rheumatology.org/

Aetiology
The cause or origin of disease.

Apoptosis
Programmed cell death.

Immune complexes
Antigen and antibody complexes which can be soluble or insoluble. This depends on the size of the complex and the presence of complement.

Pathogenesis
The origination and development of a disease.

Cross reference

Look at Chapter 4 for more information on complement.

Environmental factors such as stress and UV light may play a part in triggering disease flares in patients with the disease, but there is little evidence linking them to its induction.

Key Point

SLE is a mimic disease and may present in a number of different ways. This is a clinical problem in which autoantibody serology can be helpful in diagnosis.

CASE STUDY 5.1 Suspected SLE

A 23-year-old florist presents to her GP with increasing tiredness and a florid rash that becomes more active after sunbathing. The doctor also notices that she has some hair loss.

The doctor thinks she might have SLE and orders some blood tests. These show that the patient has a positive antinuclear antibody (ANA) test, and that antibodies to Ro60 have also been detected. He also orders lung and kidney function tests and a full blood count.

Is this serology compatible with the doctor's original diagnosis, and why has he ordered the additional tests when the patient is only exhibiting skin-related complaints?

SELF-CHECK 5.1

What specificities of ANA are found predominantly in SLE?

SELF-CHECK 5.2

Why is it important to test for all relevant autoantibodies when investigating patients with suspected SLE?

5.2 **Rheumatoid arthritis (RA)**

Multisystem disease

A disease affecting more than one component of the body. An example is rheumatoid arthritis, which can affect the joints, lungs, kidneys, and blood vessels.

Synovial membrane

The thin membrane that lines the inside of a joint. Its function is to lubricate the joint and produce synovial fluid.

Rheumatoid arthritis is a **multisystem disease**, which can affect almost all organs within the body. The principal site of inflammation is found within the joint, but the consequences of this process can cause symptoms in many other tissues, e.g. lungs, kidneys, and blood vessels, leading to the manifestations referred to as extra-articular disease, i.e. disease occurring outside the joints.

Within the joint there is a proliferation of cells within the **synovial membrane**. These cells set up an inflammatory process which causes the further influx of immune cells into the joint space and the dysregulation of the bone remodelling processes, resulting in an excess of bone loss over bone regeneration. This process leads to small cavities being formed in the bone

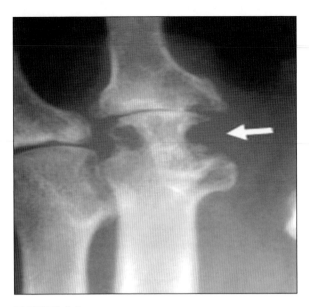

FIGURE 5.1
Erosive arthritis illustrated by plain radiography.

Reproduced by kind permission of Professor Peter Taylor,
Imperial College London.

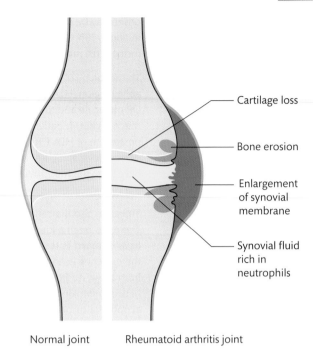

Cartilage loss

Bone erosion

Enlargement
of synovial
membrane

Synovial fluid
rich in
neutrophils

Normal joint   Rheumatoid arthritis joint

FIGURE 5.2
Pathogenesis of rheumatoid arthritis.

called erosions; over time, these erosions merge and weaken the bone, causing severe damage to the structure. Look at Figure 5.1, which is a plain radiograph showing an erosive joint.

Within this process there is evidence for an active role of T cells, macrophages, and endothelial cells. Large amounts of biologically active substances like pro-inflammatory cytokines and chemokines are found within the fluid of the joint. These potent immunoregulatory molecules ensure continued activation of cells and the recruitment of additional immunologically active cells into the joint. Look at Figure 5.2 to see the difference between a normal joint and a rheumatoid arthritis joint.

The increased levels of these immunological mediators are also found within the circulation, and presumably reflect a leakage from the joint space together with some systemic production. In addition, a number of different autoantibodies have been detected in the circulation of patients with RA and these include rheumatoid factor and antibodies to **citrullinated proteins**. Although these are useful in the diagnosis of RA, it is still unclear whether they play any role in the aetiology or pathogenesis of the disease. Other serological manifestations may include the presence of cryoglobulins and the increase of proteins associated with an acute phase response such as fibrinogen and C-reactive protein. Complement levels (C3 or C4) may appear normal or even raised due to excess production as part of the acute phase response. However, measurement of complement breakdown products (C3d or C4d) indicate that these patients often have increased levels of complement consumption as well.

Clinically the patient will often present with symptoms such as early morning stiffness and fatigue, together with joint swelling and pain. In more advanced cases there may also be symptoms in the lungs, kidneys, blood vessels, spleen, muscles, or neurological system. The

Citrullinated proteins

Citrullination is the post-translational modification of arginine within a protein to citrulline by enzymes called PADs (peptidylarginine deiminases) to form citrullinated proteins.

Cross references

You can read more about cryoglobulins in Chapter 2.

You can read more about complement in Chapter 4.

onset may be slow and symptoms will develop over a period of months and years. However, in about 20% of patients this process is accelerated and the damage occurs more rapidly. A further 20% may always have a mild disease which does not progress over time.

The aetiology of RA is unknown. There is a well-described genetic link within the histocompatability region (HLA) with a number of DRβ genes which code for a similar **epitope** on the HLA DR molecule and this is referred to as the 'shared epitope'. Frequencies of shared epitope are much higher in patients with RA than in the normal population. It has been calculated that possession of HLA DR containing the shared epitope has approximately twice the risk of any person developing RA. In addition to the shared epitope, a number of other genetic variants have been described in association with RA (e.g. PTPN22), but the contribution to the risk and the strength of the association is much lower than that for the shared epitope.

There are also indications of the effect of environmental triggers associated with the disease. There has been a long history of searching for an infective agent and prospective candidates have included Epstein–Barr virus, *Mycobacterium tuberculosis*, and *Proteus mirabilis*. However, the evidence is not strong and further work is required before any conclusion can be drawn from these studies. More recently, work from Sweden (Stolt *et al.* 2003) has suggested a link between smoking and RA, which has opened the discussion on environmental triggers to look at potential airborne pollutants as potential initiators of the immune response. It is still unclear how these environmental triggers would, in an appropriate genetically susceptible individual, lead to the production of autoantibodies and the onset of disease. The age of onset for RA is most commonly between 40 and 50 and there are four times as many cases in women as in men. However, it is important to remember that cases can occur at any time in life. There is a separate but related group of diseases which occur in children, and these may first present from the early months of life.

Epitope
The region on an antigen that is recognizable by the immune system.

CASE STUDY 5.2 Suspected RA

A 67-year-old woman presents to her doctor with joint stiffness and pain. She finds that it is worse earlier in the morning and eases as the day progresses. The doctor orders some blood tests and finds that she is anaemic, and has an IgM rheumatoid factor. He is not sure whether she has RA or not.

What further tests could the doctor order?

SELF-CHECK 5.3

What is the primary site of inflammation in RA?

5.3 Scleroderma

Systemic sclerosis is a disease in which an abnormal fibrotic process brings about changes in the structure of the skin, which lead to a decrease in permeability and flexibility. These processes may also occur in other organs of the body, which may lead to damage to kidney, lung, or digestive tract tissues.

Women are affected three to four times more often than men. The disease usually starts between the ages of 25 and 50, but occasionally it begins in children or in older people.

There are a number of variants of scleroderma, but the two most common are limited cutaneous systemic sclerosis (sometimes called **CREST syndrome)** and diffuse cutaneous systemic sclerosis.

Diffuse cutaneous systemic sclerosis combines the presence of sclerodermatous changes in the skin with those in other organs of the body. These might include blood vessels, the digestive system, lungs, and kidneys. These changes may lead to a decrease in the functioning of these organs.

The aetiology and pathogenesis of scleroderma is unknown. The connective tissue cells of patients with scleroderma can produce too much collagen. Collagen is an essential building block of the body's tissues, but if it is present in excess the tissue becomes inflexible and this may lead to an abnormal structure and consequent altered function.

These diseases are characterized by the production of specific autoantibodies that correlate well with the different disease subtypes. However, it remains unclear what role these autoantibodies play in the disease process.

> **CREST syndrome**
> A limited form of scleroderma, consisting of calcinosis (calcium deposits), Raynaud's phenomenon (a vascular defect), oesophangeal motility (problems causing difficulty with swallowing), sclerodactyly (enlarged swollen fingers), and telangiectasia (a defect of surface blood vessels in the skin).

> **Cross reference**
> The autoantibodies seen in autoimmune rheumatic diseases are discussed in section 5.8.

CASE STUDY 5.3 Suspected scleroderma

A 42-year-old nurse has noticed that her hands become painful and white when they are cold. She used to play squash, but has become increasingly breathless and now finds it difficult to climb the stairs in her house. In addition, she has also lost weight in the last 6 months.

Her GP thinks this patient could have scleroderma. Which immunological tests should he request to aid in the diagnosis?

SELF-CHECK 5.4

What are the two most common types of scleroderma and what ANA specificities are most commonly associated with them?

5.4 Sjögren's syndrome

Sjögren's syndrome is an autoimmune disease in which there is lymphocytic infiltration of the glands of the exocrine system (e.g. salivary glands and tear glands), which leads to dysfunction of the production of secretions. Other tissues of the body that may be affected include the lungs, kidneys, skin, and nervous system. It occurs mostly in women between the ages of 40 and 60 and is much less common in men than in women (only 1 in 10 of those with Sjögren's syndrome are men), and occurs only rarely in childhood. It affects all races.

There is a well-documented genetic link with genes in the HLA region. There has been much research into looking for an environmental trigger for this disease, but although a number of viruses have been proposed as candidates the story is still unclear.

SELF-CHECK 5.5

Which autoimmune rheumatic disease is associated with the dysfunction of the exocrine gland system, e.g. salivary glands or tear glands?

5.5 Polymyositis and dermatomyositis

Polymyositis is an autoimmune disease that affects mainly the large muscles of the body, such as those around the shoulders, hips, and thighs. Dermatomyositis is a related condition, which affects the skin in addition to the muscles. Polymyositis and dermatomyositis are rare diseases, affecting only 6–8 people out of every 100 000 of the population.

The disease processes that lead to the development of polymyositis and dermatomyositis are not well understood. If muscles from people with polymyositis and dermatomyositis are examined histologically, infiltrating inflammatory cells can be seen. In addition, muscle fibres can show an up-regulation of HLA molecules and the presence of deposited complement indicating an active immune process. In the case of dermatomyositis there are also pathological changes in the skin and the small blood vessels leading to the muscles.

Polymyositis and dermatomyositis are frequently associated with the presence of disease-specific autoantibodies, which can be helpful in differentiating myositic disease caused by autoimmunity from those found in cancer or in metabolic diseases. Recently, an up-regulation of autoantigen in affected tissues has been documented, although it is unclear whether this is a precursor of disease or a response to inflammation (Casciola-Rosen *et al.* 2005, Suber *et al.* 2008).

Genetic influences are seen in some variants of myositis, mostly with genes in the HLA region. There has been much research looking for potential environmental triggers in these diseases, but so far this has failed to reveal any strong associations.

5.6 Anti-phospholipid syndrome (APS)

Thrombosis

The formation of a blood clot (thrombus) within the blood vessels.

APS is a disorder in which the blood has a tendency to clot too easily. This can affect any vein or artery in the body. There are two main problems caused by APS. They are, firstly, blood clotting in inappropriate blood vessels (**thrombosis**) and secondly, in pregnant women, a tendency to miscarriage. Symptoms may include headaches, memory loss, forgetfulness and fatigue, visual disturbances, and seizures or fits. It is estimated that as many as 1 in 5 people under 40 years who suffer from strokes may have APS. Deep vein thrombosis (DVT) of the leg is the commonest type of venous thrombosis, but patients with APS may also have arterial complications. There are two main areas of the heart that can be affected: the heart valves and the coronary arteries that supply blood to the heart muscle. The heart valves may become thickened and fail to work properly. The coronary arteries may also become thicker, leading to angina. In addition, other organs such as the kidneys and lungs may also be affected.

All age groups can be affected, from infants to elderly people. However, the majority of people with APS are aged between 20 and 50 years. It seems to affect the health of women more than that of men because of its effect on pregnancy.

Like many of the autoimmune rheumatic diseases, APS may have both genetic and environmental triggers. It is characterized by the presence of circulating antibodies to phospholipids and phospholipid cofactors, but the role of the autoantibodies has yet to be fully elucidated. It can be shown experimentally that the antibodies are capable of interfering with the functioning of the clotting and fibrinolytic cascades and thus present a potential mechanism for a pathogenic role in the disease process. They may also be capable of interacting with endothelial cells and platelets to encourage conditions promoting the formation of blood clots.

In 1999 revised guidelines for the diagnostic criteria for antiphospholipid syndrome were published. These guidelines break the criteria down into three areas.

- Clinical criteria:
  - vascular thrombosis
  - pregnancy morbidity
  - laboratory criteria
- Anticardiolipin antibody
- Lupus anticoagulant.

SELF-CHECK 5.6

Which autoimmune rheumatic disease most commonly presents as either thrombosis or recurrent fetal loss?

Cross reference

You can read the Sapporo guidelines for the diagnosis criteria for antiphospholipid antibodies in more detail in Wilson *et al.* (1999).

5.7 Overlapping connective tissue diseases

Overlapping connective tissue diseases are syndromes where patients may exhibit clinical and serological features from more than one autoimmune rheumatic disease. The most common of these is mixed connective tissue disease (MCTD), in which patients exhibit symptoms of SLE, polymyositis, and scleroderma. In addition to this, there are also well described overlap syndromes between

- limited cutaneous systemic sclerosis (CREST), primary biliary cirrhosis, and Sjögren's syndrome
- polymyositis and scleroderma
- SLE and rheumatoid arthritis
- SLE and scleroderma.

In some cases, the autoantibody profiles of these diseases may reflect one or other of the diseases or in some cases both diseases. In some, however, the autoantibody profile is associated with the overlap syndrome and not with the diseases in isolation (e.g. anti-PM/Scl antibodies in polymyositis–scleroderma overlap syndrome).

Cross reference

You can read more about primary biliary cirrhosis in Chapter 8.

Key Point

Patients with overlap syndromes may appear to have different rheumatic diseases at different times, e.g. a patient with SLE/scleroderma overlap may present as SLE but develop more sclerodermatous features as the disease develops, because of the acute versus chronic nature of the two diseases.

5.8 **Autoantibodies**

This section aims to describe the autoantibodies that are tested in the clinical immunology laboratory to aid the diagnosis of autoimmune rheumatological diseases. In order to interpret the results of these tests, you need to understand the performance characteristics of the test. This applies to any of the assays performed in the clinical immunology laboratory and must be borne in mind when interpreting any result.

METHOD 5.1 Clinical Specificity and sensitivity

Sensitivity

The ability of an assay to correctly identify disease. The number of false negatives.

Specificity

Lack of interference from other elements other than the analyte being measured. The number of false positives.

Sensitivity is defined as the percentage of patients within a defined disease group who have the antibody, whereas **specificity** is defined as the percentage of positive results which are contained within the target disease group.

An ideal diagnostic assay is highly specific for the disease and occurs in the majority of patients with that disorder (high sensitivity). It must be borne in mind that diagnostic sensitivity may increase with frequent blood sampling, since the level of autoantibody (e.g. rheumatoid factor) may correlate with the activity and stage of the disease and may be affected by the drugs that are being used to treat the disease. Sensitivity may also reflect genetic heterogeneity and ethnic origins of populations under study, a notable example being the frequency of anti-Sm in SLE, which is 60% in African-Caribbean populations but only 5% in white populations. Sensitivity and specificity may also depend on the method. Thus enzyme-linked immunosorbent assays (ELISA) are more sensitive than gel precipitation techniques. However, increased sensitivity often goes hand in hand with a decrease in specificity, as increasingly small amounts of antibody are detected; thus an assay with very high sensitivity may be of little use diagnostically because of its very low specificity. The specificity of an assay may also be affected by the material used as the antigenic source, its purity, and the nature and conformation of the peptides and epitopes presented in the assay.

Specificity is usually measured in relation to a population of healthy subjects, but suitable age-matched control populations should be used, since some autoantibodies occur in healthy elderly people. It is often of greater relevance to compare the test population with others displaying clinical features which are likely to be confused (e.g. RA and SLE), or that are part of a differential diagnosis.

Anti-nuclear antibodies

Anti-nuclear antibodies (ANA) are autoantibodies directed against cellular components. The term 'ANA' is something of a misnomer, as some of these antigens are actually cytoplasmic in location. Chromosomal antigens include single- and double-stranded DNA, deoxyribonucleoprotein (DNP), and histones. Antibodies have also been described against the centromeric proteins and various nucleolar proteins. Soluble nuclear or cytoplasmic antigens which are readily extracted in phosphate-buffered saline (pH 7.2) have been termed 'extractable nuclear antigens' (ENA) or 'soluble cellular antigens'. Some of these antigens are named according to their biochemical nature (e.g. ribonucleoproteins: RNP) or according to the diseases in which they occur (e.g. Sjögren's syndrome: SS-A). ANA are usually initially tested by indirect immunofluorescence (IIF) on HEp-2 cells or on cryostat sections of rodent tissues. In addition to the strength of reaction, as either intensity or titre, the pattern of staining should be recorded as this may indicate certain specificities, such as the centromeric antigen, and those located in the nucleolus. Look at Figure 5.3 for some commonly recognized ANA patterns seen on immunofluorescence and their antigen associations.

	Pattern on HEp 2 cells	Target	Disease association
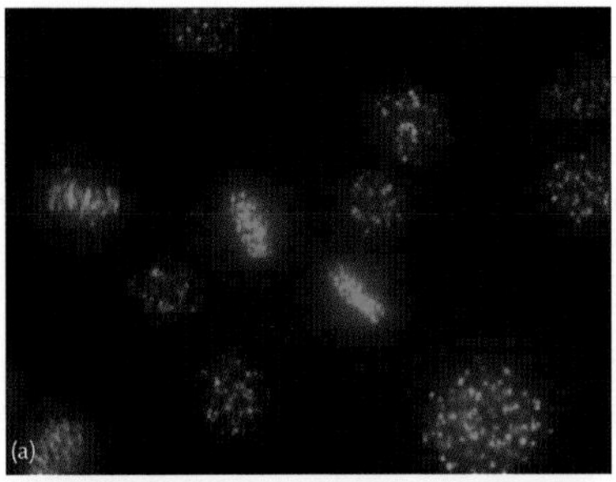	Centromere	Cenp A, B, C	Limited scleroderma / CREST (60%) Raynaud's phenomenon
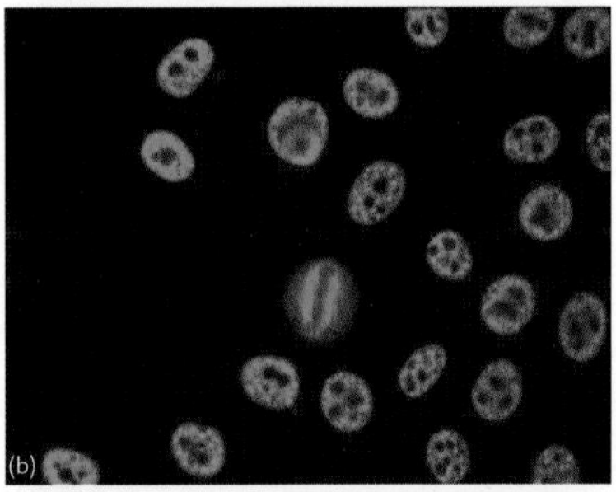	Coarse speckled	U1RNP, Sm	SLE
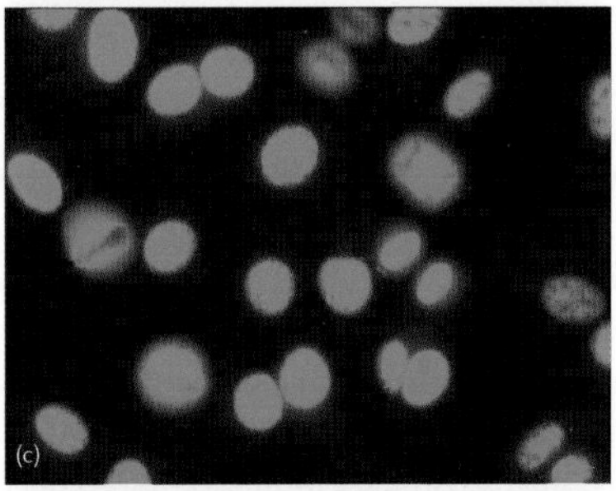	Fine speckled	Ro (SS-A), La (SS-B)	Sjögrens' syndrome (95%) SLE (40%) Scleroderma (5%)
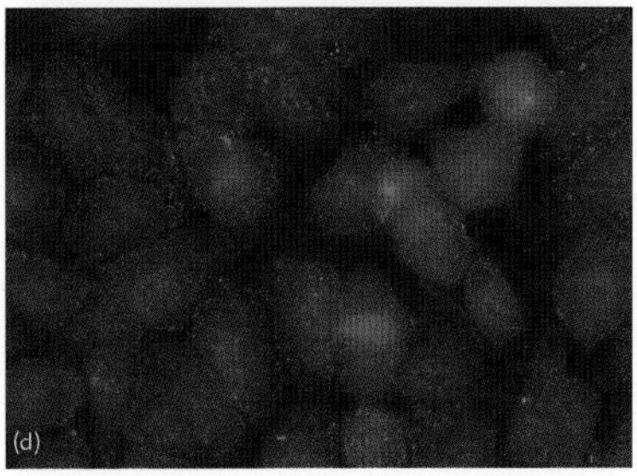	Cytoplasmic speckled	Jo-1	Polymyositis

FIGURE 5.3
Commonly recognized ANA patterns and their antigen associations.

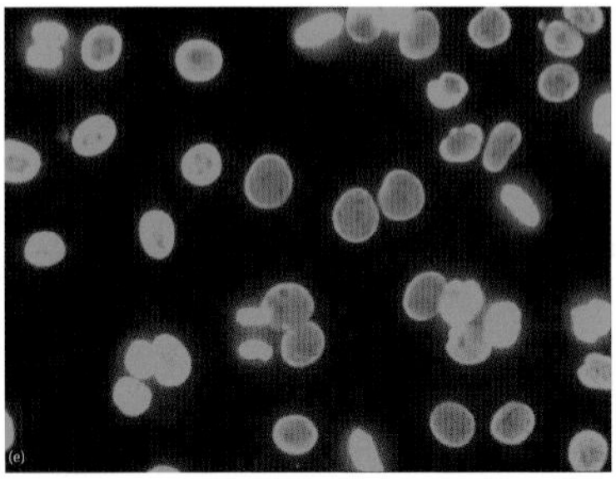	Homogenous	dsDNA, Histones	SLE (95%) Discoid lupus
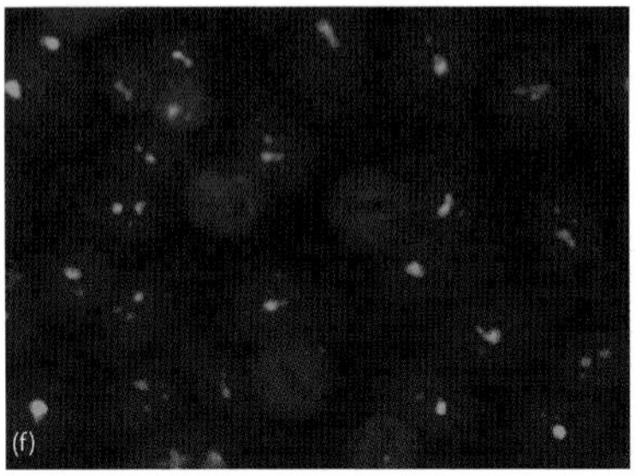	Nucleolar homogenous	Pm-Scl	Scleroderma (30%) Polymyositis/ scleroderma overlap
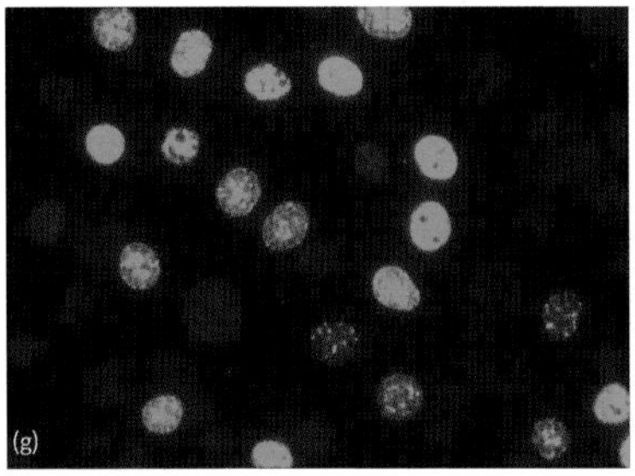	Pleiomorphic (PCNA)	Cyclin	SLE (1-3%)

FIGURE 5.3

Commonly recognized ANA patterns and their antigen associations. *(Continued)*

Other screening methods, including ELISAs using purified antigens or cell homogenates, are also gaining in popularity. These have become more popular as they do not demand the same level of expert practice as IIF in their interpretation. Although such screening techniques give an indication of the presence or absence of antibodies, it is the specificity of the antibody that is important in determining disease associations. It should be remembered that not all antigens are nuclear in cellular location, and that for certain antibodies (e.g. anti-Ro or anti-Jo-1) the ANA is not a useful test for their presence, as they may not be detected on ANA immunofluorescence.

The specificity of the antibody is determined by techniques such as radioimmunoassay, gel diffusion, ELISA, or immunoblotting. ANA with high specificity are called 'disease markers'. These antibodies are rarely found in other than their designated diseases. Look at Table 5.1 for a list of these antibodies. Certain specificities are also associated with specific clinical features and may point to future clinical developments. Look at Table 5.2 for a list of these antibodies.

Anti-dsDNA

Antibodies to DNA in SLE are directed to the double-stranded variant. These antibodies occur almost exclusively in SLE and are present in 60–70% of patients with active disease. Increasing

TABLE 5.1 Marker autoantibodies in autoimmune rheumatic diseases

Disease	Autoantibody	Sensitivity	Specificity
SLE	dsDNA	Medium	High
	Sm	Low	High
Sjögren's syndrome	La	Medium	High
Neonatal lupus erythematosus	Ro	High	High
Diffuse systemic sclerosis	Scl-70	High	High
Limited systemic sclerosis	Centromere	High	High
Polymyositis	Jo-1	Low	High
Dermatomyositis	Mi-2	Medium	High
Rheumatoid arthritis	CCP	High	High

TABLE 5.2 Associations of autoantibodies with clinico-pathological features

Clinico-pathological feature	Autoantibody	Comment
Diffuse glomerulonephritis	dsDNA	SLE with kidney disease
Membranous glomerulonephritis	Sm, Ro	SLE with kidney disease
Neonatal heart block	Ro	Maternal antibody
Raynaud's phenomenon	U1-RNP	As part of overlap syndromes
Fibrosing alveolitis	Jo-1	In polymyositis
	U1-RNP	As part of overlap syndromes
Erosive joint damage	CCP	In RA and overlap syndromes

levels may predict increasing disease activity; this rise in antibody levels is often coupled with a decrease in complement C3 and C4 levels, indicating complement consumption. Patients in remission or with inactive disease may also have very high levels of antibodies, and this has led to the suggestion that it is change in antibody level rather than absolute antibody level that may equate with changes in disease activity.

Anti-dsDNA antibodies are associated with the development of kidney failure in SLE and are associated with a specific lesion that can be seen on kidney biopsy (diffuse proliferative glomerulonephritis).

It should be noted that there are a number of different methods for the detection of anti-dsDNA and that each of these may detect a different subpopulation of antibodies. The Farr radioimmunoassay, once regarded as the gold standard assay for antibodies in SLE, detects

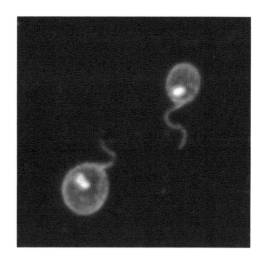

FIGURE 5.4
dsDNA antibodies on *Crithidia* substrate. Note the staining of the kinetoplast, a bundle of pure DNA.

Crithidia lucilae
A microorganism with a kinetoplast that contains only double-stranded DNA. Commercial preparations of this organism are available for test purposes.

only high-avidity-binding antibodies and has a strong association with both renal and active systemic disease. The ***Crithidia lucilae*** immunofluorescent test also has a high specificity for SLE but is less sensitive than the Farr assay. However, the *Crithidia* test is semi-quantitative and so is not useful in monitoring patients. Look at Figure 5.4 to see how dsDNA antibodies appear on *Crithidia* substrate. Generally speaking, ELISA assays for anti-dsDNA have a high sensitivity, but a lower specificity and thus some people have suggested that they have a greater role in monitoring a patient's disease activity than in diagnosis.

Anti-dsDNA may occasionally be found in diseases other than SLE. Most commonly this is connected to the patient being on certain medication such as sulphasalazine or TNF-blockers. The occurrence of these antibodies may be accompanied by lupus-like symptoms, and this is referred to as 'drug-induced lupus'. However, it is important to note that the incidence of anti-dsDNA antibodies in these patients is far higher, 10–100-fold, than the incidence of clinical symptoms of SLE in these patients. This indicates that the presence of autoantibody alone is probably insufficient to cause disease, and that maybe other factors, such as a suitable genetic or environmental background, are also necessary for the clinical expression of the disease.

Anti-Ro

Antibodies to Ro are directed to two different antigens, usually termed Ro52 and Ro60, based on their respective molecular sizes. Anti-Ro60 is detected in about 60–80% of patients with primary Sjögren's syndrome and 40% of patients with SLE. Anti-Ro52 is also found in a higher frequency in patients with SLE and Sjögren's syndrome, but in addition it is also found in systemic sclerosis, polymyositis, and overlap connective tissue disease and has little diagnostic value. Anti-Ro has also been detected in a small group of healthy adult controls.

Anti-Ro60 in all these groups may be associated with fetal congenital heart block. This condition is found in 5% of pregnant women who have circulating anti-Ro60, and rises to 25% in women who have previously had one or more affected babies. These findings suggest that the damage may be caused by a subgroup of antibodies to Ro60, probably directed against a particular epitope. Maternal anti-Ro60 is also associated with neonatal lupus, a condition in which maternal antibodies cross the placenta and cause a cutaneous disease, which regresses following birth as the maternal antibody is cleared from the baby's circulation. It is interesting to note that neonatal lupus and congenital heart block, although both associated with antibodies to Ro60, are very rarely seen occurring together in the same baby, although cases have been described where both have occurred to different babies born to the same mother.

Anti-Ro60 is also associated with a number of subsets of SLE, including the so-called ANA-negative SLE syndrome, subcutaneous lupus erythematosus, and the lupus-like syndrome associated with homozygous complement C2 and C4 deficiency.

Anti-La

Antibodies to La are found in approximately 50% of patients with primary Sjögren's syndrome. In the absence of SLE-associated antibodies, anti-La is a diagnostic marker for primary Sjögren's syndrome, particularly in patients with extraglandular features of the syndrome. In general, patients with lupus and anti-La have a later age of onset and a lower incidence of nephritis than other SLE patients.

Anti-U1RNP and anti-Sm

This group of antibodies is directed to a group of uridine-rich ribonucleic acids and their associated proteins. The U1 RNP antigens are located exclusively on the U1 RNA particle, whereas the antigenic targets for anti-Sm are found on the U2, U4, U5, and U6 RNPs. Antibodies to U1 RNP react with the 71-kDa A and C peptides, whereas anti-Sm react with the B, B1, and D peptides. The E, F, and G proteins are rarely targets for antibodies in the autoimmune diseases.

Anti-Sm

Anti-Sm is found almost exclusively in SLE. Antibodies to Sm show a marked variation in frequency. In white populations it occurs in less than 5% of SLE patients, but the reported prevalence rises to 40–60% in African-Caribbean populations. Anti-Sm and anti- U1 RNP antibodies are often found in combination, although rarely monospecific anti-Sm antibodies can occur.

Anti-U1 RNP

Anti-U1 RNP is found in 80% of patients with MCTD, one of the overlap syndromes, and in 10% of patients with SLE or scleroderma. The presence of this antibody is associated with Raynaud's phenomenon and fibrosing lung disease.

Anti-Jo-1

Antibodies to Jo-I (histidyl tRNA synthetase) are present in 20% of patients with primary polymyositis, especially in those with pulmonary fibrosis and arthritis. Antibodies to five other tRNA synthetases—thryonyl (PL7), alanyl (PLI2), isoleucyl (OJ), glycyl (EJ), and lysyl—have also been described. All appear to be associated with a clinical syndrome similar to Jo-I, but are rare, each occurring in less than 4% of polymyositis patients.

Anti-Scl-70

Antibodies to Scl-70 are directed against the enzyme DNA topoisomerase 1 and are found in 30% of patients with systemic sclerosis. They are most commonly found in patients with the diffuse variant and are much less frequently seen in patients with limited disease. Their presence in patients with Raynaud's phenomenon or limited scleroderma may indicate that the disease is becoming more aggressive.

Anti-centromere

Mitosis
Division of a somatic cell to form two genetically identical daughter cells.

This antibody gives a characteristic pattern visualized in an immunofluorescent test using cells in **mitosis**. Antibodies are directed against the A, B, and C proteins of the centromeric complex. It appears that the B protein is the immunodominant epitope and antibodies to this are found in >95% of sera containing anti-centromere antibodies. However, occasional patients are seen whose antibodies will react with only the A or C proteins. The antibody is found in approximately 30% of patients with systemic sclerosis, and in 80–90% of patients with the limited cutaneous variant. Occasionally, anti-centromere antibodies may also be present in other autoimmune diseases such as primary biliary cirrhosis or SLE, where it may identify patients who will subsequently develop features of scleroderma.

Anti-phospholipid

Lupus anticoagulant
An autoantibody which interferes with blood coagulation, as well as *in vitro* tests of clotting function, causing elevation in the partial thromboplastin time.

Antibodies directed against negatively charged phospholipids occur in SLE and other connective tissue diseases. They are responsible for false-positive syphilis serology and for the **lupus anticoagulant** reaction. In patients with SLE, anti-phospholipid antibodies (APL) have been associated with vascular thrombosis, recurrent fetal loss, and thrombocytopenia. In some patients with a similar clinical syndrome, the only serological abnormalities are the presence of anti-phospholipid antibodies and occasionally a weak ANA. This syndrome has been termed 'anti-phospholipid syndrome' (APS). Anti-phospholipid antibodies have also been detected in infections and other diseases and may reflect part of the immune response to phospholipid antigens within the membranes and cell walls of infective agents. However, the association with thrombosis, fetal loss, and thrombocytopenia has frequently not been found in these groups. It has been suggested that the lupus anticoagulant test, a functional measure of coagulation activity, is a more reliable predictor of risk for fetal loss, thrombosis, and thrombocytopenia.

Some assays for APL give variable results and may give false-positive reactions due to non-specific binding. Co-factors may be required for the binding of anti-cardiolipin to its antigen, such as β2GP1, and it is important that these are included in assay systems. Because of these variations, it is difficult to compare the many studies of APL in different diseases.

Rheumatoid factor

The association of IgM rheumatoid factor and the diagnosis of RA is well known, but rheumatoid factors are also found in other immunoglobulin classes. IgA rheumatoid factor levels correlate with cartilage loss and bone erosion in RA, and correlate well with disease activity. IgG rheumatoid factors have been associated with vasculitis, but have not, so far, found a useful role in diagnosis and management.

IgM rheumatoid factor is not specific for RA and is also found in high levels in Sjögren's syndrome and in ANCA-related vasculitis. Lower levels may also be found in SLE, systemic sclerosis, polymyositis, and in patients with infections. The diagnostic specificity of IgM rheumatoid factor is therefore quite low, and when the appropriate control groups are tested may only be about 50%.

Anti-CCP

Anti-CCP (cyclic citrullinated peptide) antibodies were first described in 1998. The current anti-CCP antibody (CCP2) assay uses a synthetically formed CCP which shows no homology to tissue proteins, and was generated using RA sera to screen citrullinated peptide libraries. The benefit of synthetic peptide production and purification is that it is cheap and reproducible, with homogeneous citrullination of the peptides.

The anti-CCP2 assay has been reported with a sensitivity as high as 81% and specificity of 91%. It has been found to identify IgM rheumatoid factor-negative (so-called seronegative) patients and offer prognostic value. However, while IgM RF concentrations have been found to decrease with treatment, anti-CCP antibody concentrations do not appear to change, limiting the use of anti-CCP as a marker of disease activity or as an indicator of response to treatment. There is increasing evidence that anti-CCP antibodies are also detected in patients with other connective tissue diseases including Sjögren's syndrome, SLE, systemic sclerosis, MCTD, and idiopathic inflammatory myositis, and may be linked to the occurrence of joint erosions in these conditions. Several studies have observed the detection of anti-CCP antibodies many years prior to disease onset (Rantapää-Dahlgvist *et al.* 2003, Nielen *et al.* 2004).

Overall, anti-CCP antibodies are a useful marker for aiding the diagnosis of early RA, especially in seronegative patients, and aid the identification of patients needing aggressive treatment for future erosive disease.

Other autoantibodies

Antibodies to ribosomal RNP (rRNP) or ribosomal P protein are present in approximately 15% of patients with SLE. They were originally described as a marker for neuropsychiatric SLE, but more recent studies suggest that they are more likely to be a marker for active generalized disease.

Anti-nucleolar antibodies react with diverse antigens located within the nucleolar region of the cell. These include anti 6–7S RNA, RNA polymerase-I, fibrillarin, and U3 RNA, which are all present in low frequencies in scleroderma. Another nucleolar specific antibody, PM-I or PM/Scl, is found in patients with overlapping features of polymyositis and scleroderma. Anti-nucleolar antibodies in low titre are occasionally seen in other connective tissue diseases.

Antibodies to Ku are found in patients with SLE, MCTD, Sjögren's syndrome, scleroderma, and myositis.

Anti-proliferating cell nuclear antigen (PCNA) antibodies are a specific marker for SLE, and are found in approximately 5% of patients. There is no known association with clinical features.

METHOD 5.2 Methods used in detecting autoantibodies in rheumatic diseases

Anti-nuclear antibodies (ANA)

- IIF using cultured cells, e.g. HEp-2
- IIF using rodent tissue sections, e.g. rat liver
- ELISA using mixtures of purified or recombinant antigens
- ELISA using cell homogenates

Traditionally ANA screening has been performed using IIF. However, many laboratories have switched in recent years to using ELISA-based assays as these require less interpretative skill and produce objective results, rather than a subjective opinion.

Anti dsDNA

- ELISA using biochemically pure mammalian DNA
- FPIA using biochemically pure mammalian DNA
- Radioimmunoassay using biochemically pure mammalian DNA
- IIF using *Crithidia luciliae*

Radioimmunoassay and *Crithidia* IIF tend to have a lower sensitivity and a higher specificity than ELISA-based assays. Quantitative results obtained from ELISA and radioimmunoassay are useful in monitoring disease activity in patients following diagnosis.

Anti-ENA (e.g. Ro, La, U1-RNP, Sm, Jo-1, Scl-70)

- ELISA using purified or recombinant antigens
- FPIA using purified or recombinant antigens
- Immunodiffusion using purified or recombinant antigens

- Dot or line blotting using purified or recombinant antigens
- Western blotting using cell homogenates
- Addressable bead immunoassay using purified or recombinant antigens

The many different techniques that are available for the detection and identification of antibodies to ENA can be confusing. The variations in technology and in the antigen sources can lead to discrepancies in the results obtained between different technologies. Some laboratories operate a system whereby a serum must be positive in two different technologies before the antibody is assigned to a patient. This avoids the problems of both false-positive and false-negative results, which may arise due to the technological variations.

Anti-phospholipid

- ELISA using biochemically purified cardiolipin or other phospholipids

IgM rheumatoid factor

- Particle agglutination using beads coated with IgG
- Nepholometry
- ELISA
- Addressable bead immunoassay

Anti-CCP

- ELISA
- FPIA

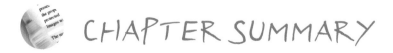

CHAPTER SUMMARY

- Autoantibodies are useful tools in the diagnosis and management of autoimmune rheumatic diseases.

- SLE is a systemic autoimmune disease which may affect many organs within the body.

- Rheumatoid arthritis is an inflammatory disease of the joints, which may have systemic features.

- Scleroderma (systemic sclerosis) is a disease in which an abnormal fibrotic process causes changes in the structure of the skin and other organs.

- Sjögren's syndrome is an autoimmune disease which results in a dysfunction of the exocrine glands (e.g. salivary and tear glands).

- Polymyositis is an autoimmune disease which results in tissue destruction and weakness.

- Anti-phospholipid syndrome is a disease which is characterized by an increase in thrombosis and recurrent fetal loss.

- Overlapping connective tissue diseases are syndromes in which patients show the features of more than one autoimmune rheumatic disease:

  — anti-dsDNA antibodies occur in 60–70% of patients with SLE and levels are commonly correlated to disease activity

  — anti-Ro antibodies are detected in SLE and Sjögren's syndrome

  — anti-La antibodies are detected in SLE and Sjögren's syndrome

  — anti-Sm antibodies are detected in SLE

  — anti-U1 RNP is detected in 80% with MCTD

  — anti Jo-1 is detected in patients with polymyositis

  — anti-Scl 70 is detected in patients with diffuse systemic sclerosis

  — anti-centromere is detected in patients with limited systemic sclerosis

  — anti-CCP is a specific and sensitive marker for the diagnosis of RA.

FURTHER READING

- **Wilson WA, Gharavi AE, Koike T, *et al*. (1999) International consensus statement on preliminary classification criteria for definite antiphospholipid syndrome.** *Arthritis Rheum*, **42**, 1309–1311.

DISCUSSION QUESTIONS

5.1 Describe the symptoms and laboratory findings included in the ACR diagnostic criteria for SLE. How many need to be present for a diagnosis to be made?

5.2 Describe the methods for detection of ANA and comment on their relative advantages and disadvantages.

5.3 Discuss the immunological mechanisms which may play a part in the pathogenesis of rheumatoid arthritis.

Answers to these questions are provided in the book's Online Resource Centre; visit www.oxfordtextbooks.co.uk/orc/ahmed/

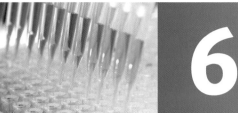

6

Autoimmune kidney disease

Learning Objectives

After studying this chapter you should be able to:

- outline the common features of autoimmune kidney diseases
- explain the clinical features of Goodpasture's disease, Wegener's granulomatosis, and microscopic polyangiitis
- outline the assays and techniques used to test for anti-neutrophil cytoplasmic antibodies (ANCA) and glomerular basement antibodies
- discuss the limitations of these techniques

Introduction

Autoimmune kidney diseases can be broken into two major disease groups. The diseases associated with antibodies to neutrophil cytoplasmic antibodies (ANCA) and those associated with antibodies to the glomerular basement membrane (GBM). Although these represent distinct syndromes, it must also be recognized that there is some commonality in symptoms, which means that in an acute presentation of a patient in renal failure, it is not easy to distinguish them. Therefore in most cases antibodies for both groups will be tested in these patients.

In all these diseases there is strong evidence that the degree of kidney damage at the time of onset of treatment is the biggest factor in determining long-term kidney survival, emphasizing the need for early recognition, diagnosis, and treatment. The immunology laboratory has an important role to play in this.

In terms of the kidney pathology, these syndromes can all present as a rapidly progressive **glomerulonephritis**. However, it is also important to realize that although the renal symptoms may represent the major immediate threat to recovery, these syndromes may also form part of a systemic inflammation of vascular organs (**vasculitis**) throughout the body. Especially in the case of diseases associated with one of the ANCA antigens, proteinase 3, they may

Glomerulonephritis
Inflammation of the glomeruli of the kidney.

Vasculitis
Inflammation of the blood vessels.

present predominantly with vasculitis of organs other then the kidney and in some patients kidney disease is totally absent.

6.1 Goodpasture's (anti-GBM) disease

Goodpasture's disease, sometimes known as anti-GBM disease, is a vasculitic syndrome predominately affecting the basement membranes of the kidney and in some patients (approximately 25%) the lung. For this reason it is sometimes called a vasculitic renopulmonary syndrome. It is almost exclusively a vasculitis of capillaries. It has two peaks of occurrence, one in the twenties and thirties and a second in patients over the age of 60. Although there is some evidence of pre-presentation disease, it is usually seen as an acute presentation, more often than not when the patient has overt kidney failure.

There is a clear genetic association in that approximately 75% of patients are HLA-DR 2 positive (compared to 25% of the normal population). The disease rarely occurs before the onset of puberty and there does not seem to be a sex bias in its distribution.

Although it has long been regarded as an autoantibody-mediated disease and the transfer of immunoglobulin from an affected individual can transfer disease in animal models, only a mild inflammation is seen. It requires the additional transfer of T cells or a T-cell reactive peptide from the glomerular basement membrane to initiate a disease that resembles that seen in the human.

SELF-CHECK 6.1

What is another name for Goodpasture's syndrome?

6.2 Wegener's granulomatosis

Wegener's granulomatosis is a systemic vasculitic disease of the small arteries, capillaries, and venules. It is predominantly a disease found in older age groups and has a roughly equal sex distribution. It is thought to be a disease of white populations, but even within this group it shows a considerable geographical distribution. It is approximately 2–3 times more common in northern European populations than in those from southern Europe.

Unlike Goodpasture's disease and microscopic polyangiitis, Wegener's granulomatosis can present in many different variants. Although the most acute presentation is that which involves a kidney lesion and deteriorating kidney function, Wegener's granulomatosis can also present as a lung disease (due to **granulomas** in the lung), as a rheumatic disease (due to the commonly associated arthritis), or as an upper airways disease (due to granulomas in the nasal cavity).

Granuloma
A mass of immune cells (lymphocytes, macrophages) that accumulates at sites of inflammation, injury, or infection.

There does not appear to be an association between HLA genes and Wegener's granulomatosis; however, there is some evidence that there may be a genetic component to disease susceptibility involving the genes governing diversity of the Fcγ receptor on neutrophils and the intracellular enzyme PTPN22, although the exact role of these molecules in the disease remains unclear.

There is good evidence that antibodies to proteinase 3 are pathogenic and play a direct role in the disease process. Antibody titres in many patients show a direct relationship to disease activity. They are capable of binding to primed neutrophils and initiate a respiratory burst, which leads to degranulation and the release of proteolytic enzymes that are capable of causing damage to surrounding tissues. These antibodies may also bind directly to endothelial cells and thus render them susceptible to damage by cell-mediated or complement-mediated cytotoxicity.

SELF-CHECK 6.2

What three areas of the body are most commonly associated with Wegener's granulomatosis?

6.3 Microscopic polyangiitis (MPA)

MPA is a systemic vasculitic disease of the small arteries and capillaries. It is predominantly a disease found in older age groups and has a roughly equal sex distribution. It has a wider ethnic distribution than Wegener's and is found commonly in both white and Asian races. Within the white population its prevalence shows a considerable geographical distribution. It is approximately 3–4 times less common in northern European populations than in those from southern Europe. MPA is a rare disease, with an incidence of approximately 2 cases per 100 000 persons in the United Kingdom.

Haematemesis
Vomiting blood.

Patients who have MPA often present with generalized symptoms (fatigue, fevers, loss of weight). They may also have shortness of breath or **haematemesis**. In addition, they may also show rashes, muscle, and joint pain. The kidney disease may not always be evident until there is a significant deterioration in renal function.

CLINICAL CORRELATIONS 6.1

Symptoms and findings commonly seen in autoimmune kidney disease

General

- **Weight loss**
- **Night sweats**
- **Fatigue**
- **Arthritis**

Specific

Haematuria
Blood in urine.

Haemoptysis
Coughing up blood.

- **Changes in blood biochemistry indicating decreasing kidney function:**
  increased urea
  increased creatinine
- **Haemoptysis**
- **Haematuria**
- **Kidney biopsy showing damage to glomeruli with crescent formation. Immunochemistry shows no immunoglobulin or complement present (in ANCA-associated diseases) or linear IgG staining of the glomerular basement membrane sometimes accompanied by associated complement deposition (anti-GBM disease)**
- **Radiograph showing infiltrates (granulomas)**

Key Points

The clinical features of Goodpasture's disease, Wegener's granulomatosis, and microscopic polyangiitis can be similar and so all should be considered in a patient presenting with acute kidney failure.

Evidence suggests that outcome, in terms of both kidney function and survival, is linked to early diagnosis and treatment.

6.4 Autoantibodies in autoimmune kidney diseases

Anti-glomerular basement membrane (GBM)

Anti-glomerular basement membrane (GBM) antibodies are strongly associated with a form of severe rapidly progressive kidney vasculitis known as Goodpasture's disease. There is some evidence that the antibodies are more closely associated with the kidney disease, as they are rarely seen in patients with lung haemorrhage alone.

Anti-GBM antibodies can be found in association with anti-myeloperoxidase (MPO) antibodies (approximately 20% of cases) and occasionally with anti-proteinase 3 (PR3) antibodies. The antigenic target of anti-GBM is the α_3 chain of collagen type IV. Anti-GBM antibodies in the absence of Goodpasture's disease are reactive with other epitopes found on the α_3 chain of type IV collagen, the other α chains, entactin, and laminin.

False-positive antibodies are most commonly found in sera from patients with other autoimmune diseases and in chronic inflammatory diseases. It is estimated that approximately 1% of normal sera may contain antibodies to these non-Goodpasture's antigens. Because of this it is important that when assessing an assay for anti-GBM antibodies, close attention is paid to the nature of the antigen and that appropriate control groups are used to determine the specificity of the assay.

Since prognosis is closely associated with prompt diagnosis and treatment, requests for anti-GBM antibodies are usually urgent, and positive results should be notified to the requesting clinician as soon as possible.

Anti-proteinase 3 (PR3)

Proteinase 3 (PR3) is a multifunctional protein found in the primary granules of neutrophils, as well as in other phagocytic cells. It is serine protease enzyme. Antibodies to PR3 are most commonly found in Wegener's granulomatosis (>95%). It has been reported, however, that this frequency may depend on the extent of the disease. In patients where the granulomatous disease is restricted to the nasal cavity, the frequency of positivity may be as low as 10%, whereas in patients with renal involvement the frequency will exceed 90%. Antibodies to PR3 may also be found in other forms of systemic vasculitis and in systemic infections, although the frequencies in these diseases are low.

Levels of anti-PR3 correlate in many patients with disease activity and thus can be used as a surrogate marker on which to monitor therapeutic needs. However, this relationship is not clear. It has been reported that patients with persistently positive anti-PR3 levels are more likely to suffer clinical relapse, and that the change from negative to positive anti-PR3 also has a high risk of predicting relapse, but that changes in level can be seen in many patients without any change in clinical activity.

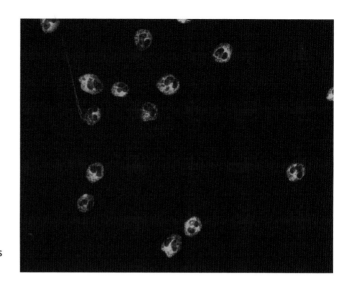

FIGURE 6.1
Cytoplasmic c-ANCA staining pattern on neutrophils fixed with ethanol.

Antibodies to PR3 produce a cytoplasmic staining pattern (c-ANCA) when tested by indirect immunofluorescence on ethanol-fixed or formalin-fixed granulocytes. It should, however, be noted that this pattern-specificity association occurs in only 90–95% of sera and that some p-ANCAs can be due to anti-PR3. Look at Figure 6.1 to see the c-ANCA pattern on neutrophils.

Anti-myeloperoxidase (MPO)

Myeloperoxidase (MPO) is an enzyme found in the primary cytoplasmic granules of neutrophils, and is involved in peroxidation reactions within the cytoplasmic vacuoles associated with the killing of ingested microorganisms.

Antibodies directed against MPO are found most commonly in microscopic polyangiitis (about 70–80% of patients). They are also associated with destruction of the glomeruli within the kidney in a condition termed rapidly progressive glomerulonephritis (RPGN). This may occur as part of a systemic vasculitis or in a form where the vasculitis is limited to the kidney.

Antibodies to MPO may also be found in Wegener's granulomatosis (approximately 5% of cases) and rarely in other forms of systemic vasculitis and autoimmune rheumatic diseases such as rheumatoid arthritis and systemic lupus erythematosus (SLE). In addition, they have also been found in up to 20% of patients with Goodpasture's disease in conjunction with anti-GBM antibodies.

Antibodies to MPO produce a perinuclear-staining pattern (p-ANCA) when tested by indirect immunofluorescence on ethanol-fixed granulocytes. This is an artefact caused by the fixation process and if other fixatives are used, e.g. formaldehyde or formalin, then antibodies to MPO give the same staining pattern as those to PR3. This differential staining pattern may be of limited use in classifying the reactive antibody on indirect immunofluorescent testing. It should, however, be noted that this pattern–specificity association occurs in only 90–95% of sera and that some p-ANCAs can be due to anti-PR3, whilst some c-ANCAs can be due to anti-MPO. Look at Figure 6.2 to see the p-ANCA pattern on neutrophils.

Cross reference
The international guidelines for ANCA testing can be found in Savige et al. (1999, 2003).

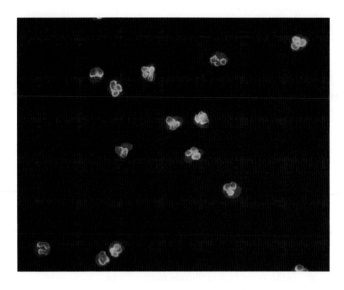

FIGURE 6.2
Perinuclear p-ANCA staining pattern on neutrophils fixed with ethanol.

Key Point

The international guidelines on ANCA testing recommend that antibodies to proteinase 3, myeloperoxidase, and glomerular basement membrane be tested in all patients in whom a diagnosis of Goodpasture's disease, Wegener's granulomatosis, or microscopic polyangiitis is suspected.

SELF-CHECK 6.3

What specificities of ANCA are associated with systemic vasculitic syndromes?

SELF-CHECK 6.4

Why is it important to test for ANCA and anti-GBM urgently in patients presenting with acute kidney failure?

6.5 Aetiology and pathogenesis of ANCA antibodies

There are a number of different hypotheses that attempt to explain the mechanisms by which ANCA antibodies arise and by which they may play a role in the mechanism of the associated diseases.

These include studies that have linked Wegener's granulomatosis and staphylococcal infections, either during active infection or bacteria carriage. It has therefore been suggested that there may be a role for bacterial proteins to act as a superantigen that is capable of stimulating and immune response in susceptible individuals (Popa *et al.* 2002, 2003; Thomas *et al.* 2005). Alternatively, in common with many other autoimmune diseases, it has also been suggested that defective apoptosis may lead to the circulation of ANCA proteins which are inappropriately processed by the immune system, leading to the antibody response seen in these patients (Esnault 2002).

6.6 **Methods of detection**

METHOD 6.1 *Methods used in detecting autoantibodies in autoimmune kidney diseases*

Indirect immunofluorescence (IIF)

- IIF using ethanol-fixed human granulocytes
- IIF using formalin-fixed human granulocytes or promyelocytic cell

Anti-PR3

- ELISA using biochemically pure proteinase 3 or recombinant protein using either direct or capture ELISA methodology
- FPIA using biochemically pure proteinase 3
- Dot or line blotting using purified or recombinant antigens
- Western blotting using cell homogenates
- Addressable bead immunoassay (ABIA) using purified or recombinant antigens

Anti-MPO

- ELISA using biochemically pure MPO
- FPIA using biochemically pure MPO

- Dot or line blotting using purified MPO
- Western blotting using cell homogenates
- Addressable bead immunoassay (ABIA) using purified MPO

Anti-GBM

- ELISA using biochemically pure antigen
- FPIA using biochemically pure antigen
- Dot or line blotting using purified antigen
- Addressable bead immunoassay using purified antigen

The many different techniques that are available for the detection and identification of these antibodies can be confusing. The variations in technology and in the antigen sources can lead to discrepancies in the results obtained between different technologies.

Indirect immunofluorescence (IIF)

The first described technique for the detection of ANCA antibodies used alcohol-fixed human granulocytes as a substrate. It was noted that most positive sera gave one of two patterns, which were termed c-ANCA (classical or cytoplasmic; Figure 6.1) and p-ANCA (perinuclear; Figure 6.2). This differentiation between staining patterns is, in fact, an artefact of fixation since *in vivo* both MPO and PR3 are found in the cytoplasmic granules. Indeed, if the cells are fixed with an alternative fixative such as formalin, then no difference in pattern is seen between anti-PR3 and anti-MPO. Initially the reactive antigens were unknown and it was noted that c-ANCA was found more commonly in Wegener's granulomatosis and that p-ANCA was more common in other forms of systemic vasculitis such as microscopic polyangiitis. In time it was reported that anti-PR3 corresponded to c-ANCA and anti-MPO corresponded to p-ANCA. However, although this relationship holds true in most patients, it is possible to find sera which give a p-ANCA on IIF that react with PR3 and c-ANCA sera which react with MPO. Thus it is important to note that this discrepancy means that it is unwise to assign specificity to the antibodies based on their IIF staining pattern. In addition, further antibodies have been described which react with a p-ANCA or 'p-ANCA like' pattern on IIF and which do not react with MPO. These patterns have been classified by some investigators as atypical ANCA (a-ANCA or x-ANCA). Yet it is often difficult in a routine laboratory setting to differentiate these from p-ANCA, and it would seem unwise to exclude sera from further testing based on these subtle differences. Antibodies which may give these 'p-ANCA like' patterns on IIF include those directed against cathepsin G, lactoferrin, and lysozyme. These other antibodies are found in a number of different conditions including rheumatic diseases, autoimmune diseases, and infections.

METHOD 6.2 Fixation of ANCA immunofluorescent slides

The **fixative** used for ANCA slides is important in the determination of the immunofluorescent pattern. It is common practice to screen on ethanol-fixed slides. The ethanol causes the cationic neutrophil granule proteins, e.g. MPO and lactoferrin, to migrate to the negatively charged nuclear membrane. This produces the artefact of fixation, the p-ANCA pattern. The PR3 granules are not **cationic** and therefore do not migrate. This produces the granular pattern seen in the cytoplasm of the neutrophils, the c-ANCA pattern.

If formalin is used as the fixative, the granules are fixed in the cytoplasm, therefore both p-ANCA and c-ANCA have the same appearance on immunofluorescence—that of a c-ANCA pattern. This is useful in distinguishing a true p-ANCA from an anti-nuclear antibody, as the anti-nuclear antibody will continue to stain the nucleus, whilst the true p-ANCA will show cytoplasmic staining.

Fixative

A compound (such as ethanol or formaldehyde) that preserves or stabilizes tissues and cells for microscopic study.

Cationic

Referring to a positively charged molecule.

In addition, it should be remembered that other autoantibodies reacting with cellular antigens may also be detected. These include antibodies to certain nuclear antigens and other cellular structures that may also be observed when reading immunofluorescent tests using neutrophils. This may be particularly confusing when a homogeneous ANA pattern is present and it may be difficult to distinguish this from a p-ANCA pattern. Figure 6.3 shows anti-nuclear antibody (ANA) staining on neutrophils. It has been suggested that an ANA test should be done in conjunction with all ANCA testing to control for this. Alternatively, some people have suggested that instead of using a pure neutrophil suspension, a whole white cell suspension which contains lymphocytes should be used for IIF testing. The lymphocytes will act as a control,

Cross reference

You can read in more detail about anti-nuclear antibodies (ANA) in Chapter 5.

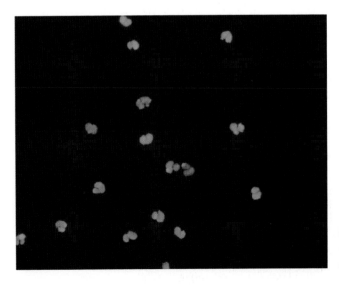

FIGURE 6.3

Homogenous anti-nuclear antibodies as seen on neutrophils fixed with ethanol.

since they will be stained by ANA but will not react with ANCA antigens as lymphocytes do not contain these enzymes. However, although these approaches may help in the differentiation between a pure ANA and a pure p-ANCA, it is likely they will be of little use in the cases where both sets of antibodies coexist. Many workers therefore take the pragmatic approach of testing all positive sera for specific antibodies, thus reducing the risk that positive sera will be missed due to the interpretation of the immunofluorescent pattern.

Anti-GBM antibodies can also be detected by indirect immunofluorescence using primate kidney sections as a substrate. The major problem with this technique is that it is well recognized that a number of potential **autoantigens** exist within the glomerular basement membrane and it is not possible to differentiate between them using IIF. Given that only one of these antigens is associated with Goodpasture's syndrome, this leads to the possibility that positive reactions may be assigned to non-Goodpasture's antigen reactivity. Given this, it is sensible that IIF testing should only be regarded, at best, as a preliminary screen to eliminate negative sera prior to more extensive testing on more specific systems.

Autoantigen

A self-antigen that is the target of an immune response, such as in autoimmune disease.

Although IIF was the original technique for the detection of both ANCA and GBM antibodies, the advent of assay systems for the detection of specific antibodies has reduced its importance in arriving at the final characterization of the antibody. The primary usage of IIF tests today is to exclude negative samples from further testing.

It has been reported that some antibodies to PR3 may give a negative result on IIF. These, in my experience, are usually seen in patients with Wegener's granulomatosis who are undergoing treatment. However, this should be borne in mind and in cases where there is a high suspicion of Wegener's granulomatosis it may be justified to measure anti-PR3, even if the IIF is negative.

Specific testing systems

Anti-PR3 and anti-MPO can be measured specifically using a number of different systems including ELISA, fluorescent polarization immunoassay (FPIA), and addressable bead laser immunoassay (ALBIA). Each of these techniques relies on the coating of the purified antigen to a solid phase and the subsequent binding of circulating antibodies and the detection of these bound antibodies using a labelled **conjugate**.

Conjugate

The term generally used to describe an immunoglobulin that has a marker attached, such as an immunofluorescent label or an enzyme. These immunoglobulins are used to label human antibodies in techniques such as IIF or ELISA.

All of these techniques are capable of producing assay systems which will give clinically valid results. The most critical aspect of these assays is probably the integrity of the antigen and it has been noted that PR3 in particular is prone to degradation, which affects its antigenicity. The effect of this on assay systems can be seen by studies which have shown considerable variation in the frequency of these antibodies in a group of patients with clinically defined Wegener's granulomatosis. One study showed variations in sensitivity from 13.3 to 66.7% in anti-PR3 ELISA kits using the same cohort of samples in different assays (Holle et al. 2005). This is an important aspect of the selection of an assay for clinical use, as a poorly reactive antigen will lead to false-negative results.

In addition to this aspect, anti-PR3 ELISA assays have been formulated in two different ways. Most commonly these assays use a direct binding format where the antigen is bound directly to the surface of the plate. Some assays, however, use a sandwich format where monoclonal antibodies are bound to the plate and antigen subsequently bound to these via the antigen binding sites. It has been argued that these assays present the antigen in a different plane and thus different epitopes are visible to the circulating antibodies. Studies comparing these two formats of assays have indicated that capture ELISAs may be more sensitive in relation to diagnosis and more informative in relation to the monitoring of disease activity (Csernok et al. 2004).

CASE STUDY 6.1 ANCA: Anti-neutrophil cytoplasmic antibodies

A 57-year-old man presented to and the hospital Emergency Department with a 3-week history of fever, fatigue, muscle pain, night sweats, and a weight loss of 6 kg. On admission it was noted that his urine contained blood and a chest radiograph showed evidence of lung granuloma formation.

The initial laboratory tests showed:

- Creatinine 115 µmol/L (reference range 32–94 µmol/L)
- Urea 12 mmol/L (reference range 2.5–7.0 mmol/L)
- ANCA (immunofluorescent test): positive (+++) perinuclear pattern
- Anti-MPO 3 U/mL (reference range <25 U/mL)
- Anti-PR3 167 U/mL (reference range <25 U/mL)
- Anti-GBM: 2 U/mL (reference range <25 U/mL).

What is the most likely diagnosis in this patient?
What would you expect the kidney biopsy to show?
Why do the international guidelines suggest that all patients presenting with these features are tested for antibodies to PR3, MPO, and GBM?
Why is it important that the results of the serological tests are available as soon as possible?

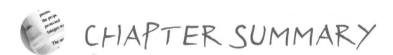

CHAPTER SUMMARY

- Goodpasture's syndrome and ANCA-associated vasculitic syndromes often present with similar symptoms.

- In Goodpasture's syndrome, kidney survival is directly related to the time between disease onset and the commencement of treatment.

- Wegener's granulomatosis is a systemic vasculitic disease which predominantly affects the upper airways, lungs, and kidneys.

- Microscopic polyangiitis is a systemic vasculitic disease of small arteries and capillaries.

- Care must be taken in selecting GBM antigen for assay systems to avoid false-positive reactions.

- Anti-GBM antibodies are found in patients with Goodpasture's syndrome.

- Anti-PR3 antibodies are usually associated with a c-ANCA pattern on indirect immunofluorescence and are found most commonly in Wegener's granulomatosis.

- Anti-myeloperoxidase antibodies are usually associated with a p-ANCA on IIF pattern and are found most commonly in microscopic polyangiitis and rapidly progressive glomerulonephritis.

- Levels of anti-GBM and ANCA are usually correlated with disease activity.

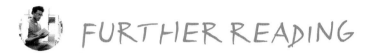

FURTHER READING

- **Savige et al. (1999) International consensus statement on testing and reporting of antineutrophil cytoplasmic antibodies (ANCA).** *Am J Clin Pathol*, **111**, 507–513.

- **Savige et al. (2003) Addendum to the international consensus statement on testing and reporting of antineutrophil antibodies.** *Am J Clin Pathol*, **130**, 312–318.

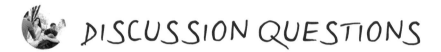

DISCUSSION QUESTIONS

6.1 Describe the methods for detection of ANA and comment on their relative advantages and disadvantages.

6.2 Describe the symptoms and laboratory findings associated with ANCA and anti-GBM-related diseases.

6.3 Describe the evidence that suggests that anti-proteinase 3 may play a role in the pathogenesis of Wegener's granulomatosis.

Answers to these questions are provided in the book's Online Resource Centre; visit www.oxfordtextbooks.co.uk/orc/ahmed/

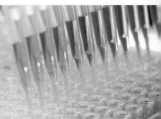

7

Organ-specific autoimmunity

Learning Objectives

After studying this chapter you should be able to:

■ outline the common features of organ-specific autoimmune diseases

■ explain the clinical features of the organ-specific autoimmune diseases

■ outline the assays and techniques used to test for organ-specific autoimmune diseases

■ discuss the limitations of these techniques

■ outline the treatment of organ-specific autoimmune diseases

Introduction

During development the body learns what is 'self' and either eliminates any immune cells recognizing 'self' or turns them off, a process called tolerance.

You should note that not all self-reactive mechanisms are eliminated, but in normal circumstances they are strictly controlled. There are a number of situations where self-reactivity is useful. These include tumour surveillance and clearing infection. A good example of the latter function is the presence of 'natural' IgM antibodies (coded by germ-line genes) which recognize apoptotic cell-associated molecular patterns on cell surfaces resulting in deposition of complement and the phagocytosis of the apoptotic cell.

For convenience, autoimmune diseases can be broken down into those that are organ specific and those that are organ nonspecific, the latter also being referred to as systemic autoimmune diseases. This division is more apparent than real, as many patients have diseases from both categories. This chapter focuses on some of the more common diseases which are related to specific organs within the body.

In order to develop autoimmune disease, three criteria need to be fulfilled. First, the patient needs to be genetically susceptible to the disease. Often there are associations between a

Cross references

You can read in more detail about the mechanisms of tolerance in a core immunology textbook, such as Janeway CA *et al.* (2001), Male *et al.* (2006), or Goldsby *et al.* (2003).

You can find more examples of organ-specific autoimmune diseases in Chapter 8.

Human leukocyte antigen (HLA)

A genetically determined series of markers (antigens) present on human white blood cells (leukocytes) and on tissues that are important in histocompatibility.

Epitope

The region on an antigen that is recognizable by the immune system.

Cross reference

You can read in more detail on the structure and function of the major histocompatibility complex and HLA in the *Transfusion and Transplantation Science* textbook of this series.

Cytokines

Proteins produced by cells of the immune system that act as regulatory proteins and intercellular mediators facilitating the immune response.

Cross reference

For an example of pathogenic autoantibody, see anti-TSH receptor, and for a marker autoantibody see anti-thyroglobulin antibody in section 7.1.

particular disease and specific **human leukocyte antigen (HLA)** genes. Also within this sphere are endogenous factors such as hormone balance. Women are more often affected by autoimmune disorders than men. The exact mechanism is not yet understood, but oestrogen appears to effect gene expression that alters the activation and survival of B cells, which in turn predisposes to the breaking of tolerance. Thus the higher oestrogen levels found in women may explain why women are more often affected by autoimmune disorders than men. Secondly, the patient requires some form of trigger to break tolerance. Often this trigger is unknown, but infections are commonly thought to be involved. Evidence for this has been hard to acquire in humans. However, there are animal models that show an antibody response developing to a part of a protein in the virus (an **epitope**) can also react with a similar epitope on a native protein (sometimes called 'molecular mimicry'). A good example of molecular mimicry can be seen in rabbits immunized with a peptide derived from hepatitis B virus polymerase, which then develop a response to rabbit myelin basic protein and subsequent inflammation of the central nervous system. Finally, the patient requires an element of bad luck, as even identical twins brought up in the same environment do not always both get the disease.

Autoimmune diseases are mediated in most cases by T cells. T-cell responses are difficult to evaluate in the laboratory because there are no routine assays for T-cell responses that equate directly to looking at the product of B cells (i.e. antibody). To assess specific T-cell responses, the isolated T cells must be incubated with stimulating antigen. Evidence of T-cell stimulation is provided either by measurement of **cytokine** production (e.g. interferon) or, after several days, cell proliferation. Although there are assays that can determine the presence of T cells reactive to some infections, there are as yet no routinely available assays for autoimmune T cells. Therefore, we often have to rely on indirect evidence of autoimmunity. The presence of self-reactive antibodies (autoantibodies) is a useful way of demonstrating autoimmunity. Sometimes the antibodies are directly pathogenic, i.e. they cause the disease. Sometimes the antibody is just a 'marker': the presence of the antibody indicates autoimmunity without itself actually causing harm.

You should also be clear about the difference between autoimmune phenomena and auto-immune disease. Autoantibodies may be detected in some members of the normal, healthy population. It is important, therefore, to interpret any laboratory findings carefully, taking note of the clinical context in which they are found. Also note that the transient appearance of autoantibodies, particularly during and after a viral infection, is a common occurrence. Most patients do not go on to develop autoimmune disease, although some do. After the infection and associated cell destruction has been cleared, tolerance is re-established and the autoanti-bodies again become undetectable. Where this balance is not restored the patient may go on to develop autoimmune disease. Those with persistent antibody on re-testing are more likely to develop the associated autoimmune disease in the future.

In the rest of this chapter we will look in more detail at autoimmune diseases that involve a number of different organs: the thyroid gland, small intestine, stomach, pancreas, and adrenal glands. In each case we will consider the clinical features, the immunobiology of the disease, and the laboratory tests which may be of help in the diagnosis or monitoring of the disease.

Key Points

Detection of autoantibodies is not a guarantee of an autoimmune disease.

Autoantibodies are frequently an effect of autoimmune disease, not the cause.

SELF-CHECK 7.1
What are the three requirements that need to be fulfilled to acquire an autoimmune disease?

7.1 Autoimmune thyroid disease

Thyroid function

To understand the different autoimmune thyroid diseases you must first understand the thyroid's central role in controlling metabolism. The thyroid gland produces hormones that are released into the bloodstream and affect most, if not all, organs and tissues in the body. These effects include the control of the rate at which the body utilizes energy, the growth and structure of bones, and sexual development.

In disease the thyroid may become overactive (**hyperthyroidism**), leading to a 'fast metabolism' or underactive (**hypothyroidism**), leading to a 'slow metabolism'.

The production of the thyroid hormones thyroxine (T_4) and triiodothyronine (T_3) are critical to thyroid function. Thyroxine is formed on tyrosine residues of a thyroid protein, thyroglobulin. Iodine is bound to tyrosine by the action of an enzyme (thyroid peroxidase, TPO). Two iodinated tyrosine residues are combined to make to make T_3 or T_4. Look at Figure 7.1 to see how the structures of tyrosine, T_3, and T_4 are related. Production of thyroid hormones is regulated by another hormone (thyrotropin/thyroid stimulating hormone, TSH), which is released from the pituitary. There is a self-regulatory feedback loop to the pituitary by T_4 to suppress TSH release. Look at Figure 7.2 to see how these pathways work. Thyroglobulin, TPO, and the receptor for TSH on the thyroid may all be targets for autoimmune reactions.

Hyperthyroidism
Excessive production of thyroid hormones caused by overactivity of the thyroid gland.

Hypothyroidism
A reduction in the production of thyroid hormones caused by underactivity of the thyroid gland.

Cross reference
For more information on the symptoms of thyroid disease see Clinical correlations box 7.1.

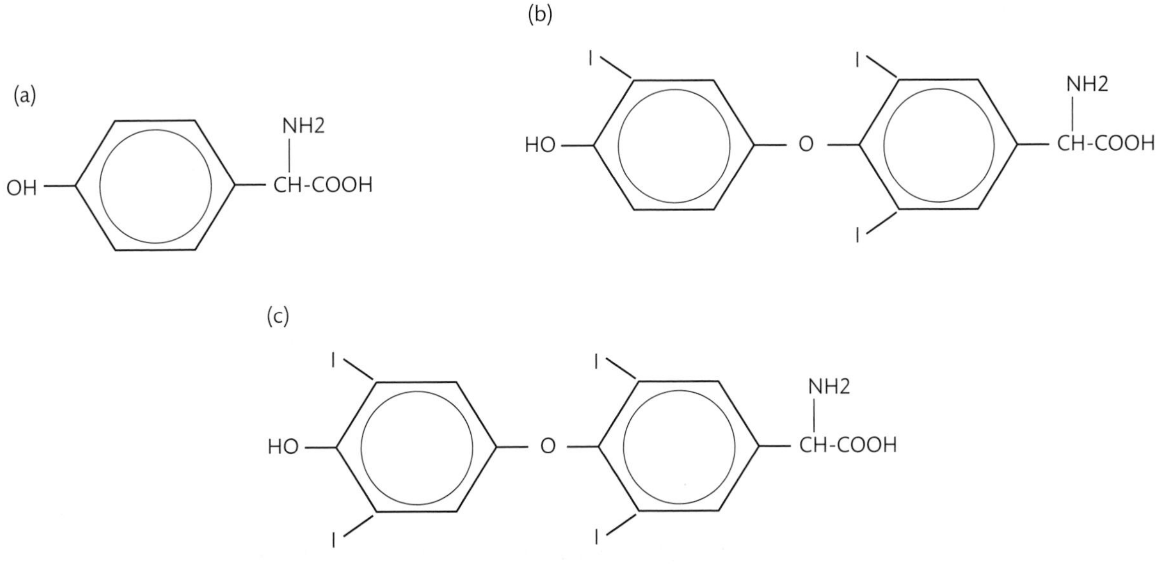

FIGURE 7.1
Chemical structures of (a) tyrosine; (b) tri-iodothyronine (T_3); and (c) thyroxine (T_4).

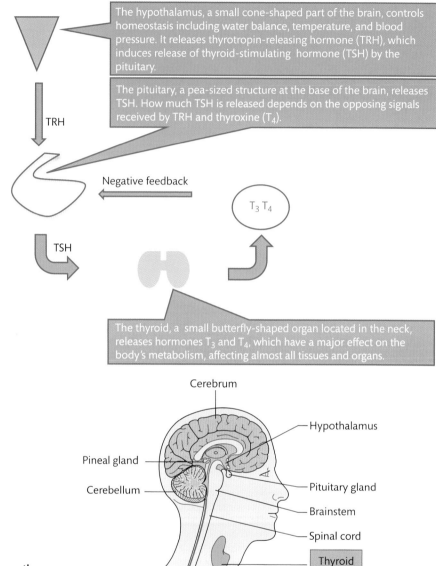

The hypothalamus, a small cone-shaped part of the brain, controls homeostasis including water balance, temperature, and blood pressure. It releases thyrotropin-releasing hormone (TRH), which induces release of thyroid-stimulating hormone (TSH) by the pituitary.

The pituitary, a pea-sized structure at the base of the brain, releases TSH. How much TSH is released depends on the opposing signals received by TRH and thyroxine (T_4).

TRH

Negative feedback

T_3 T_4

TSH

The thyroid, a small butterfly-shaped organ located in the neck, releases hormones T_3 and T_4, which have a major effect on the body's metabolism, affecting almost all tissues and organs.

Cerebrum

Hypothalamus

Pineal gland

Cerebellum

Pituitary gland

Brainstem

Spinal cord

Thyroid

FIGURE 7.2
Thyroid hormone regulation pathways.

Epidemiology

In this section we will consider the biology of thyroid disease and the factors that predispose toward autoimmune thyroid disease.

The most common causes of thyroid dysfunction are autoimmune. Less frequent causes of hyperthyroidism include thyroid tumours, rare pituitary tumours, infection, drugs, and hyperactive nodular disease (which may be a genetic defect in the TSH receptor). Less frequent causes of hypothyroidism include birth defects, infection (De Quervain's thyroiditis), secondary hypothyroidism (e.g. due to pituitary disease), and tertiary hypothyroidism (due to a problem with the hypothalamus).

SELF-CHECK 7.2

Why would diseases of the pituitary or hypothalamus cause thyroid disease?

Autoimmune thyroid disease may result in hypothyroidism or hyperthyroidism. Approximately 2% of the population in Europe and North America are affected with an autoimmune thyroid disease. Autoimmune thyroid diseases are five to ten times more common in women than in men. The most common are autoimmune hyperthyroidism (Graves' disease) and autoimmune hypothyroidism (Hashimoto's and atrophic thyroiditis). Look at Clinical Correlation box 7.1 for more detail.

Key Point

Women are more likely to develop autoimmune diseases than men.

CLINICAL CORRELATIONS 7.1

Autoimmune thyroid diseases

Hyperthyroidism

Hyperthyroidism leads to a 'fast metabolism'. Symptoms include nervousness, insomnia, palpitations, warm, moist skin and intolerance to heat.

Graves' disease is characterized by a diffuse goitre (swelling of the thyroid gland) with hyperthyroidism or ophthalmopathy (eye involvement, often resulting in bulging eyeballs (exophthalmus)) or both. Smoking increases the risk of developing the ophthalmopathy.

Hypothyroidism

Hypothyroidism leads to a 'slow metabolism'. Symptoms of hypothyroidism include fatigue, weight gain, coarse dry hair, dry skin, hair loss, and intolerance to cold. There are several subtypes of autoimmune hypothyroidism.

Hashimoto's thyroiditis and atrophic thyroiditis

These two forms of chronic autoimmune thyroiditis differ only in the presence or absence of goitre; Hashimoto's thyroiditis (with goitre) and atrophic thyroiditis (without goitre). Together these are the most common form of hypothyroidism.

Postpartum thyroiditis

Silent thyroiditis is a transient disorder which presents with hyperthyroidism or hypothyroidism. This may present as postpartum thyroiditis in approximately 5% of women during the first year after parturition. However, around 20% of these women develop permanent hypothyroidism over the next decade.

Subclinical hypothyroidism

Subclinical hypothyroidism is a laboratory-based diagnosis. Subclinical hypothyroidism is characterized by high TSH (usually 5–10 mU/L (reference range typically <5 mU/L)) with normal serum-free T4. It is primarily a disease of older women. In patients who also have anti-thyroid peroxidase antibodies there is a high risk of progression to overt hypothyroidism.

Focal thyroiditis

Focal thyroiditis (infiltration by lymphocytes) is seen in 30% of thyroid glands at autopsy. Focal thyroiditis is often asymptomatic but may develop into hypothyroidism in some individuals.

Juvenile lymphocytic thyroiditis

Juvenile lymphocytic thyroiditis presents as a chronic disorder, often with nontoxic goitre but with subclinical hypothyroidism and growth retardation in some. Spontaneous recovery occurs in some children.

Apoptosis
Programmed cell death.

Pathogenesis
The origination and development of a disease.

Idiopathic
Of unknown cause.

Thyrotoxicosis
The condition resulting from an excess of thyroid hormones.

In autoimmune thyroiditis the thyroid is infiltrated with T cells. These appear to damage the thyroid through several mechanisms: direct cytotoxicity, cytokine production, and induction of **apoptosis** via the interleukin-1-induced Fas ligand expression on thyroid cells. Whether autoantibodies also have a role in the disease process (**pathogenesis**) in autoimmune thyroiditis remains uncertain. However, in Graves' disease the main function of CD4$^+$ T cells infiltrating the thyroid, after antigen recognition, appears to be to help B cells produce pathogenic autoantibodies.

Most cases are **idiopathic**, but some are induced by drugs. A good example of this is an iodine-containing drug, amiodarone, used for the treatment of heart disease. Up to 20% of patients on amiodarone get drug-induced **thyrotoxicosis**. Other drugs that may induce thyroid disease include lithium (for psychiatric disorders) and α-interferon. Patients with pre-existing anti-TPO antibodies are particularly susceptible to developing thyroid disease.

High iodine intake is a further environmental factor known to increase the risk of both Graves' disease and hypothyroidism. Tobacco smoking is a minor risk factor for Graves' disease.

CLINICAL CORRELATIONS 7.2

Diseases associated with autoimmune thyroid disease

Autoimmune thyroid disease is often found together with other autoimmune diseases. Some are chance findings. Many are found more often than expected by chance alone and these are listed here. Figures (where they are given) are estimates of the frequency of the associated disease. The presence of the related antibodies is often much higher. For example, parietal cell antibodies (seen in pernicious anaemia) are found in 20–40% of patients with autoimmune thyroid disease and anti-nuclear antibodies (seen in connective tissue diseases) in 20–30%.

- Pernicious anaemia (5–20%)
- Addison's disease (1–2%)
- Systemic lupus erythematosus
- Rheumatoid arthritis
- Primary biliary cirrhosis
- Coeliac disease (3–5%)
- Myasthenia gravis (an autoimmune disease in which autoantibody-mediated destruction of acetylcholine receptors at the neuromuscular junction leads to profound weakness and fatiguability)
- Lymphocytic hypophysitis (lymphocytes infiltrating the pituitary gland resulting in an underactive pituitary)
- Autoimmune polyglandular syndromes (about 4% of type 1 and 75% of type 2 have autoimmune thyroid disease)

Cross reference

You can find out more about diabetes, Addison's disease, and autoimmune polyglandular syndromes in section 7.4.

The genetic predisposition in thyroid disease is less clear. The major association in Graves' disease in white people is with the class II HLA protein, HLA-DR3. Expression of HLA-DR3 is also a risk factor for other autoimmune diseases. Studies in twins indicate that other genes must also play a role. The *CTLA4* gene (coding for a protein (CTLA-4, also called CD152) which inhibits costimulation of T cells) is the only other confirmed susceptibility gene so far. *CTLA4* polymorphisms are also associated with hypothyroidism and other related disorders, including type 1 diabetes and Addison's disease. We know therefore that several autoimmune diseases share the same genetic predispositions and, as a consequence, several autoimmune diseases may be found together in the same patient. The best example of this is autoimmune polyglandular syndrome. You can see examples of other autoimmune diseases associated with autoimmune thyroid disease in Clinical correlations box 7.2.

What are hyperthyroidism and hypothyroidism? What is the effect of each on the body's metabolism?

Testing for autoimmune thyroid disease in the clinical laboratory

We have seen how the various types and subtypes of autoimmune thyroid disease present clinically, and that some of these have characteristic autoantibodies. In this section we will explore how the laboratory is able to help in making the diagnosis and the limitations of the assays available.

Initial screening in many cases is by serum analysis for serum TSH to indirectly assess thyroid function. TSH is raised in hypothyroid disorders and suppressed in hyperthyroidism. If TSH is abnormal, a further test of thyroid hormones, usually free T_4, is performed. Most T_4 is bound to proteins, but free T_4, the metabolically active fraction, is not. However, there are other causes of disrupted thyroid function tests, including pituitary dysfunction and severe disease such as sepsis. The autoimmune nature of the disease will only be confirmed by the presence of circulating autoantibodies or by biopsy of the thyroid gland. Look at Method 7.1 for a breakdown of the autoantibodies seen in thyroid disease. Biopsy of the thyroid gland shows infiltration by lymphocytes.

METHOD 7.1 Autoantibody testing for autoimmune thyroid disease

Three main anti-thyroid antibodies have been described: anti-TSH receptor antibody (TSHRAB), anti-thyroglobulin, and anti-thyroid peroxidase (anti-TPO). Many techniques have been used to detect anti-thyroid antibodies, including immunofluorescence (now rarely used for anti-thyroid antibodies), particle agglutination, radioassay, and ELISA. Of these, ELISA has become the most widely used for anti-TPO and anti-thyroglobulin assays. ELISA has distinct advantages over the agglutination and immunofluorescence assays in that it is less subjective, easier to automate, and gives fully quantified results.

■ TSHRAB mimics the effect of TSH on the thyroid, thus causing hyperthyroidism. This is one of the occasions when the antibody is pathogenic, i.e. it causes disease. The most widely used assay for TSHRAB measures the inhibition of binding of iodine-125-labelled thyrotropin to soluble TSH receptors by the antibodies. These thyroid-binding inhibition assays have a sensitivity of 70–90% and a specificity of 90–95% for untreated Graves' disease. Most TSHRAB assays on the market cannot distinguish between thyroid-stimulating and thyroid-inhibiting antibodies. Results need to be interpreted with care in a clinical setting.

Cross references

For details of testing for thyroid disease, see Demers and Spencer (2002).

See Chapter 5 for further information on anti-nuclear antibodies.

■ Anti-thyroglobulin antibodies are rarely seen in the absence of anti-TPO antibodies. For this reason they are generally not used in the diagnosis of autoimmune thyroid disease. Anti-thyroglobulin antibodies may interfere in assays for thyroglobulin in serum. Serum thyroglobulin measurement is used to monitor patients with differentiated thyroid cancer. In this group of patients it is therefore important to know whether they have anti-thyroglobulin antibodies. Anti-thyroglobulin antibodies are found in about 20% of patients with thyroid carcinoma.

■ Anti-TPO antibodies are found in 60–80% of patients with Graves' disease and 90–95% of patients with Hashimoto's or atrophic thyroiditis. You should note that this antibody may be found in both hyper-and hypo-thyroid disease and again the result requires interpretation in the clinical setting.

■ Other antibodies may be seen in autoimmune thyroid disease. Forty per cent of patients will have antinuclear antibody. Anti-thyroid antibodies may also be seen in other organ-specific autoimmune disease, such as type 1A diabetes and pernicious anaemia.

SELF-CHECK 7.4

What are the three protein targets for autoantibodies in autoimmune thyroid disease?

Treatment for autoimmune thyroid disease

We have seen how the laboratory can help in determining the type and cause of the thyroid disease. We have also noted that this is limited by the sensitivity and specificity and that knowing the clinical context is crucial to interpretation of the results. Treatment is then tailored to correct the disrupted metabolism.

In Graves' disease the purpose of therapy is to reduce the activity of the thyroid; there are a number of therapeutic options. Radioactive iodine has been used effectively. However, it can have the side effect of destroying too much of the thyroid, resulting in hypothyroidism. Indeed, a few patients, mostly elderly, actually get worse after treatment with radioactive iodine.

Anti-thyroid drugs (propylthiouracil, carbimazole) interfere with thyroid hormone production by preventing the binding of iodine to tyrosine. Anti-thyroid drugs also have an immunomodulatory action which reduces the release of proinflammatory molecules from thyroid cells.

The treatment of the ophthalmopathy associated with thyroid disease has proved difficult. In the future, it is possible that anti-inflammatory drugs that have proved effective in other autoimmune diseases, such as anti-TNF, might have a role here also.

Anti-thyroid receptor antibodies can be used to monitor response to anti-thyroid drugs. Declining concentration of TSHRAB in patients on long-term anti-thyroid drugs suggests remission. Patients with very low or undetectable TSHRAB at the end of treatment are likely to have long-term remission. However, those patients with positive TSHRAB at the end of therapy are only three times more likely to relapse than those patients in whom the antibody is undetectable. As a result, using the criterion of positive TSHRAB to predict relapse is likely to misclassify 25% of patients with regard to their subsequent outcome.

In future, there may be scope for use of more directed therapy, particularly in the ophthalmopathy of Graves' disease, which has a significant inflammatory component. New anti-inflammatory monoclonal antibodies such as those used in rheumatoid arthritis (e.g. anti-TNF) might also be of benefit here.

For most patients with hypothyroidism, treatment is relatively simple: the deficient hormone is replaced. For most levothyroxine, a synthetic form of T$_4$, taken orally is effective. Fluctuating requirements for levothyroxine may be a result of problems with absorption and could indicate the presence of coeliac disease.

The development of other autoimmune diseases is common in patients with autoimmune thyroid disease. The patient should be watched carefully for these and annual testing for relevant antibodies might be appropriate. This is particularly true for pernicious anaemia, where anti-gastric parietal cell antibodies provide a sensitive screen.

CASE STUDY 7.1 *A troubled infant*

A 24-year-old woman known to have Graves' disease gave birth at 38 weeks to a male child. She was on therapy with an anti-thyroid drug. After a week the baby, underweight at birth, became more fractious. A diagnosis of neonatal Graves' disease was considered a strong possibility.

How do you think the baby has acquired Graves' disease?

The doctors adopted a 'watch and wait' policy.

How long do you think it will be before the baby shows significant improvement?

Summary

Autoimmune thyroid disease is common. It may result in over-activity (e.g. Graves' disease) or under-activity (e.g. Hashimoto's thyroiditis). Thyroid dysfunction is assessed first by TSH and thyroxine measurements. Autoantibody analysis may help to confirm the diagnosis, although sensitivity is only 70–95%. Treatment for hyperthyroidism is by anti-thyroid dugs. Treatment for hypothyroidism is by hormone replacement.

7.2 **Coeliac disease**

Coeliac disease is a gluten-sensitive **enteropathy**. Coeliac disease is an immunologically mediated **hypersensitivity** response (type IV) to gluten, a complex of gliadin and glutelin proteins, found in wheat. The disease manifests as an atrophy of the small-intestinal villi, giving a classic 'flat mucosa'. The patient has an inability to absorb nutrients, leading to malabsorption. Classic symptoms are weight loss, fatigue, diarrhoea, and anaemia.

Epidemiology

Coeliac disease is a common disease in Europe and the USA, affecting all age groups. The incidence varies geographically from 1:4000 in southern Europe to 1:100 in North Europeans and is

Cross reference
You can see more information on pernicious anaemia in section 7.3.

Enteropathy
A disease of the intestinal tract.

Hypersensitivity
The reaction that causes reproducible signs or symptoms, following exposure to a defined stimulus, in a susceptible individual.

Cross reference
You can read more about the four types of hypersensitivity in Chapter 3.

twice as common in females as in males. It is seen in 5–15% of family members. This rises to 70% in identical twins. The disease can manifest at any age, with a peak onset in early childhood.

Coeliac disease is HLA-associated, with over 95% of patients expressing the HLA-DQ2 protein. However, the association of DQ2 with coeliac disease is complex, as there are several isoforms of DQ2, of which DQ2.2 and DQ2.5 are strongly associated with coeliac disease. The DQ2.5 isoform is able to bind and present deamidated gliadin. The DQ2.2 isoform does not have both the required subunits but, in combination with DQ7.5, can express a protein on the cell surface almost identical to that expressed by DQ2.5. Almost all the remaining 5% of patients with coeliac disease express HLA-DQ8. You should note that this genetic background provides a susceptibility to coeliac disease but does not predict who will eventually develop the disease. For example, about 25–30% of North American and European white populations carry the HLA-DQ2.5 isoform but only 1% of the population develops coeliac disease.

Cross reference

Further detail on the genetics of coeliac disease (including allelic data) may be found in Sollid et al. (2000).

Coeliac disease and the closely related disorder dermatitis herpetiformis are unusual when compared to many other autoimmune diseases because we know the environmental antigen that triggers the disease. The trigger is the α-gliadin fraction of gluten found in cereals, in particular in wheat. Other proteins from cereals (e.g. hordein from barley, avenin from oats) may cause similar problems but much less frequently.

Tissue transglutaminase is an enzyme thought to be involved in tissue repair. Tissue transglutaminase cross-links glutamine residues to lysine or, at low pH or when there is no recipient amino acid, removes NH_2 groups (deamidation) from glutamine residues. The reaction is shown in Figure 7.3. α-Gliadin is rich in the amino acid glutamine. There are some peptides of gliadin that are resistant to breakdown and are also rich in glutamine. You can see the structure of these peptides in Figure 7.4. Once deamidated by tissue transglutaminase the peptides bind strongly to the HLA-DQ2 or HLA-DQ8 molecules on antigen-presenting cells. $CD4^+$ T cells recognize these gliadin peptides and subsequently produce pro-inflammatory cytokines,

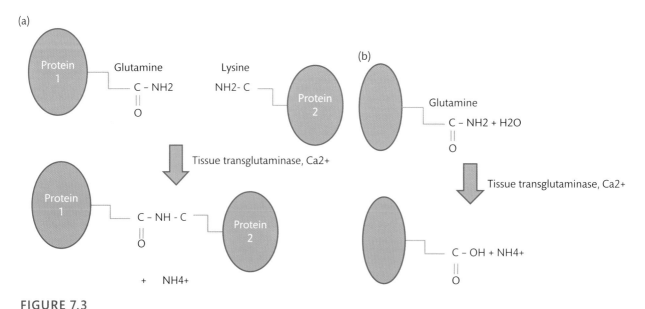

FIGURE 7.3

Deamidation of glutamine residues by tissue transglutaminase: (a) crosslinking of two proteins; (b) deamidation of proteins when no lysine acceptor is available.

31 L-G-Q-Q-Q-P-F-P-P-Q-Q-P-Y 43
31 L-G-Q-Q-Q-P-F-P-P-Q-Q-P-Y-P-Q-P-Q-P-F 49
44   -P-Q-P-Q-P-F-P-S-Q-Q-P-Y 55

FIGURE 7.4

Immunogenic peptides derived from breakdown of α-gliadin. Gliadin is rich in glutamine and proline (as seen in the peptides shown) and very resistant to degradation by gut enzymes. Peptides pass intact across the epithelial barrier where they are deamidated by tissue transglutaminase. The deamidated peptides are processed by macrophages and presented to the immune system. L, leucine; G, glycine; Q, glutamine; P, proline; F, phenylalanine; Y, tyrosine.

including γ-interferon. The ensuing inflammatory response releases other tissue-damaging molecules and ultimately induces the changes in the crypts and villi (which you will find illustrated in Figure 7.7 later in the chapter).

Clinically, there are three types of disease onset:

- classical (typical) form:
  - childhood onset of symptoms
  - failure to thrive
  - bloating
  - diarrhoea
- atypical forms:
  - adult onset
  - anaemia (especially in women of childbearing age)
- asymptomatic (silent) form.

It is not unusual for a disease to express itself in different ways in different patients. It appears from various studies that autoantibodies and other autoimmune phenomena may be present in people for many years before the onset of symptoms. The patients give the impression of being 'primed' and only when a second stress on the immune system occurs (e.g. infection) does tolerance get broken. Hence some patients present with the classical symptoms in childhood yet others are not detected until their ninth decade. The phenomenon whereby many people have undetected disease and a few have severe symptoms is sometimes referred to as 'the coeliac iceberg'. Figure 7.5 shows how this works. A similar model could equally well be applied to other diseases where there is a long time between onset of the disease and onset of symptoms. It is worth reiterating here the point made in the introduction, that some patients with autoantibodies never go on to develop clinical disease.

Like autoimmune thyroid disease, coeliac disease is frequently found in association with other diseases, many of which are also autoimmune in nature. Look at Clinical Correlations 7.3 for a detailed list of other diseases associated with coeliac disease.

Key Point

It is a common feature of autoimmunity to have diseases that overlap.

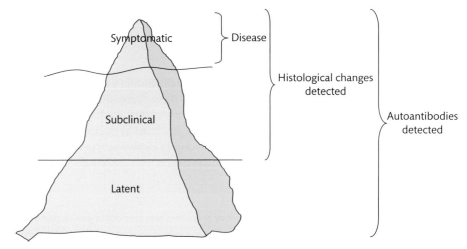

FIGURE 7.5

The 'iceberg theory' of coeliac disease presentation. There are many more people with detectable disease than present with symptoms.

CLINICAL CORRELATIONS 7.3

Diseases associated with coeliac disease

Coeliac disease is often found together with other autoimmune and non-autoimmune diseases. These include:

- Dermatitis herpetiformis
- Type 1A diabetes
- Autoimmune thyroid disease
- Systemic lupus erythematosus
- IgA nephropathy
- IgA deficiency
- Primary biliary cirrhosis
- Common variable immune deficiency
- Down's syndrome

Testing for coeliac disease in the clinical laboratory

Cross reference

We look at autoimmune diabetes type 1A in more detail in section 7.4.

We have seen that coeliac disease results from an interaction between gliadin and the immune system. In this section we look at the antibodies and autoantibodies generated as a part of that response and the use of these antibodies in the diagnosis of coeliac disease. We will also explore the use of biopsy to visualize the morphological changes that take place in coeliac disease.

There are a number of serological techniques available for the testing of coeliac disease, of which three are still in general use. Some laboratories still offer all three antibodies, but as sensitivity and specificity improves for the newest markers, the older ones (such as anti-reticulin antibody) are being replaced. The three key techniques are:

- endomysium antibodies
- gliadin antibodies
- tissue transglutaminase antibodies.

You will notice that there are two categories of antibody detected; those to an external antigen (anti-gliadin) and those to internal antigens (autoantibodies: anti-endomysium, anti-tissue transglutaminase). In addition to the mechanisms we saw earlier, CD4+ T cells also control B-cell responses. The major immune response in coeliac disease takes place in the gut, a site where mucosal immunity is most important. For this reason IgA responses predominate and are the more important in diagnosis. Anti-gliadin antibodies are a result of the normal immune response to a foreign antigen. Why the autoantibodies arise is less well understood. One proposed mechanism is that the deamidated gliadin peptides may become covalently bound to tissue transglutaminase, thus creating a new antigen (**neoantigen**) which is then seen as foreign by the immune system. It has been shown that the major antigen contributing to anti-endomysium (and indeed, anti-reticulin and anti-jejunum antibodies, which are not used routinely but are described, particularly in the older literature) is in fact tissue transglutaminase. Thus, tissue transglutaminase is the major autoantigen of coeliac disease.

Details of the three most widely used methods are given in Methods 7.2.

Neoantigen

A newly acquired and expressed antigen; often present after a cell is infected by an oncogenic virus.

METHOD 7.2 *Serological testing of coeliac disease*

There are three main serological markers for coeliac disease. We will look at each in turn. IgA class antibodies have a much higher **specificity** for coeliac disease than the corresponding IgG class antibodies. There are guidelines for the investigation of coeliac disease in children, and more recently guidelines from the National Institute for Clinical Excellence referring to both children and adults; these are outlined in Clinical Correlations box 7.4.

In recent years, anti-tissue transglutaminase has become the preferred screening test for a number of reasons. As an ELISA it has the benefit of being fully automated. This has become important as demand for coeliac disease testing has increased. It can be made fully quantifiable, although there is no agreed international standard as yet. Some commercial ELISAs are oversensitive and so positive results may be confirmed by anti-endomysium. The specificity of anti-tTG is greatly superior to the older anti-gliadin ELISA.

Specificity

Lack of interference from other elements other than the analyte being measured. The number of false positives.

Endomysium antibodies

These are the most reliable marker, and were first described by Chorzelski in 1983. Endomysium is connective tissue found between microfibrils. The test has high **sensitivity** and specificity.

IgA antibodies to endomysium are detected by indirect immunofluorescence. As such it is a labour-intensive, subjective assay requiring specially trained staff to interpret the results. It is also susceptible to false-negative results when in high titre or when found with anti-smooth muscle antibodies. Look at Figure 7.6 for examples on different tissue substrates

Sensitivity

The ability of an assay to correctly identify disease. The number of false negatives.

	Sensitivity	Specificity
IgA Endomysium antibody	84–100%	94–100%

Gliadin antibodies

Gliadin antibodies, which can be detected using ELISA, are less sensitive and specific. For this reason they are no longer recommended for screening for coeliac disease (see Clinical Correlations box 7.4). You should note, however, that there are newer assays to deamidated gliadin which have promise for the future.

	Sensitivity	Specificity
IgA anti-gliadin	84–100%	70–90%
IgG anti-gliadin	50–70%	60–75%

Tissue transglutaminase antibodies

Tissue transglutaminase (tTG) is the major auto-antigen in coeliac disease and is the target for endomysium antibodies. It is a protein cross-linking enzyme, which upon wounding is released from cells to aid in tissue repair. Antibodies to tissue transglutaminase were first described by Dieterich in 1997. IgA antibodies to tTG are measured by ELISA.

Antibodies to tissue transglutaminase have higher sensitivity (>95%) and specificity (>90%) than do gliadin antibodies. Quantified levels of anti-tTG correlate well with coeliac disease activity. Transglutaminase antibodies are therefore useful to monitor response to therapy.

Cross reference

For details of tissue transglutaminase testing, see Hill and McMillan (2006).

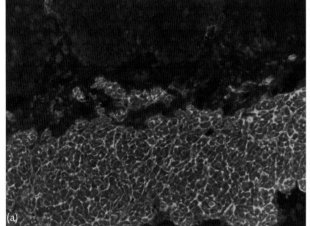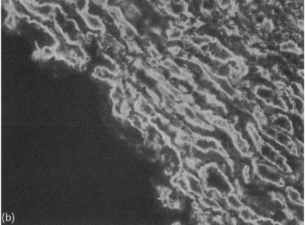

FIGURE 7.6

Indirect immunofluorescence staining of anti-endymysium antibodies on (a) monkey oesophagus; and (b) human umbilicus. Magnification ×400.

CLINICAL CORRELATIONS 7.4

Guidelines for coeliac disease

In 2005 guidelines were published by the North American Society for Pediatric Gastroenterology and Nutrition for the diagnosis and treatment of coeliac disease in children. The guidelines recommend that coeliac disease 'be an early consideration in children with FTT (failure to thrive) and persistent diarrhoea'. The recommended testing strategy was to screen with IgA class tissue transglutaminase antibody and confirm with biopsy.

This has led to a move away from gliadin antibody testing, previously used in the diagnosis of coeliac disease in children.

In 2009, NICE recommendations were issued for services in the United Kingdom. The key recommendations for immunology laboratories were that initial screening should be by IgA anti-tissue transglutaminase; anti-endomysium antibodies should be used to confirm equivocal anti-tTG; and anti-gliadin should no longer be used.

Cross reference

See Hill *et al.* (2005) and NICE (2009) for detailed guidelines.

The current final tool for diagnosis is an intestinal biopsy, as described in Method 7.3. This is still considered to be the 'gold standard' test. There are advantages and disadvantages to this technique. The main advantage of biopsy is that you can look directly at the affected tissue rather than relying on indirect indications of disease. The disadvantage is that the technique is invasive and can be uncomfortable for the patient, who needs to be sedated. There are always risks of adverse reactions to drugs, although these are small. Care must be taken, particularly in small children, not to pass the tube into the trachea.

METHOD 7.3 *The intestinal biopsy*

The intestinal biopsy is still considered the gold standard technique to confirm a diagnosis of coeliac disease.

- A tube is passed down the patient's throat and through the stomach to the small bowel (usually the duodenum).
- A device is then fed through this tube that can snip off a small piece of bowel and be withdrawn.
- The biopsy is snap frozen in liquid nitrogen.
- The biopsy is cut into thin sections (4–6 μm).
- Sections are stained and examined under a microscope to look for changes that are seen in coeliac disease.

In normal small bowel there are villi, finger-like projections, which increase the surface area available for the absorption of nutrients. In severe coeliac disease these are absent over much of the small bowel mucosa (also called coeliac sprue). There are intermediary states. One popular system for grading the damage to the small bowel is the Marsh classification. There are also variants of this system. See Figure 7.7 for more detail of the original classification. The disease can be focal or patchy, and so multiple biopsies should be obtained.

Although this is considered the gold standard technique, you should remember that other disorders can also lead to a 'flat gut'. These include infection, e.g. by *Giardia lamblia* (a protozoan) and some immunodeficiency syndromes. In order to be certain that the patient has coeliac disease, the patient must be put on a strict gluten-free diet. After about 3 months the gut should have largely recovered. Until recently, guidelines recommended that a second biopsy was required to prove this. However, it is now not thought necessary, provided that the autoantibodies (endomysium antibodies, tissue transglutaminase antibodies) are no longer detectable in the serum.

IgA deficiency in coeliac disease

We have seen how the most useful serologic tests look for IgA class antibodies. We also saw (in Clinical Correlations box 7.3) that coeliac disease is associated with IgA deficiency. Clearly, IgA-deficient patients will not develop IgA-class immune responses to gliadin. In this section we explore the extent of the problem and the implications of this association for the diagnosis of coeliac disease.

IgA deficiency is a common finding in the United Kingdom. About 1 in 500–700 blood donors are IgA-deficient. In most people this does not cause any obvious problems. However, people with IgA deficiency are more prone to develop autoimmune disease. Genetic studies

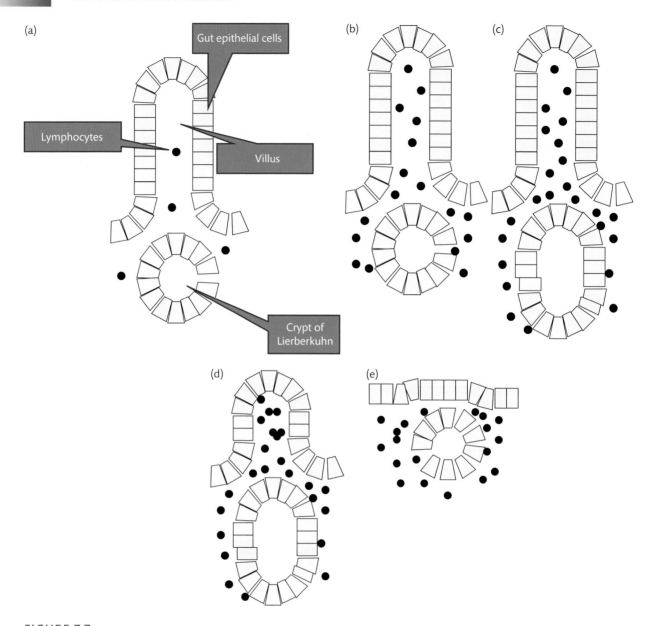

FIGURE 7.7

Histological changes seen in the small bowel of patients with coeliac disease. The diagrams show increasing severity from normal to total villous atrophy (the Marsh classification). (a) Marsh grade 0 (pre-infiltrative). The mucosa is normal; note the tall villus and the shallow crypt of Lieberkuhn. Very few lymphocytes are present (<25 per 100 enterocytes). (b) Marsh grade 1 (infitrative). The overall architecture is essentially unchanged, but infiltrating intraepithelial lymphocytes are present. There are more than 25 lymphocytes per 100 enterocytes. (c) Marsh grade 2 (infiltrative hyperplastic). Lymphocytic infiltration and proliferation of crypts can be seen. Note that the crypts are now deeper as cell proliferation increases (crypt hyperplasia). (d) Marsh grade 3 (flat destructive). The villus is now shorter or even absent in places (subtotal or total villus atrophy). Crypts are still plentiful and deep but damage to enterocytes is evident. This appearance is commonly seen in untreated coeliac disease. (e) Marsh grade 4 (atrophic hypoplastic). Destruction of the normal mucosa is almost complete. This is the classic 'flat gut' of coeliac disease. Notice that crypts are small and reduced in number or even absent. Lymphocytes are numerous.

have shown that the HLA-A1: C7: B8: DR3: DQ2 haplotype confers a susceptibility to develop selective IgA deficiency, although the reasons for this are unclear. As we have seen, most coeliac disease patients also express HLA-DQ2. Thus individuals with the HLA-DQ2 phenotype are more susceptible to both disorders than those without HLA-DQ2. IgA deficiency is about 10 times more common in patients with coeliac disease than in the general population.

IgA-deficient coeliac patients will not have IgA-class antibodies to gliadin, endomysium, or tissue transglutaminase. However, most IgA-deficient coeliac patients will have IgG-class anti-bodies. Despite the lower specificity, it is helpful in IgA-deficient patients to check for IgG-class antibodies and this has been recommended by NICE.

Treatment of coeliac disease

We have seen how the diagnosis of coeliac disease is confirmed by the laboratory. In theory, treatment is relatively simple.

The treatment for coeliac disease is to remove the gluten from the patient's diet. By removing the stimulus the whole inflammatory process in the gut can be reversed and normal gut mucosa restored. Furthermore, the autoimmune phenomena all die away. Look at Case Study 7.2. This is an example of how, by removing the gluten stimulus from the patient's diet, the sero-logical markers can be affected. In practice, as wheat is used in many manufactured food products, complete avoidance is sometimes difficult to achieve.

Patients with coeliac disease are twice as likely to get cancer as the general population. In particular, enteropathy-associated T-cell lymphoma is a rare but important complication of coeliac disease. This immune system cancer is most likely to arise in the jejunum but may be found elsewhere. The risk of getting this cancer is much lower if the patient keeps to a gluten-free diet. One way of checking if the patient is keeping to their diet is to monitor the autoantibodies. Autoantibodies return after the immune system is re-challenged with gluten. If the patient is suspected of noncompliance, or if new symptoms develop, the autoantibody test should be repeated.

CASE STUDY 7.2 Gluten-free diet

A 31-year-old woman visited her GP complaining of bloating, abdominal cramps, and general lassitude. However, since booking the appointment with the GP she has started a new diet plan to lose weight for her holidays and has cut all carbohydrates from her diet. She has noticed a dramatic improvement. The GP takes routine bloods for haemo-globin, vitamin B_{12}, folate, iron status, serum albumin, and calcium and also includes a 'coeliac screen' (anti-tissue transglutaminase antibody). How do you think changes to her diet may affect the results of the coeliac screen? If the coeliac screen results were inconclusive, what advice could you give to the GP if they were still concerned about coeliac disease?

Summary

Classically, coeliac disease presents as a gluten-sensitive enteropathy in young children with failure to thrive, often with diarrhoea. More often now it presents more subtly in adults, often with anaemia as a feature. Characteristic antibodies are present to gliadin, endomysium, and tissue transglutaminase. Of these, IgA anti-endomysium has the best diagnostic reliability. However, anti-tissue transglutaminase antibodies are technically easier and provide a quantified answer which may be useful in monitoring treatment. Therefore, anti-tissue transglutaminase is likely to take over as the standard first-line investigation. Treatment is by removal of gluten from the diet.

7.3 **Pernicious anaemia**

Vitamin B_{12} is an essential requirement for the production of red blood cells. In pernicious anaemia absorption of vitamin B_{12} is impaired. Normally, a cofactor, intrinsic factor, is released from parietal cells in the stomach. This binds to vitamin B_{12}. Further down the gut the vitamin B_{12}–intrinsic factor complex binds to receptors in the terminal ileum, leading to active transport of vitamin B_{12} across the gut epithelium (see Figure 7.8 for more detail). In individuals with pernicious anaemia, parietal cells are destroyed. Consequently, intrinsic factor is deficient and so vitamin B_{12} is not absorbed. The patient develops a form of anaemia with large red cells (macrocytes) low in haemoglobin (megaloblastic anaemia). The most common presenting symptom is fatigue. A further complication seen in some patients is numbness or tingling

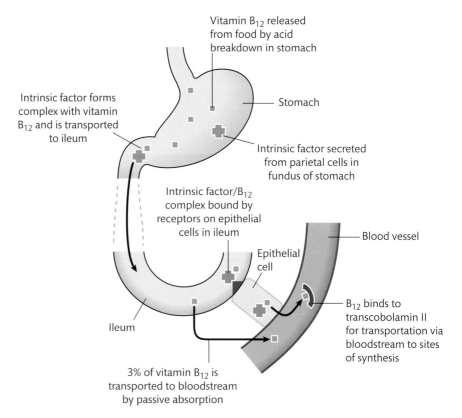

Vitamin B_{12} released from food by acid breakdown in stomach

Intrinsic factor forms complex with vitamin B_{12} and is transported to ileum

Stomach

Intrinsic factor secreted from parietal cells in fundus of stomach

Intrinsic factor/B_{12} complex bound by receptors on epithelial cells in ileum

Blood vessel

Epithelial cell

Ileum

B_{12} binds to transcobolamin II for transportation via bloodstream to sites of synthesis

3% of vitamin B_{12} is transported to bloodstream by passive absorption

FIGURE 7.8
The importance of intrinsic factor in the absorption of vitamin B_{12}.

in the hands and feet (peripheral neuropathy). This occurs because a lack of vitamin B_{12} leads to nerve damage.

Epidemiology

In this section we will look at the biology of disease of pernicious anaemia and atrophic gastritis.

Pernicious anaemia is the end stage of autoimmune **gastritis** (also called type A chronic atrophic gastritis). Autoimmune gastritis affects the corpus of the stomach, which contains the parietal cells. It is characterized by an inflammatory infiltration by lymphocytes of the main body of the stomach. Parietal cell antibody is a marker for autoimmune gastritis. It is most commonly seen in individuals over 60 years of age. In North America and Europe, pernicious anaemia is said to be the most common cause of vitamin B_{12} deficiency. Pernicious anaemia is found in 2% of individuals over 60 years of age. It affects women twice as often as men. It may take 20–30 years for atrophic gastritis to develop into pernicious anaemia.

The anaemia is caused by a deficiency of vitamin B_{12}. This results from two mechanisms. Primarily, the destruction of parietal cells in the stomach leads to a lack of intrinsic factor, which, as we have seen in Figure 7.8, is necessary for efficient vitamin B_{12} absorption. As a secondary mechanism, intrinsic factor autoantibodies can further impair the absorption of vitamin B_{12}, either by preventing B_{12} binding to intrinsic factor or by interfering with the binding of intrinsic factor to receptors in the ileum.

There is a second form of atrophic gastritis (type B) caused by *Helicobacter pylori*. It is interesting to note that antibodies to parietal cells are found in 20–30% of patients with *H. pylori* infection. This has led to the hypothesis that *H. pylori* might be the environmental trigger for the development of pernicious anaemia.

Gastritis
Inflammation of the stomach lining.

Testing for pernicious anaemia in the clinical laboratory

We now consider the tests available to confirm the diagnosis of pernicious anaemia.

Given that the key feature of the disease is anaemia, we must first establish that we are looking at the right sort of anaemia. Many patients suffer from iron-deficiency anaemia and this usually results in small red cells being made in the bone marrow (**microcytic anaemia**). In both B_{12} deficiency and folate deficiency, large red cells are made (**macrocytic anaemia**). This is as a result of delayed DNA synthesis, as both B_{12} and folate are required for thymidylate synthesis. However, RNA synthesis is unaffected and cytoplasmic development continues; a larger than normal cell results. Most modern blood count analysers allow the distinction to be made very easily.

If the patient has macrocytic anaemia, tests for folate and vitamin B_{12} are performed. Deficiencies, particularly folate, may be due to poor diet. However, vitamin B_{12} deficiency may also be due to autoimmune disease—the pernicious anaemia we are considering here. Characteristic autoantibodies are found in pernicious anaemia; anti-parietal cell antibody and anti-intrinsic factor antibody. Look at Method 7.4 for details of the serological tests used in the diagnosis of pernicious anaemia. You will see that, although they may provide supporting evidence, serological tests are not sufficiently sensitive or specific for us to be sure of the diagnosis.

Microcytic anaemia
An anaemia in which the red blood cells are smaller in volume than normal (reduced mean cell volume).

Macrocytic anaemia
An anaemia in which the red blood cells are larger in volume than normal (raised mean cell volume).

METHOD 7.4 *Serological testing for pernicious anaemia*

Two tests are commonly used to support a diagnosis of pernicious anaemia: anti-parietal cell antibody and anti-intrinsic factor antibody.

Anti-parietal cell antibodies are most commonly detected by indirect immunofluorescence using rat or mouse stomach as substrate.

Look at Figure 7.9 to see what anti-parietal cell staining looks like. As the antigen is now defined (H^+,K^+-ATPase), it is also possible to use ELISA. However, ELISA is more expensive than immunofluorescence and is not yet widely used in the United Kingdom.

Parietal cell antibodies are found in more than 90% of persons with pernicious anaemia. However, this percentage decreases with disease progression, possibly due to reduced antigen drive as the parietal cells are destroyed. Parietal cell antibodies are found in about 50% of patients with only atrophic gastritis. Parietal cell antibodies are also found in 30% of nonanaemic first-degree relatives of patients with pernicious anaemia.

There are two types of **intrinsic factor antibody**. Type 1 (blocking) antibodies recognize the vitamin B_{12} binding site, whereas type 2 (binding) antibodies recognize a remote site. Type 1 antibodies affect transport of vitamin B_{12}, whereas type 2 antibodies do not. ELISA is most commonly used to detect intrinsic factor antibody. ELISA detects both type 1 and type 2 antibodies.

Intrinsic factor antibodies have higher specificity for pernicious anaemia but lower sensitivity, being found in 40–70% of patients, depending on study. Type 1 antibodies are found in around 70% of patients with pernicious anaemia and type 2 in about one-third. They are rare in patients with only atrophic gastritis.

The presence of both antibodies is strong support for a diagnosis of pernicious anaemia. You should note, however, that the two antibodies are not always found together. Some patients with pernicious anaemia will have only one of the two antibodies. Furthermore, most commercial kits do not recognize the difference, so this distinction is somewhat academic in routine practice.

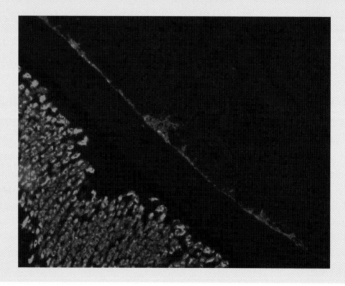

FIGURE 7.9
Indirect immunofluorescence staining of anti-parietal cell antibody in mouse stomach.

It is also possible to look directly at vitamin B_{12} absorption using an assay called the Schilling test. This assay compares the absorption of radioactive vitamin B_{12} (labelled with radioactive cobalt) with and without intrinsic factor by looking for vitamin B_{12} excretion in the urine. The ability to absorb more of the B_{12}-intrinsic factor complex, compared to free vitamin B_{12} indicates pernicious anaemia. Poor absorption of both would indicate malabsorption for another reason (e.g. coeliac disease). It is no longer popular as a test, as poor renal function may affect the result and the results of the test rarely affect management of the disease.

Treatment of pernicious anaemia

We have seen how the laboratory can help in confirming the diagnosis of pernicious anaemia. The treatment is simple and cheap.

The key to treatment of pernicious anaemia is to replace the missing vitamin B_{12}. This may be either by oral replacement (pills) or by injection. Before replacement therapy was discovered this disease was invariably fatal. High-dose oral vitamin B_{12} works because a small amount of vitamin B_{12} is passively absorbed across the gut wall (as we have seen in Figure 7.8). This takes place even in the absence of intrinsic factor. Most patients receive injections to start with and then take high-dose vitamin B_{12} to keep stores replenished. Provided that treatment is started early enough and continued lifelong, the patient should have a normal lifespan. However, some patients may have permanent nerve damage before treatment is started.

Summary

Pernicious anaemia is caused by the destruction of parietal cells by T-cell infiltration and subsequent cytokine excretion (as described above). The destruction of parietal cells in the stomach leads to lack of intrinsic factor and hence to vitamin B_{12} deficiency. Pernicious anaemia is the end result of atrophic gastritis. It may take many years for pernicious anaemia to develop. Antibodies to parietal cells are seen in both atrophic gastritis and pernicious anaemia. Antibodies to intrinsic factor are more specific but less sensitive for pernicious anaemia. Treatment is by vitamin B_{12} replacement.

7.4 **Autoimmune endocrinopathies**

Any organ in the body may be a target for autoimmunity. In this part of the chapter we will look at some examples where hormone-secreting organs are involved.

Diabetes

Diabetes mellitus is a disorder of carbohydrate metabolism. It is characterized by high blood glucose (hyperglycaemia). Normally, glucose is controlled by insulin, a hormone released from the pancreas. Look at Figure 7.10 for detail on the structure and function of the pancreas. As we will see, diabetes may be autoimmune in nature, but many cases are not autoimmune. In this section we will be concentrating on the major autoimmune variant of diabetes, looking at the biology of the disease, the serological tests that help to confirm the autoimmune nature of the disease, and therapy.

Epidemiology

Diabetes is broken down into subtypes according to the aetiology of the disease. Look at Clinical Correlations 7.5 for details on the clinical findings seen in diabetes.

- Type 1A (the subject of this part of the chapter) is immune-mediated diabetes (formerly 'juvenile onset' or 'insulin-dependent diabetes mellitus'). This is the major autoimmune subtype of diabetes. It tends to present in younger people (under the age of 40 years) and accounts for about 10–15% of all diabetes. In type 1A, the β cells in the islets of the pancreas

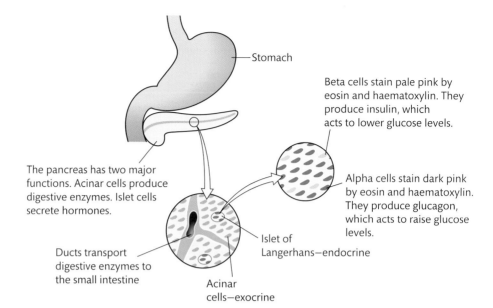

Stomach

Beta cells stain pale pink by eosin and haematoxylin. They produce insulin, which acts to lower glucose levels.

The pancreas has two major functions. Acinar cells produce digestive enzymes. Islet cells secrete hormones.

Alpha cells stain dark pink by eosin and haematoxylin. They produce glucagon, which acts to raise glucose levels.

Islet of Langerhans—endocrine

Ducts transport digestive enzymes to the small intestine

Acinar cells—exocrine

FIGURE 7.10

Structure of the pancreas, showing the exocrine and endocrine areas and the location and function of α and β cells in the islets of Langerhans.

are destroyed. The exact mechanism in humans is still not completely understood. By the time patients present, the disease has been established for months or years, with some 80% of β cells being destroyed. Extensive mononuclear cell infiltrates can be seen. These infiltrating cells include CD8$^+$ cytotoxic T cells with specificity for β-cell antigens, which are thought to be an important mechanism of β-cell destruction.

- Type 1B is nonimmune-mediated diabetes with severe insulin deficiency.

- Type 2 is late-onset (formerly non-insulin-dependent) diabetes. It is much more common in Western populations than type 1 diabetes, accounting for 85–90% of all cases. Most cases of type 2 diabetes are not mediated by immune mechanisms. Onset of type 2 diabetes is usually in older people (>40 years old), often in association with obesity. In this form of diabetes the mechanisms are metabolic, rather than autoimmune. The pancreas does not produce sufficient insulin for the body's needs. In addition, insulin is not used efficiently (so-called 'insulin resistance').

- There is a subgroup (about 10%) of type 2 diabetes in which antibodies to islet cells are found (i.e. autoimmunity is a feature of this subgroup). This subgroup is sometimes called 'latent autoimmune diabetes of adults' (LADA). LADA is similar in many ways to type 1A diabetes. Patients with LADA often become insulin-dependent over time.

- There are also forms of diabetes associated with other conditions (examples include pregnancy, pancreatitis, and drug-induced (e.g. steroids)). These are not immune-mediated.

There is a genetic disposition to type 1A diabetes. Over 90% of patients have HLA-DR3:DQ2 or DR4:DQ8, whereas in population studies only 40–50% of whites have one or other phenotype. In contrast, DQA1:01:02:DQB1:06:02 is protective, being found in 20% of the background population, compared with less than 1% of children with type 1A diabetes. Many non-HLA susceptibility genes have also been described but only the *IDDM2* gene has been identified with certainty in this context.

The prevalence of all forms of diabetes mellitus in the United Kingdom is 3.5–4.5%, with about 15% of these being type 1 diabetes or about 600 per 100 000 persons. In family studies, concordance in identical twins is 50%. The risk to a first-degree relative for developing type 1A diabetes is 5%.

In terms of environmental factors, only congenital rubella infection has been proven to be associated with type 1A diabetes. Other potential triggers, such as bovine milk ingestion or enteroviral infection, remain unproven.

CLINICAL CORRELATIONS 7.5

Clinical findings in type 1A diabetes

■ The main problems seen in diabetes stem from damage to blood vessels. Glucose binds to proteins, increasing rigidity. Endothelial progenitor cells, essential for blood vessel repair, become too rigid to move to sites of damage. Damage to small blood vessels (microvascular damage) may lead to renal disease and blindness. Damage to large blood vessels (macrovascular disease) may lead to atherosclerosis (hardening and narrowing of the arteries). Atherosclerosis in turn may cause strokes or coronary heart disease.

■ Early symptoms are related to the high blood sugar and low insulin. Patients pass large amounts of urine and have increased thirst. The low insulin levels affect metabolism and patients do not store fat or protein properly. So, despite an increased appetite, patients lose weight. They become fatigued and are prone to infections of the bladder and skin.

■ Infection can increase the requirement for insulin.

■ The most severe complication is diabetic coma. This can happen when the blood sugar falls too low. This form of coma results from low blood sugar when the patient is over-treated with insulin. It is treated with infusion of glucose or glucagon.

■ Coma can also happen when the blood sugar gets too high and the patient becomes dehydrated. In these circumstances the patient's metabolism becomes deranged. Ketones are generated and the blood pH falls (ketoacidosis). It is a life-threatening condition. The patient requires prompt treatment: fluids to rehydrate the patient and insulin to reverse the ketoacidiosis.

Testing for type 1A diabetes in the clinical laboratory

In this section we consider some of the assays that confirm the presence of diabetes in general and then the autoimmune tests that can confirm the presence of autoimmune diabetes specifically.

Diabetes is a disorder of glucose metabolism and therefore the most useful first-line test is a measurement of blood glucose. It is also possible to challenge the patient with a solution of glucose and monitor blood glucose over a period of hours (the 'glucose tolerance test'). In a normal person blood glucose becomes elevated but rapidly returns to normal. In a diabetic patient the glucose rises higher than normal and takes longer to return to normal.

Measurement of blood glucose is key to monitoring response to therapy. There are home monitors available for patients to check their control of glucose levels. A second useful monitoring tool is the glycosylated haemoglobin (HbA_{1c}). The more circulating glucose, the more will be bound to haemoglobin. HbA_{1c} levels fluctuate less than glucose and give a better measure of overall glucose load. Good control is indicated when the HbA_{1c} is less than 7.5%, that is less than 7.5% of total haemoglobin has glucose bound to it. The range for a normal nondiabetic person is about 3.5–5.5%.

Many autoantibodies have been linked to type 1A diabetes. Only a few have so far proved to be useful in clinical practice. Although autoantibodies are frequently found in type 1A diabetes there is no evidence to suggest they are causative of the disease. For details on testing for these look at Method 7.5.

METHOD 7.5 Autoantibody testing for type 1A diabetes

Islet cell autoantibodies (ICA)

In practice, this is the only test readily available in general pathology laboratories. It was first described in 1974 using human pancreas as substrate in an indirect immunofluorescence test. Now it is more usual to use monkey pancreas, as this is commercially available. The Juvenile Diabetes Foundation (JDF) developed an international standard for this assay. Look at Figure 7.11 to see what anti-islet cell staining looks like.

Cross reference

You can look up the use of positive and negative predictive values in the *Biomedical Science Practice* textbook of this series.

At the onset of type 1A diabetes approximately 70–75% of white individuals are ICA-positive (sensitivity 70%) with a specificity of >95%. With destruction of the β cells, and thus the concomitant depletion of antigen, ICA levels fall and are rarely found after the first year of disease. The positive predictive value for type 1A diabetes is 85% for ICA above 40 units of the JDF standard.

These antibodies can also be seen in patients with an overlapping neurological disorder called stiff person syndrome. In stiff person syndrome, the autoantibodies are directed against GAD (see below).

Glutamic acid decarboxylase (GAD) antibodies

GAD is an enzyme involved in the control of release of insulin. It is also found in tissues other than pancreas, including the cerebellum and sympathetic ganglia. Antibodies to GAD are common in type IA diabetes, with a sensitivity of about 80–85%. They are most often detected by ELISA or radioassay. Anti-GAD can also be detected by indirect immunofluorescence, and may be the dominant ICA reactivity. GAD antibodies are found mostly in adult patients. The antibodies to GAD found in type 1A diabetes and in stiff person syndrome are directed against different isoforms of the GAD molecule.

IA-2 (insulinoma-like antigen-2, also called ICA512) antibodies

IA-2 is a tyrosine phosphatase-like molecule. IA-2, like GAD, is found in nervous tissue and pancreas. Sensitivity for type 1A diabetes is about 75%. It is detected by radiobinding assay.

Insulin antibodies

Autoantibodies to insulin may be present for many years before the onset of type 1A diabetes. Insulin autoantibodies are more often seen in children than adults and are often the first antibody seen in young children. They may be detected by either ELISA or radioassay. These assays do not measure the same population of antibodies. The radioassay results are better at predicting development of type 1A diabetes.

FIGURE 7.11
Indirect immunofluorescence staining of anti-islet cell antibody on monkey pancreas.

Insulin autoantibodies are also found in many other autoimmune diseases including Graves' disease, Hashimoto's throiditis, Addison's disease, and pernicious anaemia.

All of these autoantibodies may be present for years before the onset of disease. Studies of family members have shown that the more autoantibodies you have, the more likely you are to develop type 1 diabetes.

Treatment of type 1A diabetes

In this section we consider the treatment of autoimmune diabetes. Note that other therapies are used in diabetes generally.

The key to treatment of type 1A diabetes is insulin replacement. In the past this has been by porcine insulin. Some patients reacted to this nonself-antigen by making antibodies specific to porcine insulin. These antibodies made the insulin ineffective. Notice that these anti-porcine insulin antibodies (to an extrinsic antigen) are different from the *auto*antibodies directed against human insulin (an intrinsic antigen). Nowadays most therapeutic insulin is human recombinant insulin, largely avoiding this problem. It is administered by injection. For some patients with poor control, an insulin pump is used to provide a more constant supply of insulin. Different formulations (fast-, medium-, or long-acting) are used, e.g. to balance the need for more insulin at mealtimes against the lesser requirement of sleep. One recent development is the use of inhaled insulin, which may be used instead of injections before meals.

In future, transplantation may be a therapeutic option. Some patients have had successful pancreas transplants; others have been transplanted with isolated islets. However, there are drawbacks to this approach. First, the patients need immunosuppression to prevent transplant rejection. Second, there is a lack of suitable donors. Finally, many patients have only partial success in that their need for insulin is reduced but they do not fully recover.

As with other organ-specific autoimmune diseases there is an increased risk of developing further disorders, particularly autoimmune thyroid disease, pernicious anaemia, and coeliac disease. For these reason many clinics now monitor diabetes patients annually for the development of antibodies seen in these disorders.

Summary

Autoimmune type 1A diabetes is a disorder of glucose metabolism. It is caused by lack of insulin due to destruction of beta cells in the pancreas. Treatment is by replacement of insulin, usually by injection.

Autoimmune Addison's disease

Addison's disease is caused by a failure of the adrenal glands. The classic feature of Addison's disease is hyperpigmentation (darkening of the skin). This is most noticeable on the knuckles, knees, ankles, and creases in the palm of the hand. Salt craving is common.

Epidemiology

In this section we consider the biology of Addison's disease and the factors that predispose towards autoimmune Addison's disease.

Addison's disease is characterized by deficient production of adrenocortical hormones, both mineralocorticoids and glucocorticoids. There is a concomitant increase in secretion of adrenocorticotropic hormone (ACTH) from the pituitary. In the Western world, autoimmunity is the most common cause of adrenal failure, accounting for 70–80% of cases. The next most common cause is tuberculosis. Addison's disease affects approximately 1 in 10 000 persons. Other rare causes include adrenal cancer, fungal infections, and haemorrhage (e.g. after trauma). There are also cases of secondary adrenal insufficiency caused by disease of the pituitary (particularly pituitary cancer). The pituitary, as well as controlling thyroid function (as we saw in Figure 7.2) controls cortisol release by release of ACTH. ACTH triggers cortisol production in the adrenals. In pituitary disease ACTH levels are reduced, leading to low levels of corticosteroid release from the adrenals.

Addison's disease may be an isolated disease, but is often found with other autoimmune diseases in the autoimmune polyendocrine or polyglandular syndromes. Many patients with autoimmune Addison's disease (50–60%) develop other autoimmune diseases, such as type 1A diabetes or autoimmune thyroid disease. Other disease associations are shown in Clinical Correlations 7.6. The disease mechanism is not fully understood but, as with many other autoimmune diseases, is thought to be T-cell mediated. In autoimmune Addison's disease the autoantibodies seen are not thought to contribute to the destruction of the adrenal gland.

The main clinical feature is hyperpigmentation. This results indirectly from the increase in levels of ACTH. ACTH derives from the same pro-hormone as melanocyte-stimulating hormone (MSH). MSH stimulates production of melanin, the dark pigment in the skin.

Other symptoms include low blood pressure, anorexia, salt craving, weight loss, and fatigue. Why do we see salt craving as a symptom? Salt balance relies on another hormone released by the adrenal glands, aldosterone. When aldosterone falls too low the kidneys do not function properly to retain sodium and maintain blood pressure. It is the low aldosterone levels that lead to salt craving.

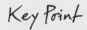

Key Point

Patients with Addison's disease frequently go on to develop other autoimmune endocrine disorders.

The main genetic association is with HLA-B8; DR3. Patients with HLA-DR3;DQ2 and HLA-DR4; DQ8 have a risk as high as 1 in 200–500. An atypical HLA molecule, MIC-A (to be exact the MICA-5.1 allele), is also strongly associated with Addison's disease.

CLINICAL CORRELATIONS 7.6

Diseases associated with Addison's disease

Addison's disease is very often found together with other autoimmune and nonautoimmune diseases. These include:

- autoimmune thyroid disease (10–30%)
- type 1A diabetes (5–15%)
- pernicious anaemia
- autoimmune polyglandular syndromes
- hypoparathyroidism
- poor ovarian or testicular function

Hypoparathyroidism
Underactivity of the parathyroid, the gland that controls calcium levels in both blood and bone.

Testing for autoimmune Addison's disease in the clinical laboratory

We now consider the tests available to confirm the diagnosis of Addison's disease. There are two approaches. First, we need to confirm that the adrenal gland is not producing enough hormones. This is proven biochemically by artificially stimulating the adrenal gland and seeing how it reacts. Secondly, we need to show there is an autoimmune component. For details on testing for Addison's disease, see Method 7.6.

Treatment for autoimmune Addison's disease

The treatment for autoimmune Addison's disease focuses on hormone replacement. Both glucocorticoids and mineralocorticoids need to be replaced. Oral replacement is preferred where possible. In acute situations (e.g. patient collapse) intravenous hydrocortisone is used. Hydrocortisone is used to counter glucocorticoid deficiency. When the patient has an infection, has an accident, or is stressed, the dose of hydrocortisone needs to be increased to cope with this. Fludrocortisone is used to replace mineralocorticoid deficiency. The dose is adjusted according to the amount of salt craving and the blood pressure changes seen.

It is important to monitor patients regularly for other endocrine disorders which may develop during the course of the disease.

Summary

Autoimmune Addison's disease results in adrenal failure. Both glucocorticoid and mineralocorticoid hormones are reduced. Adrenal failure is confirmed by ACTH challenge and the effect

METHOD 7.6 Laboratory testing for autoimmune Addison's disease

Electrolytes

- Low serum sodium is found in 90% of primary adrenal insufficiency cases.
- Elevated serum potassium is found in 65%.
- Low serum calcium is found in 50% of chronic cases

Short Synacthen test

We can look at adrenal function by challenging the patient with synthetic adrenocorticotrophic hormone (Synacthen, Tetracosactrin).

Serum samples are taken before injection of Synacthen and then at 30 minutes and 60 minutes after injection. Serum cortisol is measured. In a normal subject there will be a predictable increase in cortisol output. In patients with Addison's disease the output of cortisol is suppressed.

This can be a difficult test to interpret. If the patient has been taking glucocorticoids the response may be suppressed. In addition there are variations, depending on the time of day the test is done (diurnal variation).

Adrenal cortex antibodies

Indirect immunofluorescence is still a popular method for looking for adrenal antibodies. It is positive in about 60% of patients with Addison's disease. Look at Figure 7.12 to see what anti-adrenal gland staining looks like.

Recently, the steroid 21-hydroxylase (P450c21) was shown to be an important autoantigen in Addison's disease. Using radioassay, antibodies to 21-hydroxylase are found in >90% of patients with Addison's disease. False-positive results are rarely seen.

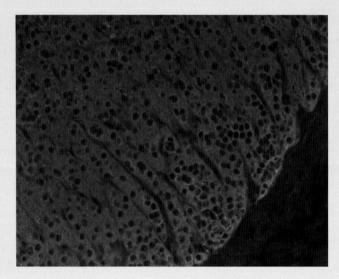

FIGURE 7.12
Indirect immunofluorescence staining of anti-adrenal gland antibody on monkey adrenal gland.

this has on cortisol release. Autoantibodies may be found to confirm the autoimmune nature of the disease. Treatment is by hormone replacement.

Cross reference

Look at Clinical correlations 7.2, 7.3, and 7.6 for examples of the multiple associations seen in autoimmune diseases.

Autoimmune polyglandular syndromes

As we have seen above, it is common for a patient to have more than one organ-specific autoimmune disease. In this part of the chapter we look at those syndromes where the disease associations are so strong that they are considered as a single entity.

Epidemiology

There are two main autoimmune polyglandular (or polyendocrine) syndromes (APS), called type 1 (APS-1) and type 2 (APS-2). In this section we look at the clinical features found in APS-1 and APS-2, the genetic predispositions of each, and the associations with other autoimmune disorders.

APS-1 is a rare autosomal recessive disorder, which presents in childhood. APS-1 also has several other names, including **APECED**. About 500 cases have been described worldwide. Look at Clinical Correlations 7.7 for details of the clinical features of APS-1.

APS-1 is caused by mutation in the autoimmune regulator gene (*AIRE*) on chromosome 21q22.3. Over 50 different genetic variants have been described in APS-1 patients. *AIRE* expression is highest in the thymus. The AIRE protein is thought to have a role in transcription. Mouse models suggest that AIRE is a critical regulator of self-antigen expression in the thymus. Alterations in this gene disrupt self-recognition. APS-1 was the first systemic autoimmune disorder to be found to be due to defects in a single gene.

APECED

Autoimmune polyendocrinopathy, candidiasis, ectodermal dystrophy.

CLINICAL CORRELATIONS 7.7

Clinical features of APS-1

The most frequent findings are mucocutaneous candidiasis (infection of the mucous membranes and skin with a fungus, *Candida*), hypoparathyroidism, and Addison's disease. At least two of these three are should be present to make the diagnosis. Typically the disease presents in early childhood, with mucocutaneous candidiasis as the first manifestation.

- Mucocutaneous candidiasis is found in nearly all cases.
- Hypoparathyroidism (under-activity of the parathyroid glands) is found in 70–80% of patients with APS-1. This leads to disordered metabolism of calcium and phosphorus and therefore bone metabolism.
- Addison's disease is found in 70–80% of patients with APS-1.
- Other endocrine features include:
  - premature ovarian failure in 60% of affected women
  - testicular failure in men (though this is less common)
  - type 1A diabetes in 5–20% patients with APS-1
  - autoimmune thyroid disease in 10–15% of patients with APS-1.
- Nonendocrine features include:
  - alopecia (hair loss), vitiligo (loss of melanin), autoimmune hepatitis, pernicious anaemia, corneal opacity, and enamel hypoplasia of teeth.

Cross reference

For more detail, look at section 7.1 for autoimmune thyroid disease, 7.3 for pernicious anaemia, and earlier in 7.4 for type 1A diabetes and Addison's disease.

APS-2 is much more common than APS-1, being found in about 1 in 20 000 individuals. In contrast to APS-1, it usually presents in adulthood. The key features are Addison's disease, autoimmune thyroid disease, and type 1A diabetes. However, it is rare for APS-2 to present with several diseases simultaneously. More often the patient presents with one of the key disorders and the others develop with time. Look at Clinical Correlations 7.8 for more details of the clinical features of APS-2.

Studies on susceptibility genes in APS-2 have produced variable results depending largely on the population studied. HLA-DRB1:03:DQB1:02 and HLA-DRB1:04:DQB1:03 appear to be associated with Addison's disease in APS-2, whereas HLA-DRB1:01:DQB1:05 confers protection from Addison's disease in APS-2. *AIRE* gene mutation is not found in this disorder.

CLINICAL CORRELATIONS 7.8

Clinical features of APS-2

In order to be classified as having APS-2, the patient should have two of type 1A diabetes (55%), Addison's disease (45%), and autoimmune thyroid disease (75%), either autoimmune hypothyroidism or Graves' disease.

Other autoimmune disorders seen in this complex include vitiligo (20%), pernicious anaemia (5%), hypogonadism, coeliac disease, and myasthenia gravis.

Treatment for autoimmune polyglandular syndromes

The treatment of APS-1 includes replacement of deficient hormones and antifungal agents for the *Candida* infection. Hypoparathyroidism is treated with oral calcium and 1,25-dihydroxy-vitamin D.

The treatment for APS-2 is based on the treatments for the individual components of the syndrome found in any given patient. The treatment can be complicated by the side effects of the drugs used. For example, thyroxine has an effect on liver to enhance liver production of corticosteroids. This can mask problems with the adrenal glands. Conversely, TSH secretion is inhibited by glucocorticoids from the adrenal gland. So treating one component of the disease may affect the therapy for another part.

In both APS-1 and APS-2 careful follow-up is required, as patients may develop further autoimmune diseases with time.

Summary

There are two main types (APS-1 and APS-2). APS-1 is caused by mutations in the autoimmune regulator gene (*AIRE*); APS-2 is not.

- APS-1 is characterized by candidiasis, hypoparathyroidism, and Addison's disease.
- APS-2 is characterized by Addison's disease, autoimmune thyroid disease, and type 1A diabetes.

Treatment for both APS-1 and APS-2 addresses the individual components of the disease.

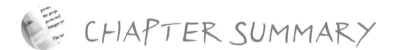 CHAPTER SUMMARY

- Organ-specific autoimmune diseases are common disorders.
- Organ-specific autoimmune diseases are more common in females than males.
- The presence of one autoimmune disease increases the risk for developing other autoimmune diseases.
- In part the overlap seen in organ-specific autoimmune disease is because certain genetic predispositions (HLA genes) are common to many.
- Characteristic antibodies ('disease markers') are often found.

- The characteristic antibodies may be pathogenic but more often are not.

- Indirect immunofluorescence and ELISA are the main laboratory tools for detecting autoantibodies.

- Autoimmune disease requires an environmental trigger, but for most this is unknown.

- Coeliac disease is an exception, as gluten is known to be the trigger.

- Treatment is directed at replacing the lost factors (e.g. insulin in diabetes or vitamin B_{12} in pernicious anaemia) or modifying the immune response (e.g. removing the antigen (gluten) in coeliac disease).

 FURTHER READING

- Demers LM, Spencer CA (eds) (2002) *Laboratory medicine practice guidelines. Laboratory support for the diagnosis and monitoring of thyroid disease.* National Academy of Clinical Biochemistry, http://www.nacb.org/. A comprehensive guide to testing for thyroid disease for both laboratory and medical personnel.

- Goldsby RA, Kindt TJ, Osborne BA, *et al.* (2003) *Kuby's Immunology*, 4th edition. W.H. Freeman, New York.

- Hill ID, Dirks MH, Liptak GS, *et al.* (2005) Guideline for the diagnosis and treatment of celiac disease in children: recommendations of the North American Society for Pediatric Gastroenterology, Hepatology and Nutrition. *J Paediatr Gastroenterol Nutr*, **40**, 1–19.

- Hill PG, McMillan SA (2006) Anti-tissue transglutaminase antibodies and their role in the investigation of coeliac disease. *Ann Clin Biochem*, **43**, 105–117. A comprehensive review of the use of this recently introduced test.

- Janeway CA, Travers P, Walport M, Shlomchik M (2001) *Immunobiology. The Immune System in Health and Disease*, 5th edition. Garland Science, New York.

- Male D, Brostoff J, Rith D, Roitt I (2006). *Immunology*, 7th edition. Mosby, St Louis.

- NICE (2009) *Coeliac disease: recognition and assessment of coeliac disease*. Clinical Guideline 86, http://www.nice.org.uk

- Sollid LM, Spurkland A, Thorsby E (2000) HLA and gastrointestinal diseases. Chapter 17 in Lechler R, Warrens A (eds) *HLA in Disease and Health*, pp. 249–262. Academic Press, London.

 DISCUSSION QUESTIONS

7.1 What three criteria are needed to develop autoimmune disease?

7.2 What is the difference between an autoimmune phenomenon and an autoimmune disease?

7.3 What are the autoimmune diseases associated with hypothyroidism and hyperthyroidism?

7.4 Why is it so important to know a patient's serum IgA level when performing tests for coeliac disease?

7.5 What are the two mechanisms that cause anaemia as a result of pernicious anaemia?

Answers to these questions are provided in the book's Online Resource Centre; visit www.oxfordtextbooks.co.uk/orc/ahmed/

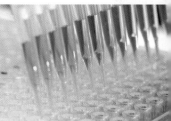

8

Autoimmune liver diseases

Learning Objectives

After studying this chapter you should be able to:

- outline the common features of autoimmune liver diseases
- explain the clinical features of autoimmune hepatitis, autoimmune sclerosing cholangitis, and primary biliary cirrhosis
- outline the assays and techniques used to test for autoimmune liver diseases
- discuss the limitations of these techniques
- outline the treatment of autoimmune hepatitis, autoimmune sclerosing cholangitis, and primary biliary cirrhosis

Introduction

The main autoimmune liver diseases are autoimmune hepatitis (AIH), autoimmune sclerosing cholangitis (ASC), and primary biliary cirrhosis (PBC). AIH and ASC are rare and may not be encountered in every laboratory.

Data on the incidence of the above diseases tend to be regional rather than national. The rarity of both AIH and ASC makes the gathering of incidence and prevalence data difficult. However, some data are available; a report from a group in Oslo (Boberg *et al.* 1998) gives a mean annual incidence of AIH as 1.9/100 000 of the specific Norwegian population studied. It must be remembered that this is a regional figure and cannot be extrapolated to a Europe-wide or global population. The reason for this is that autoimmune disease is closely linked to genetic make-up and the huge variation seen in the human genome suggests an equally huge variation in incidence geographically. AIH is found in two serologically distinct forms, known as type 1 and type 2. In studies on northern European populations possession of the human leukocyte antigen (HLA) DRB1*03 is associated with type 1 and DRB1*07 is associated with type 2. In the United Kingdom population susceptibility to ASC in children is associated with the possession of HLA DRB1*1301.

PBC is now included in the autoimmune group, although this was not always the case. This is a far more frequently encountered disease than either AIH or ASC and will be seen in most laboratories in the United Kingdom. The association of PBC and HLA DRB1*0801 was confirmed in a large-scale study of well-characterized PBC patients from the United Kingdom and Italy (Donaldson *et al.* 2006). This is not the case in China, where the associated allele is HLA DRB1*0701 (Liu *et al.* 2006).

Key Point

The autoimmune liver diseases are autoimmune hepatitis (AIH) types 1 and 2, primary biliary cirrhosis (PBC), and autoimmune sclerosing cholangitis (ASC).

8.1 Autoimmune hepatitis (AIH)

Hepatitis
Inflammation of the hepatocytes in the liver.

Cirrhosis
Irreversible change in liver tissue that results in the degeneration of functioning liver cells and their replacement with fibrous connective tissue.

Epiphenomenon
A secondary symptom that appears during the course of a disease, secondary to the existing disease symptoms.

Immunosuppression
A suppression of the immune system with a reduction in number, reactivity, expansion, or differentiation of T and/or B lymphocytes.

AIH is an inflammatory liver disease characterized by a mononuclear cell infiltrate with interface **hepatitis**. This leads to the death of hepatocytes and their subsequent replacement by connective tissue, a process known as **cirrhosis**. The loss of hepatocytes leads in turn to the loss of hepatic function and ultimately hepatic failure. The adjective 'autoimmune' derives from the presence of autoantibodies that accompany the disease process. The antigen specificity of these autoantibodies is used in a classification of AIH into types 1 and 2. Interestingly, these autoantibodies are not liver-specific, with the exception of anti-liver cytosol 1 (LC1). The current view is that such autoantibodies are **epiphenomena** and not directly responsible for hepatocyte damage. The treatment for AIH is **immunosuppression**, usually starting with corticosteroids and using more potent immunosuppressive agents as required. If this therapeutic approach fails then liver transplantation is the next option.

Incidence

AIH is a disease with a biphasic incidence; the first peak is seen in children and young adults and the second in the sixth and seventh decades of life. Type 1 AIH is found in both phases of the disease, while type 2 is more commonly seen in children. As is seen in many autoimmune diseases, there is a female preponderance, with as many as 4/5 cases being female across both types. As a disease of childhood the incidence is some 7:1, female to male.

Histopathology

Necrosis
Unprogrammed cell death.

The histopathology of both type 1 and type 2 AIH is identical and shows a mononuclear cell infiltrate of the hepatic portal tracts with interface hepatitis (inflammation of the hepatocytes) and hepatocyte **necrosis** (hepatocyte death); see Figure 8.1. As the necrosis intensifies, the dead hepatocytes are replaced with fibrous tissue, ultimately leading to cirrhosis. As a result of the loss of hepatocytes the liver enters a functional decline, terminating in liver failure.

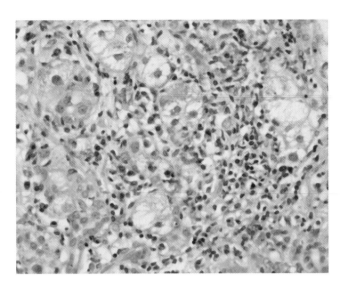

FIGURE 8.1
Margin of portal tract in autoimmune hepatitis. (Reproduced by kind permission of Professor Bernard Portmann.)

METHOD 8.1 *Measuring autoantibodies for autoimmune liver disease*

■ Most commonly, the screening for autoantibodies in autoimmune liver disease is performed by indirect immunofluorescence (IIF), using an LKS substrate. This triple block consists of liver, kidney, and stomach sections from either mouse or rat. There are arguments about which tissue is the best to identify the different patterns seen using this technique. The conjugate used is an anti-human polyclonal IgG isotype.

■ The screening dilution varies from laboratory to laboratory, but is usually at 1/40 for adults. It is recommended to screen at 1/10 for children, as low-titre antibodies can be clinically significant in this population.

■ Commercial ELISAs are available for some of the liver autoantibodies, such as M2 mitochondrial autoantibodies and F-actin autoantibodies. However, many laboratories are now moving towards confirming liver autoantibodies using immunoblot techniques. The immunoblot strips contain many of the clinically significant antigens, such as M2, LKM1, LC 1, SLA, and F-actin.

Serology—the autoantibodies

The two serologically distinct forms of AIH present differently in the laboratory.

Type 1 is characterized by the presence of anti-smooth muscle antibody (SMA) and/or anti-nuclear antibody (ANA). At one time AIH was known as 'lupoid hepatitis', mainly because the presence of ANA.

The presence of anti-liver kidney microsomal antibody-1 (LKM 1) defines type 2 AIH. In addition to the anti-LKM 1, the classical indicator autoantibody of type 2 AIH, there is another autoantibody of relevance, anti-liver cytosol-1 (LC 1). Anti-LC 1 is present in some 40% of anti-LKM-1 positive cases but is never detected in IIF because it is masked by the brighter fluorescence of the anti-LKM 1. It cannot be stressed too frequently that anti-LC 1 can and does occur without any other autoantibody. Failure to detect this lone autoantibody represents a crucially missed diagnostic opportunity.

Not all autoantibodies are detected by the use of IIF. One such case pertinent to liver disease is that of anti-soluble liver antigen (SLA). It has been suggested by some authorities that the presence of anti-SLA establishes yet another type of AIH, type 3. As anti-SLA is found in both types of AIH and in PBC/AIH overlaps, this classification is rarely used. Other assays are needed for the demonstration of anti-SLA.

Cross reference

See section 8.4 for more on AIH and PBC overlap syndromes.

Key Point

AIH types 1 and 2 are differentiated by their autoantibody profiles.

Anti-smooth muscle antibody (SMA)

There is a group of IIF patterns associated with the autoantibody known as SMA. This alone indicates that there is probably more than one target autoantigen. The original classifcation of SMA by Bottazzo *et al.* (1976) describes three predominant patterns seen in rat kidney alone:

- vessel wall staining alone (SMA-V)
- glomeruli with some vascular staining (SMA-G)
- both vessels and glomeruli with intracellular fibres of renal tubules (SMA-T).

The group found that sera from patients with 'lupoid hepatitis' and 'chronic active hepatitis ANA negative' (both now described as AIH type 1) were positive for anti-SMA-G and anti-SMA-T antibodies. This positivity was lost in most cases after absorption with actin, indicating actin as a target autoantigen. We now know that autoantigenic target to be F-actin, and antibodies to F-actin to be typical of AIH type 1. This is not to say that anti-F-actin is the only SMA found in AIH type 1, or that it is unique to AIH type 1.

The routine use of rodent LKS sections in IIF allows one to go beyond the Bottazzo classification (which is kidney-based) and to look at smooth muscle autoantibodies in the other tissues. The stomach is particularly useful in this respect. The staining of the transverse and longitudinal muscle bands of the stomach along with the staining of intragastric fibres is another manifestation of SMA seen in AIH type 1. This staining pattern is associated with anti-F-actin but not uniquely so. In some cases there is staining only of the longitudinal and transverse muscle bands, which is not anti-F-actin but nevertheless is associated with AIH type 1. Also in AIH type 1 there is staining of the vessels of the kidney only, with nothing seen in the stomach. Such a pattern is also seen in viral hepatitis and other viral infections and is usually of low titre. Anti-F-actin is the major SMA seen in AIH type 1 but accounts for only some 80% of the SMA positivity. The patterns are predominantly VGT, which is taken to be anti-F-actin and VG, nonanti-F-actin. Hence, there is by implication more than one antigen responsible for the SMA pattern.

The nonanti-F-actin antibody patterns have been associated with desmin, vimentin, and myosin antibodies. Desmin, myosin, and vimentin are described as intermediate filaments. The

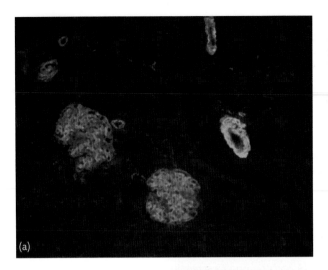
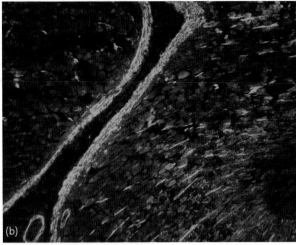
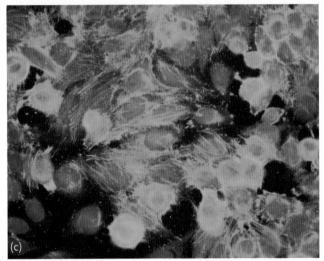

FIGURE 8.2

(a) Anti-smooth muscle antibody from the serum of an 8-year-old girl with AIH type 1. The section of rat kidney shows positive staining in both the glomeruli and blood vessels. This is anti-F-actin. (b) Anti-smooth muscle (serum from the same patient as Figure 8.2a). The section of rat stomach shows positive staining of one of the three major muscle bands of the stomach (bottom left to top centre) and two small vessels in the connective tissue between the bands. Note also the staining of the fine, smooth muscle fibres within the mucosal area (right). (c) Smooth-muscle antibody seen as a microfilamentous pattern on HEp2.

use of antigen-specific assays such as ELISA and immunoblot for anti-F-actin does not give 100% positivity in histologically proven AIH where SMA has been detected by IIF. This may be seen as further evidence that not all anti-smooth muscle antibody associated with AIH type 1 is anti-F-actin. Another substrate frequently used in IIF is the HEp-2 cell line, and this shows anti-F-actin particularly well. When a strong positive anti-F-actin antibody is detected in HEp-2 cells it becomes self-evident as to why F-actin is described as a microfilamentous form of SMA.

Look at Figure 8.2 to see what smooth muscle antibodies look like on kidney and stomach substrate and Hep-2 cells using IIF.

Cross reference

You can read in more detail about the HEp-2 cell line in Chapter 5. This cell line is commonly used in the detection of anti-nuclear antibodies.

Key Point

Anti-smooth muscle antibody has several molecular targets, hence the different patterns seen in IIF.

Anti-nuclear antibody (ANA)

Cross reference

Read Chapter 5 to find out more about anti-nuclear antibodies.

ANA are the most commonly seen autoantibody in clinical immunology. The usual substrate for the detection of ANA is the HEp-2 cell line or one of its derivatives. However, when searching for autoantibodies relating to liver disease, the substrate of choice is the rodent liver, kidney, and stomach (LKS) composite section. At the time of the serological classification of AIH it was the LKS substrate and not the HEp-2 cell line that was used to define ANA positivity. However, the International Autoimmune Hepatitis Group (IAHG) in a consensus statement recommended the use of HEp-2 cells 'to assess the pattern of nuclear staining'. This is to be done after finding a positive ANA reaction on LKS screening. There is not an absolute correlation between ANA positivity found on rodent substrate and that found on the HEp-2 cell line. The protocol in our laboratory is to use both substrates at the screening point and thus avoid the problem. A possible explanation may be found in the serum dilutions used on LKS and HEp-2. A dilution of the order of 1/40 is generally used with LKS, but for HEp-2 1/100 or more is the norm. Thus a weak ANA seen at 1/40 on LKS is not likely to be detected on HEp-2 at 1/100 or greater. Added to this possibility is the difference in the antigens expressed in the two substrates, one rodent and the other human. It is not beyond comprehension that they will not be identical.

Cross reference

You can read the consensus statement from the committee for autoimmune serology of the International Autoimmune Hepatitis Group in Vergani *et al.* (2004).

In connective tissue disorders the detection of ANA positivity is a trigger to investigate further. This is because ANA has low disease specificity and in order to elucidate the potential disorder other investigations are required. The use of assays for nuclear-related autoantibodies such as anti-extractable nuclear antigens (ENA) and anti-double-stranded DNA are very useful in this respect. However, in AIH type 1 there appears to be no unique specificity of the ANA associated with the disease. A study by Gregorio *et al.* (1995) on a small paediatric population with both AIH type 1 and 2 showed 20% of the cases to have a variety of anti-ENA specificities. It is of interest that the majority of the anti-ENA-positive patients belonged to the anti-LKM 1-positive group, type 2 AIH. This raises some questions as this group were ANA-negative by definition. One (heretical) possibility is that any ANA present would be hidden by the anti-LKM-1 in IIF if of lower titre than the anti-LKM 1. This study was done on unfixed LKS sections and did not use HEp-2 cells.

Anti-liver kidney microsomal antibody (LKM)

Anti-LKM was first described in 1973 by Rizzetto and colleagues. Subsequently, other forms of anti-LKM have been found, having a pattern in IIF identical to that of the autoantibody of Rizzetto's group but having different molecular targets. A numerical postscript has been added to the descriptive 'anti-LKM' to facilitate identification. The numbering reflects chronological discovery, hence the anti-LKM of Rizzetto is designated anti-LKM 1.

APECED

Autoimmune polyendocrinopathy, candidiasis, ectodermal dystrophy.

The occurrence of anti-LKM 2 was associated with a hepatitis caused by the use of a diuretic agent known as tienilic acid. This was withdrawn from clinical use in 1980 and hence will not be found currently. Anti-LKM 3 has been described in small groups of hepatitis D virus (HDV)-infected patients. Anti-LKM 4 may be seen in AIH type 2 associated with **APECED**.

Key Point

Anti-LKM 1 is not unique to AIH type 2; it is also found in some cases of hepatitis C virus infection.

CLINICAL CORRELATIONS 8.1

APECED

APECED is caused by a mutation of the *AIRE* (autoimmune regulator) gene, which is located on chromosome 21q22.3. The essential features of the disorder are as given in its name. However, the endocrine disorders are primarily hypoparathyroidism and adrenal insufficiency; many other autoimmune disorders may be seen, including AIH type 2, which occurs in approximately 20% of cases. APECED is also known as autoimmune polyendocrine syndrome 1 (APS1), but APECED is preferred in order to avoid confusion with anti-phospholipid syndrome (APS).

Cross reference

You can read more about APECED in Chapter 7.

A further complication can arise in the case of anti-liver microsomal antibody (anti-LM). The staining pattern of anti-LM is indistinguishable in the rodent liver from anti-LKM 1. However, again as the name suggests, no reaction is seen in the kidney. This autoantibody is found rarely; it may be seen in cases of dihydralazine-induced hepatitis and there are reports of its presence in AIH. The molecular target of anti-LM is a P450 cytochrome, P450 1A2.

As can be seen in Table 8.1, many of the molecular targets of anti-LKM belong to the P450 cytochrome family. The current naming system of the P450 family, as designated by the Human Cytochrome P450 (CYP) Allele Nomenclature Committee (Ingelman-Sundberg *et al.* 2000), is shown in brackets.

AIH type 2 is a rare disorder and hence its marker autoantibody anti-LKM 1 is unlikely to be seen with great frequency in all laboratories. This does not, however, mean that any laboratory using the LKS substrate is absolved from failing to recognize the IIF pattern. Anti-LKM 1 detection forms part of the United Kingdom National External Quality Assurance Scheme (NEQAS) in General Autoimmune Serology, and as such all participants must be competent in its detection. Recent data from the scheme indicate that a sizeable minority of participants still fail to report the presence of anti-LKM 1 correctly. The IIF pattern of anti-LKM 1 is sometimes mistaken for the more commonly seen anti-mitochondrial M2 pattern. There are several reasons for this failure, which will be addressed in section 8.3. The successful identification of any autoantibody seen in IIF is obviously based on pattern recognition. It is useful to consider the individual components that constitute any particular pattern; it is by dissecting out these components that correct identification is made.

Cross reference

The report from NEQAS on reporting of anti-LKM 1 can be found at http://www.immqas.org.uk/docs/LKM%20 Commentary.pdf

TABLE 8.1 The molecular targets of anti-LKM

LKM 1	P450 2D6 (CYP2D6)
LKM 2	P450 2C9 (CYP2C9)
LKM 3	UDGT (uridine diphosphate glucuronosyl transferase)
LKM 4	P450 1A2 and P450 2A6

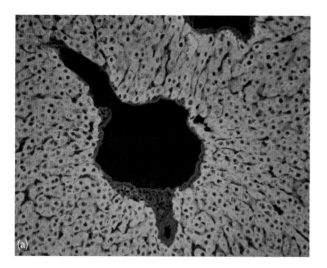
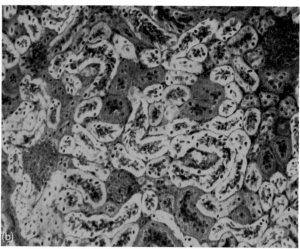

FIGURE 8.3

(a) Anti-LKM 1 on rat liver. Anti-LKM 1 stains all hepatocytes. Note that the portal tract is unstained, unlike anti-M2, which stains the portal tract in a granular fashion. (b) Anti-LKM 1 on rat kidney. Anti-LKM 1 preferentially stains the proximal tubules of the kidney. Also note that the glomeruli remain unstained; this is not the case in the presence of anti-M2, where they are again stained in a granular fashion.

What are the components that signify the presence of anti-LKM 1?

Look at Figure 8.3. The cytoplasm of the hepatocytes of the rodent liver stain, usually very intensely, but the nuclei are spared. They appear as dark holes in the hepatocytes. The staining quality is an important factor and in the case of anti-LKM 1 the staining is homogenous, 'flat' and nongranular. Another striking feature is the nonstaining of the hepatic portal tracts. These appear as black irregular shapes among a mass of bright green tissue. No other autoantibody produces this pattern in the rodent liver.

The staining seen in the rodent kidney presents more of a problem. The proximal renal tubules are selectively stained and the distal tubules remain unstained. The differentiation of the renal tubules is difficult when seen in IIF. The appearance obviously depends on the plane of section but when the tissue is correctly orientated the proximal tubules are more elongated than the distals, which themselves are more circular and generally smaller. Perhaps an easier means of deciding whether or not you are seeing anti-LKM 1 is to ask the question, 'Are all the tubules stained, or only some of them? If the answer is 'Only some of them', then it is more likely that you are seeing anti-LKM 1.

The third tissue of the LKS substrate is the stomach and this remains unstained by anti-LKM 1, as the name of the autoantibody suggests. There is, however, the possibility that staining of the gastric parietal cells may occur. To reiterate, this is not due to anti-LKM 1 but to anti-gastric parietal cell antibody which may found in some cases of type 2 AIH. In particular, anti-gastric parietal cell antibody may be seen in cases of APECED associated with type 2 AIH. It is the joint incidence of the two autoantibodies that gives rise to the confusion of the IIF pattern with that of anti-mitochondrial M2 antibody. Anti-M2 stains the gastric parietal cells because they contain the target autoantigen.

Cross references

Mitochondrial antibodies are discussed further in section 8.3.

Parietal cell antibodies are discussed in more detail in Chapter 7.

CASE STUDY 8.1 Anti-LKM 1 antibodies

Patient history

- 8-year-old female
- GP visit 7 days previous; loss of appetite, tiredness, slight elevation of temperature
- GP thought viral illness, patient sent home to rest
- Mother called GP. Child very sleepy, dark urine noted.

The GP visited, and on seeing the deterioration in the child called an ambulance. The child was admitted to the local hospital under the paediatricians and investigations ordered. The laboratory investigations included viral hepatitis screen, coagulation studies, liver function tests (LFTs), immunoglobulins, C3, C4, and autoantibodies.

Results

- Hepatitis virus screen negative
- LFTs show transaminitis, aspartate aminotransferase (AST) 800 IU/L (normal range 10–50)
- IgG 57.50 g/L, IgA 0.06 g/L, IgM 1.44 g/L
- C3 0.96 g/L, C4 0.06 g/L
- International normalized ratio (INR) 4.2
- Anti-LKM 1 positive 1/5120.

Significance of the results

- Negative screen for hepatitis viruses; basically removes viral infection from the diagnostic possibilities (the differential).
- AST 800 IU/L; AST is one of the components of the LFTs and elevated concentrations are indicative of hepatocyte death.
- The IgG is elevated (normal range 5.4–16.1 g/L). This is a common finding in autoimmune hepatitis; some 80% of cases present with elevated IgG.

- The IgA is decreased (normal range 0.5–2.4 g/L). A subset of patients with AIH is IgA deficient (more type 2 AIH than type 1 AIH).
- The C4 is decreased (normal range 0.15–0.58 g/L). The C4 has not been consumed by classical pathway activity, nor has the liver damage prevented its synthesis; it was never there in the first place. Again, a subset of patients lacks an allele at the C4 locus and has a partial C4 deficiency.
- INR is a coagulation parameter; ideally it should be 1.0. In this case the abnormal INR reflects the liver damage (clotting proteins are hepatic in origin) and rules out liver biopsy (haemorrhage would occur during such a procedure).
- The high-titre anti-LKM 1 antibody is diagnostic of AIH type 2 in this case, as hepatitis virus C and B have been excluded.
- Anti-LKM 1 is not unique to AIH type 2 and may be seen in a small percentage of cases with viral hepatitis.

Subsequent to the finding of anti-LKM 1 by IIF the patient's serum was assayed by immunoblot to confirm the presence of anti-P450 2D6 (cytochrome P450 2D6 is the anti-LKM 1 molecular target). This is our normal laboratory practice for all newly found liver-related autoantibodies where a confirmatory (antigen-specific) assay exists. In this case the immunoblot also detected anti-liver cytosol 1 (anti-LC 1). This autoantibody is also characteristic of AIH type 2 but was not seen in IIF due to its being masked by the high-titre anti-LKM 1.

The patient responded well to corticosteroid therapy and when the INR returned to within normal limits a liver biopsy was performed. The histology was consistent with AIH.

Anti-liver cytosol 1 (LC1)

Anti-LKM 1 is not the only marker of AIH type 2. Anti-LC1 is the second marker of this disease and is less commonly found for two reasons: it is hidden by anti-LKM 1, and its appearance as the sole autoantibody marker is rare. Also, because of its rarity it may well be overlooked. It is not the

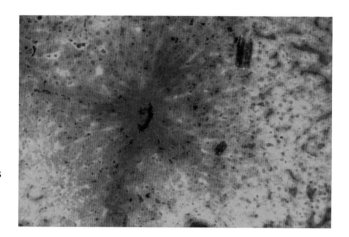

FIGURE 8.4

The molecular target of anti-LC 1 is formiminotransferase cyclodeaminase. This enzyme is found within hepatocytes but is either absent or present in very low concentration in those hepatocytes surrounding the centrilobular vein, hence the lack of staining in these areas.

easiest of autoantibodies to detect as its pattern may be misinterpreted as a technical artefact, especially at low titre. Anti-LC1 is present in about 20% of anti-LKM 1-positive cases but because of its staining pattern it is overshadowed or outshone by anti-LKM 1 in IIF. The staining pattern is confined to the liver in the LKS sections. Like anti-LKM 1 this autoantibody stains the hepatocytes but unlike anti-LKM 1 it does not stain those hepatocytes around the centrilobular vessels. Hence the appearance in the liver is one of 'patchy' staining with both bright and dark areas visible under low to intermediate power. It is this appearance that is sometimes seen as being a technical artefact, inasmuch as it seems that conjugate has not been applied evenly to the whole section. The molecular target of anti-LC 1 is the enzyme formiminotransferase cyclodeaminase (FTCD). Figure 8.4 shows immunofluorescent staining of antibodies to LC-1.

> **SELF-CHECK 8.1**
>
> Why is it vital to differentiate between viral hepatitis and autoimmune hepatitis?

Anti-soluble liver antigen

Unlike the liver disease-related autoantibodies described above, antibodies to SLA are not detectable by IIF on LKS substrate. The anti-SLA antibody was described in 1987 by Manns *et al.*, and in 1993 Stechemesser *et al.* described anti-liver pancreas (LP) antibodies. The two autoantibodies are now known to be directed at the same target, hence the term anti-SLA/LP is sometimes used. Originally, the presence of anti-SLA was thought to define a third form of autoimmune hepatitis, AIH 3. This definition was based on clinical findings and the absence of the classical marker autoantibodies for types 1 and 2 AIH. This classification has now been abandoned as with more sensitive assay procedures anti-SLA has been found in some patients with both types 1 and 2 AIH and also in the PBC/AIH overlap syndrome.

The methodology for the detection of anti-SLA in the diagnostic setting is enzyme immunoassay or immunoblot, both of which are commercially available. In the research laboratory a radio-ligand binding assay has been described, which shows more anti-SLA positivity in both forms of AIH than either of the above assays.

Key Point

Anti-soluble liver antigen (SLA) can be seen in both types of AIH.

Liver function tests

Liver function tests mean different things to different people. Here only the 'liver enzymes' will be covered.

- AST (aspartate transferase) and ALT (alanine transferase) are found within hepatocytes. When hepatocytes are damaged the enzymes are released and enter the plasma pool, thereby increasing the plasma concentration. This condition is known as 'transaminitis' and is a feature of AIH.

- Alkaline phosphatase is found in many tissues, one of which is bile duct epithelium. Damage to this epithelium again releases the enzyme into the plasma, raising its concentration, as may be seen in PBC.

- Gamma-glutamyl transpeptidase (γGT) is found in hepatocytes and biliary epithelium. Raised concentrations of γGT reflect cholestatic and ultimately hepatocyte damage. Elevated concentrations are seen in many liver diseases.

Cross reference

You can read in more detail about liver function tests in the *Clinical Biochemistry* book of this series.

8.2 Autoimmune sclerosing cholangitis (ASC)

ASC is a disease characterized by inflammation of both intra- and extrahepatic bile ducts and hepatitis. The ducts are replaced by fibrous tissue, hence 'sclerosing', and bile flow is interrupted. Bile acids accumulate in the liver, where they are hepatotoxic. ASC may be considered an overlap syndrome, as it shares many clinical and pathological features with autoimmune hepatitis and primary sclerosing cholangitis (PSC).

PSC is a disorder primarily of adults and is thought to have an autoimmune component, in that a prime risk factor for the disease is having a relative with the disease. Unlike most autoimmune disorders there is a male preponderance in PSC. The disease may be asymptomatic for many years and is sometimes only discovered when investigating inflammatory bowel diseases such as ulcerative colitis and Crohn's disease. It is estimated that some 70% of PSC patients have such disorders. In childhood ASC the incidence of inflammatory bowel disease is approximately 45%.

The diagnosis of ASC relies heavily on **cholangiography**. In a series reported by the group of Mieli-Vergani, 25% of the children had no histological evidence of bile duct pathology; it was the cholangiography that revealed the abnormalities and ultimately the diagnosis. It is largely through the work of Professor Mieli-Vergani that ASC has been recognized as a distinct disease entity.

Cholangiography
Imaging of the biliary tract.

ASC has some of the clinical and serological features of autoimmune hepatitis. Its treatment is also like that of AIH in that immunosuppression is the first line with the use of corticosteroids and azathioprine. But unlike AIH a therapeutic agent is used to address the biliary component of the disease: this is ursodeoxycholic acid. Liver transplantation is necessary in some cases.

Incidence

As ASC is a relatively newly recognized disorder as well as a rare one, incidence and prevalence data are not abundant. The prevalence is reported to be the same as that of AIH type 1 (Gregorio *et al.* 2001) in children in the United Kingdom. No doubt in time data will appear from other geographical locations.

Histology

As stated above, histology may not give the definitive diagnosis in all cases of ASC. The histological picture is that of interface hepatitis (as in AIH) and periductal fibrosis. In the Mieli-Vergani series (Mieli-Vergani *et al.* 2008), the pathology of the bile ducts was less severe than that seen in adult PSC.

Serology—the autoantibodies

The autoantibodies associated with ASC are ANA and SMA, as found in AIH type 1. The autoantibody that occurs more frequently in ASC than in AIH is the perinuclear anti-neutrophil cytoplasmic antibody (P-ANCA). This P-ANCA is often referred to as 'atypical' as it does not demonstrate positivity to any single neutrophil cytoplasmic antigen. The 'typical' P-ANCA associated with the small vessel vasculitides is usually anti-myeloperoxidase (MPO). In ASC there may be positivity to MPO but there is also positivity to many other neutrophil antigens, including cathepsin G and lactoferrin. This atypical P-ANCA is also seen in ulcerative colitis and other inflammatory bowel disorders which also form part of the disease spectrum of ASC.

A note of caution: the high incidence of ANA in ASC can raise problems when performing ANCA by IIF, as the patterns are not totally dissimilar. Remember that ANCA and ANA are not mutually exclusive phenomena.

Other similarities exist in both ASC and AIH; elevated concentration of serum IgG (more frequent in ASC than AIH) and deranged LFTs mainly showing a transaminitis.

Key Point

ASC is clinically similar to AIH type 1 in autoantibody profile. However, the incidence of atypical P ANCA is far higher than in AIH type 1.

Cross reference

You can read in more detail about ANCA in Chapter 6.

SELF-CHECK 8.2

What other important technique is used in the diagnosis of ASC and why?

8.3 **Primary biliary cirrhosis (PBC)**

PBC is the result of the destruction of the epithelia of the small intrahepatic bile ducts. This destruction is considered to be T-cell mediated. This, along with the presence of anti-mitochondrial autoantibodies (AMA) seen in the vast majority of PBC patients, has led to the disease being designated as an autoimmune liver disease. The loss of these ducts adversely affects the normal flow of bile within the liver, known as cholestasis. The resultant accumulation of bile products is hepatotoxic and ultimately leads to the loss of hepatocytes and their subsequent replacement by fibrous tissue. If left untreated cirrhosis occurs and results in end-stage liver disease. The only remedy at this stage is liver transplantation. Unlike AIH the prime

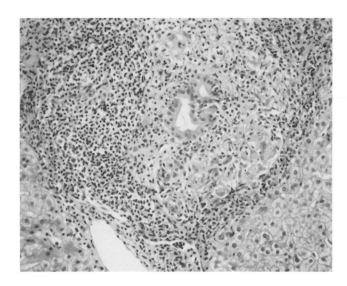

FIGURE 8.5
A case of PBC stage 1 showing mononuclear cell infiltrate (left) invading a bile duct (centre). Note eosinophils (low centre). (Reproduced by kind permission of Professor Bernard Portmann.)

treatment is not immunosuppression but is based on managing the bile acid content with the administration of ursodeoxycholic acid (less hepatotoxic than other bile acids).

Incidence

PBC has a relatively high incidence in Scandinavia and the northern British Isles compared with continental Europe; in the USA there are pockets of high incidence. It would be interesting to know whether these pockets correspond to areas of settlement by migrants from northern Europe. Annual incidence and point prevalence vary depending on geographical location and study criteria used to gather the data (Field and Heathcote 2003). The United Kingdom appears at the top of the incidence table. Again, as with many autoimmune disorders there is a female to male preponderance, which in the case of PBC is approximately 9:1. Most cases present between the ages of 40 and 60 years.

Histopathology

The loss of intrahepatic bile ducts is a prime feature of the histology of the disease (Figure 8.5). The early-stage inflammatory lesion shows a mixed infiltrate of neutrophils, lymphocytes, plasma cells, and eosinophils around the duct with hyperplasia of the duct epithelia. Multinucleate giant cells and granulomas are also prominent features of the disease. The final stages of the disease are characterized by the absence of ducts and cirrhosis.

Serology—the autoantibodies

The serological hallmark of PBC is the anti-mitochondrial antibody, more specifically the anti-M2 mitochondrial antibody. There are nine mitochondrial antibodies of varying clinical significance and conveniently these are designated anti-M1 to anti-M9. In cases of PBC anti-M2 is the major autoantibody but not the only mitochondrial antibody associated with the disease. Anti-M4 and anti-M8 are present with anti-M2 in most cases and hence the IIF

TABLE 8.2 Anti-mitochondrial autoantibodies

Antibody	Molecular target/agent	Disease association
M1	Cardiolipin	Syphilis
M2	A-ketoacid dehydrogenase complex	PBC
M3	Venocuran	Drug-induced pseudo-lupus
M4	Sulphite oxidase	PBC
M5	?Cardiolipin like complex	Unclassified rheumatological disorders
M6	Iproniazid/monoamine oxidase?	Drug-induced hepatitis
M7	Sarcosine dehydrogenase	Myocarditis
M8	Outer mitochondrial membrane	PBC
M9	Glycogen phosphorylase	PBC

pattern seen is probably a composite of all these autoantibodies. The other significant autoantibody is anti-M9. This autoantibody can be found in isolation (in the absence of anti-M2) but usually is present with anti-M2. The anti-M2/M9 combination is considered to be an indicator of a less severe disease progression, whereas the anti-M2/4/8 profile is indicative of a more aggressive form of the disease.

The target antigens associated with these M1–9 autoantibodies are listed in Table 8.2 and are based on the description of Berg and Klein (1986).

The IIF patterns of the various anti-mitochondrial autoantibodies are not dissimilar when seen in the LKS substrate. The non-PBC associated antibodies are relatively rare, but when encountered may be confused with those associated with PBC. The differential staining of the LKS component tissues is the basis for determining the type of mitochondrial antibody. This, as with all IIF, is subject to many variables and may not be definitive. The IIF patterns associated with PBC are somewhat better defined.

The obvious feature of anti-M2 in IIF using LKS substrate is its granularity. Look at Figure 8.6. This is particularly well demonstrated in the liver, where each hepatocyte appears to be a mass of green microdots. In contrast, the staining of the liver seen in anti-LKM 1 is a smooth, homogenous pattern. Another feature which is useful to differentiate the two antibodies when looking at the liver section is the staining of the portal tracts. In the presence of anti-M2 the portal tracts are not easy to see as they blend into the general fluorescence of the hepatocytes. However, when the portal tracts are located, the connective tissue matrix that supports the vessels of the tract can be seen to be stained in the typical granular pattern. This same connective tissue matrix is unstained in the presence of anti-LKM 1 and appears as a black zone in the mass of fluorescence.

It is said that the distal tubules of the kidney are preferentially stained when compared to the proximal tubules. This is not obvious at the screening dilution, where all tubules appear of equal intensity. The differential staining becomes clearer as the titration endpoint is neared. The glomeruli are another useful marker in the differentiation of anti-M2 and anti-LKM1. Again, the granularity of anti-M2 can be seen in the glomeruli, whereas in anti-LKM1 the glomeruli remain unstained. Anti-M2 also stains the gastric parietal cells (GPC), but so does anti-GPC. Again, the difference does not concern what is stained but the appearance of that

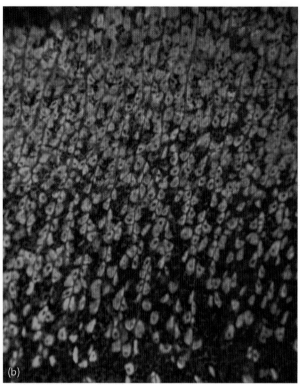

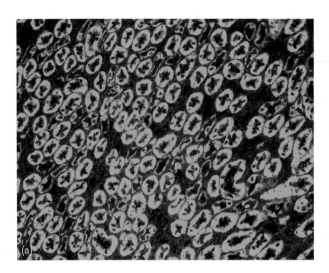

FIGURE 8.6
(a) Anti-M2 on kidney; note that all tubules stain here as this is a high titre (1/10240) seen at screening dilution of 1/40. Also note that the two glomeruli are stained in a typical granular fashion. This not seen in the case of anti-LKM 1. (b) Anti-M2 stains the gastric parietal cells of the rat stomach. Note the fine granularity here, which is absent in anti-gastric parietal cell antibody.

staining. The cytoplasm of the GPCs is granular (the nuclei are spared in the absence of a coexistent anti-nuclear antibody).

> **Key Point**
>
> Anti-mitochondrial antibody M2 may be detected many years before the onset of clinical symptoms.

Nuclear-related autoantibodies

Anti-M2 is sometimes accompanied by anti-nuclear antibodies in PBC. The anti-nuclear antibodies associated with PBC are the multiple nuclear dot (MND) pattern, the rim or peripheral pattern, and centromere antibodies.

Multiple nuclear dot pattern

One of the antigens responsible for the MND pattern is Sp-100, a 95–100-kDa nuclear protein which has been shown to be up-regulated in cell culture in the presence of interferons. This

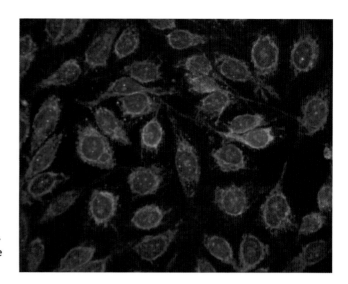

FIGURE 8.7
Anti-Sp 100 (multiple nuclear dots) on HEp-2010 cell line. Note the presence of anti-mitochondrial antibodies in the cytoplasm of the cells.

has led to speculation concerning the role of interferons in the inflammatory process surrounding the destruction of the bile duct epithelium. Although the up-regulation of Sp-100 presents a 'larger' target for the autoimmune process, it does not account for the fact that only 20–30% of PBC cases are positive for anti-Sp-100. With the use of the HEp-2 cell line or one of its derivatives, the anti-Sp-100 pattern is relatively easy to detect. Look at Figure 8.7. There appears to be a consensus that the number of dots that constitute the MND pattern is around 20 per nucleus, but a definitive definition is not readily available. A similar pattern, few nuclear dots (FND), is also seen in unclassified rheumatological disorders. This pattern usually contains less than 10 dots per nucleus in the author's experience, which is too limited to be taken as definitive. It must be remembered, however, that anti-MND is not uniquely associated with PBC and may be seen in rheumatological disorders.

Other nuclear antigens such as promyelocytic leukaemia (PML) antigen and small ubiquitin-like modifier proteins (SUMO) also give the MND pattern in IIF and have association with PBC. Antigen-specific assays are required to identify the molecular specificity of the autoantibody.

Rim or peripheral pattern

The rim or peripheral ANA pattern was detectable in rodent LKS substrate before the use of HEp-2 cell lines became commonplace. However, the presence of high-titre anti-M2 antibody can obscure the rim pattern in this substrate. The pattern is now known to be due to staining of the nuclear pore complex (NPC). Two major antigens have thus far been identified in the NPC, Gp 210 (a 210-kDa glycoprotein) and NUP 62 (a 62-kDa nucleoporin) as being associated with PBC. The rim pattern is easily detected in most cases when using HEp-2 cells. The presence of anti-Gp 210 is associated with more advanced stage of disease and a worsening prognosis, as evidenced by a higher Mayo risk score.

CLINICAL CORRELATIONS 8.3

The Mayo natural history model for PBC

This is a mathematical model for the calculation of estimated probability of survival and is based on patient age, bilirubin concentration, albumin concentration, prothrombin time, presence of oedema (yes or no), and diuretic therapy (yes or no).

Following the computation of the above data a risk score is derived in terms of years of survival. The calculation can be performed on the Mayo website for individual patients and is freely available.

http://www.mayoclinic.org/gi-rst/mayomodel1.html

Centromere antibodies

A more probable cause of confusion is the presence of centromere antibodies, which do occur in cases of PBC. The numerous dots seen in IIF of centromere antibodies can be misread for anti-Sp 100, and vice versa. The counting of individual dots is somewhat tedious and the identification of centromere antibodies relies upon the identification of the characteristic mitotic pattern seen in those cells in metaphase. The presence of anti-centromere antibody in PBC is said to be associated with a portal hypertension endpoint in the disease rather than a hepatic failure scenario. PBC and limited systemic sclerosis, previously known as **CREST syndrome**, should always be considered in the presence of anti-centromere antibody. The overlap syndrome of both disorders is known to exist.

CREST syndrome

A limited form of scleroderma, consisting of <u>c</u>alcinosis <u>R</u>aynaud's phenomenon, o<u>e</u>sophageal motility, <u>s</u>clerodactyly, <u>t</u>elangiectasia.

Key Point

Nuclear-related autoantibodies, while not diagnostic of PBC, can be of clinical significance, especially in anti-M2-negative cases.

Cross reference

You can read more about centromere antibodies in Chapter 5.

Anti-mitochondrial antibody-negative PBC

Not all cases of PBC have mitochondrial antibodies. The concept of AMA-negative PBC is now accepted. The very high association of AMA with the disease previously led to the reasoning that in the absence of AMA there could not be PBC. The histopathological and biochemical evidence in the AMA-negative PBC cases leaves little doubt that the presence of AMA is not an absolute requirement for the diagnosis of the disease.

Somewhere in the region of 95% of PBC cases are AMA-positive. This statement is based on AMA positivity determined by immunofluoresence, which was once the only tool available. The discovery of the molecular nature of the antigens responsible for the immunofluroescence pattern, combined with advances in biotechnology, has made antigen-specific assays a reality. Early evidence that IIF was not the absolute arbiter of AMA positivity came from the work of Muratori and colleagues (2003), who demonstrated AMA positivity by immunoblot in a third of their IIF AMA-negative cases. This raised the question of analytical sensitivity of IIF versus immunoblot. The antigen source used in the immunoblot was a bovine heart mitochondrial fraction and the IIF substrate was rat LKS. This may suggest that the antigen source was responsible for differences in AMA positivity. However, this group also reported that all their AMA-positive cases by IIF were also AMA-positive by immunoblot, indicating similarity of antigen. Hence a very small but significant percentage of once AMA-negative PBC cases became AMA-positive.

AMA-negative PBC does not necessarily mean autoantibody-negative PBC. The nuclear-related autoantibodies described above are strongly associated with AMA-negative PBC.

Original reports found the PBC-related anti-nuclear antibodies were present in a higher percentage in AMA-negative PBC than in AMA-positive PBC. This argues well for the inclusion of HEp-2 cells in the screening of suspected autoimmune liver diseases.

It is possible to find anti-M2 in apparently well people without any overt clinical or biochemical signs of liver disease. Such a finding is considered to be evidence of disease to come, and is known as a **prodrome**. It is important to report these cases, as therapeutic intervention may be required. The presence of anti-M2 has been reported in women with a history of urinary tract infections. These women had no evidence of liver disease and the presence of the anti-M2 is considered to be due to molecular mimicry. Epitopes present in the causative organism of the infection, *E. coli*, are also present in the pyruvate dehydrogenase complex of the M2 antigen (Bogdanos *et al.* 2004).

Prodrome
An early symptom of disease.

Key Point

A diagnosis of PBC can be made in the absence of anti-mitochondrial antibody M2.

SELF-CHECK 8.3

In what other disorders apart from those of the liver might you find anti-M2, and why?

8.4 Overlap syndromes

The term 'overlap syndromes' in the context of autoimmune liver disease refers to the coexistence of two individual disorders, one cholestatic and the other hepatitic. The most common of these overlaps is AIH/PBC, which exhibits autoantibodies associated with both disorders. The most frequent combination is anti-M2 and anti-SLA. The rim ANA (anti-Gp210) and the multiple nuclear dot pattern (anti-Sp100) tend to relate to PBC rather than act as a marker for AIH. This overlap heralds a poorer prognosis than either of the individual disorders.

The overlap between AIH and PSC occurring in adolescents is now considered to be a separate disease entity, ASC. This disorder shares ANA/SMA of AIH and the atypical P-ANCA found in inflammatory bowel disease.

The definition of overlaps in autoimmune liver disease is not yet codified.

Key Points

ASC is considered to be an 'overlap syndrome' because it has features of both primary sclerosing cholangitis and AIH type 1.

PBC/AIH is the most common overlap syndrome and is usually characterized by the presence of anti-M2 and anti-SLA.

CASE STUDY 8.2 *Anti-mitochondrial antibodies*

Patient history

- 47-year-old woman, born in Stockholm, living in London 20 years
- Visits GP complaining of indigestion not responding to over-the-counter remedies
- Also complains of 'itchiness' (pruritus) from time to time on trunk and limbs; general fatigue
- Bloods taken for investigation of possible gastric ulcer, anaemia
- No previous medical history of note

Results (1)

- Borderline haemoglobin and PCV
- WBC normal range
- Alkaline phosphatase 195 IU/L (NR 30–130)
- γGT 67 IU/L (NR 1–55)
- AST 210 IU/mL (NR 10–50)

Significance of results (1)

All the enzymes of the LFTs were abnormally high, indicating a problem with the liver. The patient gave no history of drug or alcohol abuse when questioned further by the GP. The deranged LFTs prompted the GP to order further investigations, namely autoantibodies and immunoglobulins.

Results (2)

- IgG 25.9 g/L, IgA 3.10 g/L, IgM 5.52 g/L
- AMA positive 1/1280 by IIF

Significance of results (2)

- IgG increased (reference range 6.34–18.11 g/L), not unusual in inflammatory liver disease of any aetiology but AIH is worth consideration
- IgA within reference range (0.87–4.12 g/L)
- IgM increased (reference range 0.52–2.23g/L). Raised IgM is a presenting feature of the majority of PBC cases.
- Anti-M2 antibody at this titre is the strongest of indications of a case of PBC.

The AMA was confirmed by immunoblot as anti-M2. The immunoblot also detected anti-soluble liver antigen (SLA).

The patient underwent liver biopsy and cholangiography and was subsequently diagnosed as having a PCB/AIH overlap syndrome. The autoantibody profile by IIF showed only the anti-M2 but the immunoblot also revealed anti-SLA. The latter is not seen on IIF but its discovery adds to the diagnosis as this profile is typical of the overlap syndrome, the major significance being that the therapeutic regime may need to include an immunosuppressive modality, not only ursodeoxycholic acid, to manage the PBC.

Alternative assays

Anti-M2 has a characteristic cytoplasmic staining pattern on HEp-2 cells and, depending on its intensity, can mask the presence of anti-Gp 210. Antibodies to centromere and Sp 100 are not affected by such fluorescence as the antigens are situated away from the nuclear envelope. In order to overcome this particular problem and other problems associated with subjective IIF assay, other assay systems are required. These are the antigen-specific and objective assays such as immunoblot and ELISA. Not only are these assays objective, they are usually of greater analytical sensitivity. This was demonstrated in the cases of the AMA-negative PBC, some of which become positive with a more sensitive assay. Though limited, assays for anti-Gp 210, anti-Sp 100, and anti-centromere are commercially available in either ELISA or immunoblot format.

Another approach to increase the detection rate of AMA in PBC has been to bioengineer a recombinant antigen complex representing three of the major antigenic components of the M2 antigen. Peptides were synthesized conforming to the major epitopes of the pyruvate dehydrogenase complex (PDC-E2), 2-oxo-glutarate dehydrogenase complex (OGDC-E2), and the branched chain 2-oxo-acid dehydrogenase complex (BCOAD-E2) and used in both ELISA and immunoblot. Various modifications have been made to the ELISA system over time and it has now become commercially available. Reports from two studies (Field and Heathcote 2003, Mieli-Vergani and Vergani 2008) have shown that some 60% of IIF AMA-negative PBC sera were AMA-positive in this test system.

Assays for the non-PBC-related anti-mitochondrial antibodies, anti-M4, anti-M8 (always associated with anti-M2) and anti-M9 are not commercially available in any test format.

The use of in-house western blot or ELISA is a possible means to overcome the lack of commercial products. It must be remembered that if such assays are to be used clinically they must be subject to stringent validation within the current regulatory framework.

Key Point

Antigen-specific assays such as ELISA and immunoblot are useful adjuncts to IIF and may provide information not given in IIF.

8.5 **Technical notes**

The efficient demonstration of autoantibodies by IIF consists of several stages:

- the substrate
- the patient and control sera dilutions
- the second antibody conjugate
- the fluorescence microscope
- the observer/reporter.

All these variables must be incorporated into a suitable standard operating procedure (SOP).

Key Point

Indirect immunofluorescence (IIF) is a subjective assay dependent on many components for its result.

The substrate

The choice of substrate for the detection of liver disease-related autoantibodies is an important one. Historically many laboratories prepared their own sections (in house) from locally available rodent tissues. However, the number of sections required in the modern laboratory to meet the current high workload makes this impossible in most cases. The advantage of such locally prepared sections was that they were unfixed and the antigenic repertoire was in its native state. It should be remembered that the patterns originally described for the majority of autoantibodies were from such sections. There is a commercial source of unfixed rodent tissue available in the United Kingdom, but most laboratories use commercially available fixed sections. The advantage of such sections is that they have a long shelf-life when stored according to the manufacturer's instructions. The various fixation schedules used by commercial manufacturers do lead to some differences in the IIF pattern observed for a particular autoantibody.

Substrate selection

The LKS composite block is the accepted standard format for the detection of liver disease-related autoantibodies. The source is either rat or mouse and either performs well. There is a concern that the use of rat stomach may lead to the detection of **heterophile** antibodies which are of no clinical value and may be reported as anti-gastric parietal cell antibody. The pattern is readily identifiable by experienced observers but may be avoided by the use of mouse stomach.

Heterophile
An antibody against an antigen from one species that also reacts against antigens from other species. Often seen in IIF.

The fixation of tissues varies from supplier to supplier and consequently the final pattern seen under the microscope may vary. The aim of fixation is to preserve the tissue in a near a life-like state as possible. This is a definition for the histologist, but for the immunologist there is another concern. Antibodies bind to specific three-dimensional structures, epitopes. The exposure of such structures to alcohols and acetone, the commonly used fixatives, may cause alteration of the epitope and thus adversely affect antibody binding. This is not in the interest of suppliers, hence the fixation schedules they use are considered suitable for the intended purpose. The simplest approach for selection of substrate is to use a panel of known positive controls for the autoantibodies of interest and to see how they react with the different commercial substrates. Most suppliers will be pleased to offer material for evaluation at no cost. Your laboratory SOP for the introduction of a new assay may cover this, or a more specific one can be written following that format with suitable amendments.

The plane of section is of importance and should be such as to allow easy observation of the relevant tissue structures used in the identification of the autoantibody. In the case of the liver this does not matter, as the liver may be seen as a homogenous mass which appears the same regardless of plane of section. The stomach must be sectioned in a way that allows simultaneous viewing of both the mucosa and the muscle bands, avoiding the gastro-oesophageal junction. The kidney sectional plane should reveal both cortex and medulla. This is essential in the demonstration of anti-LKM and anti-mitochondrial M2 antibodies.

The patient and control serum dilutions

The International Autoimmune Hepatitis Group (IAIHG) has published a consensus statement on the detection of autoantibodies in liver disease (Vergani *et al.* 2004). Briefly, the statement advises 1/40 initial screening dilution for adults and 1/10 for paediatric cases, defined as less than 18 years old. The use of ANA-, SMA-, LKM-1-, and AMA-positive controls forms part of the recommendations. Control sera may be obtained from commercial sources or from patient samples. If using patient material there must be compliance with departmental policy and/or the local ethics committee policy. Not only does the use of positive control material conform to good practice, but it allows an instant reference in cases of uncertainty that may arise with patient sera.

Key Point

The use of well-characterized positive and negative control sera is essential to every successful autoantibody assay.

The second antibody conjugate

Anti-human IgG fluorescein isothiocyanate (FITC) is the conjugate of choice when investigating liver disease-related autoantibodies.

The use of a chequerboard titration is the only scientific means of determining the optimum dilution of the conjugate. Manufacturers' recommendations are only suggestions, but offer a central point around which to design the titration range. Again, as with all IIF the endpoint is subjective. The aim is to clearly visualize the autoantibody with as little extraneous or background staining as possible. The use of counterstains to reduce backgrounds should not be necessary if the chequerboard is performed accurately.

The fluorescence microscope

The selection of microscopes suitable for IIF work is wide and varied. The optics and the light source are the major components of any system. Modern microscopes use dichroic mirrors in conjunction with exciter and barrier filters to achieve the desired configuration for the fluorochrome of choice. Detailed information is available on the websites of the major suppliers.

There are three main light sources: mercury vapour, xenon, and light-emitting diodes (LED). The LED sources offer the advantages of longevity, up to 10 000 hours usage compared to xenon and mercury, which are in hundreds of hours. The ability to switch on and off as required, with no warm-up time, is another advantage of the LED. There are issues of safety with high-pressure lamps which are absent with the use of LED. The possibility of explosion is present, and increases as the envelope ages. The escape of mercury into the local environment is another cause for concern, though any vapour readily condenses. The centring of lamps often proves difficult and is a contributory factor in poor overall performance. The LED systems require no such centring, just an instrument-based calibration.

The observer/reporter

Training is a time-consuming process, perhaps even more so in the case of fluorescence microscopy. The correct identification of the relevant IIF patterns is a skill best acquired over time with the teaching of experienced colleagues. Photomicrographs from textbooks and websites are useful adjuncts to the learning process, but no substitute for regular sessions at the microscope. Because IIF is a subjective assay system it is advisable to use two observers to report. Any divergence of opinion can then be the subject of further investigation or subjected to the laboratory's SOP, which should cover such situations.

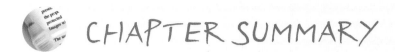

CHAPTER SUMMARY

- IIF is a subjective assay; antigen-specific assays are useful confirmatory tools.

- Type 1 AIH is defined by the presence of ANA/and or SMA.

- Type 2 AIH is defined by the presence of anti-LKM 1.

- Anti-LKM 1 also occurs in 10% of hepatitis C infection.

- Anti-liver cytosol is found in approximately 50% of type 2 AIH.

- Anti-mitochondrial antibody (M2) is the marker autoantibody of PBC, but anti-mitochondrial antibody-negative PBC exists.

- ASC is serologically like AIH type 1 but also has a high incidence of atypical P-ANCA.

- Overlap syndromes exist; PBC/AIH. ASC appears to be a PSC/AIH overlap.

- Immunosuppression is the major therapeutic, but when the biliary tree is involved a therapeutic modality is required for managing bile acids.

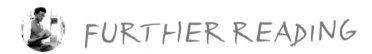

FURTHER READING

- **Vergani D, Alvarez F, Bianchi F, *et al*. (2004) Liver autoimmune serology: a consensus statement from the committee for autoimmune serology of the International Autoimmne Hepatitis Group. *J Hepatol*, 41, 677–683.**

- **Davies E (2008) LKM antibody—still a trap for the unwary. http://www.immqas.org.uk/docs/LKM%20Commentary.pdf**

DISCUSSION QUESTIONS

8.1 Discuss the factors influencing the result of an IIF assay for anti-LKM1 in a child.

8.2 You receive a request for 'mitochondrial antibodies please; clinically and biochemically PBC'. Your IIF result is negative for anti-mitochondrial antibody on LKS substrate. How would you proceed?

8.3 A known PBC (anti-M2 positive) patient has transferred to your hepatology clinic. Physicians request LFTs and note a marked transaminitis along with the expected raised alkaline phosphatase. They suspect PBC/AIH overlap and subsequently request 'AIH antibodies, please'. Your IIF reveals anti-M2 to a titre of 1/640 only. How would you proceed?

Answers to these questions are provided in the book's Online Resource Centre; visit www.oxfordtextbooks.co.uk/orc/ahmed/

9

Neuroimmunology

Learning Objectives

After studying this chapter you should be able to:

- outline the immunological mechanisms involved in autoimmunity associated with paraneoplastic neurological syndromes (PNS)
- describe why PNS are diverse
- explain why paraneoplastic neurological antibodies (PNA) are useful early diagnostic markers of PNS
- outline with examples, why some of the antibodies are pathogenic and others unlikely to be so
- explain what the characteristics of PNS-associated tumours are
- explain why there is a need for confirming specificities of PNA with other methodologies

Introduction

This chapter is intended to provide an overview of recent developments in neuroimmunology, focusing on how clinical and paraclinical (laboratory) investigations contribute to diagnosis leading to effective management and enhanced quality of life.

In view of the scope of this chapter, only selected topics of interest in this specialist field will be addressed. The major emphasis will be on paraneoplastic neurological antibodies (PNA) associated with nonmetastatic neurological complications of cancer. These neurological complications are collectively known as paraneoplastic neurological syndrome (PNS).

The list of paraneoplastic anti-neuronal antibodies has grown to double figures since the discovery, in the mid-1980s, of the first clinically relevant anti-neuronal antibody specific for paraneoplastic aetiology; an advance that assists in the definitive clinical diagnosis of PNS. Furthermore, identifying these antibodies in the absence of a specific aetiology alerts the clinician to carry out a thorough examination of the patient for the possible presence of an unidentified neoplasm. Early diagnosis of the tumour is essential as it provides an opportunity for effective treatment. See Table 9.1 for a summary of the paraneoplastic anti-neuronal antibodies that have been characterized.

In the present chapter the characteristic elements of PNS will be addressed, namely neurological disorder, neoplasm, and paraneoplastic neurological antibodies.

Terminology

The terms used in this chapter are unlikely to be found in other chapters and are different from those describing other disease processes. Furthermore, nomenclature used in the naming of these antibodies has not been standardized; consequently, an antibody may be referred to by different names, leading to confusion.

9.1 Epidemiology of paraneoplastic syndrome

Malignancy-related neurological disorders are rare, and their relative rarity makes it difficult to carry out extensive clinical, epidemiological, and experimental studies in individual laboratories. The few studies that have addressed the incidence and prevalence of PNS in the overall cancer population have found an estimated frequency of around 0.01% (1/10 000), whereas in a UK survey conducted among physicians, about 50 cases of PNS were reported in 1 year, which approximates to an incidence of only 0.0001% (Rees 2004). Such low incidences are likely to reflect under-reporting of PNS. Other studies have focused on either the association of certain cancers with PNS or on the specific PNAs, their neurological syndrome, and associated neoplasm. It is worth noting that neuromuscular abnormalities such as **Lambert–Eaton myasthenic syndrome (LEMS)** can occur in up to 1% of patients with small-cell lung cancer (SCLC). A study by Pittock et al. (2005) looked at the detection of PNA in 120 000 samples received over a 15-year period from patients suspected of neurological disorders. They found low detection frequencies of PNA, with the highest frequency of 0.4% assigned to an antibody known as ANNA1. These data are summarized in Table 9.2.

> **Lambert-Eaton myasthenic syndrome (LEMS)**
> Muscle weakness, fatigue, difficulty swallowing, and autonomic symptoms.

The patient group affected by PNS, particularly paraneoplastic cerebellar degeneration (PCD), tend to be in the latter part of life, with several studies quoting median range above 60 years.

9.2 Clinical features of paraneoplastic syndromes

The term 'paraneoplastic syndromes' refers to a collection of clinical disorders that occur at sites remote from a tumour or its metastases and can be of a nervous, cutaneous, endocrine, gastrointestinal, haematological, renal, or rheumatological nature or origin. When the nervous system is involved (central or peripheral, including the neuromuscular junction and muscle), this is known as paraneoplastic neurological syndrome and can affect any level of the nervous system. It has been known at least since the eighteenth century that certain neurological illnesses, termed the 'classical syndrome' almost always accompany a neoplasm. Neurological deficits loosely associated with the malignancy are referred to as 'nonclassical PNS'. These are shown in Table 9.3.

TABLE 9.1 Summary of paraneoplastic anti-neuronal antibodies, their staining patterns, associated disorders, common tumours, and relevant target antigens

Antibody	MW (kDa)	Staining pattern	PNS	Associated tumour(s)	Target antigen
A. Well-characterized PNA					
Hu (ANNA-1)	34–40	Nuclei of both central and peripheral neurons	PCD, PEM, SN	SCLC	HuD, PLE21/HuC, Hel-N1, 35–40-kDa nucleus and slightly cytoplasm RNA recognition motifs, translation
Yo (PCA-1)	34, 52, 62	Purkinje cell cytoplasm and axons	PCD	Ovary, breast	PCD17/CDR62 (58 kDa), cytoplasm, leucine zipper, zinc finger, transcription 34 kDa, 6 amino acid repeat
CRMP-5/CV-2	66	Oligodendrocytes cytoplasm	PEM/SN	SCLC, thymoma	POP66, 66 kDa, cytoplasmic in some oligodendrocytes
Ri (ANNA-2)	55, 80	Nuclei of central neurons	OM, PCD, BE	Breast, SCLC, gynaecological	Nova-1 (55 kDa) and 80 kDa, nucleus and slightly cytoplasm only in CNS, RNA recognition motifs, translation
Ma2 (Ta)	41.5	Neuronal nucleoli, perikaryon	BE, LE	Testicular cancer	Unknown function
Amphiphysin	128	Central presynaptic terminals	SPS, PEM	Breast cancer, SCLC	Amphiphysin, neurophil, cytoplasm doublet bands at 125–128 kDa, synaptic vesicle-associated protein
Recoverin	23, 65	Retinal photoreceptor	Retinopathy	SCLC	Recoverin, 23 kDa, calcium-binding protein
B. Partially characterized PNA					
Tr (PCA-Tr)	[??]	Purkinje cell cytoplasm with 'dots' in molecular layer	PCD	Hodgkin's lymphoma	Unknown function (found in the Purkinje cell cytoplasm)
ANNA-3	170	Purkinje cell cytoplasm and nucleus + glomerular podocytes	PCD, PEM, SN	SCLC	170-kDa protein found in cytoplasm of Purkinje cells and glomerular podocytes
PCA-2	280	Purkinje cell cytoplasm and other neurons	PEM, PCD, LEMS	SCLC	280-kDa Purkinje cell cytoplasmic protein
Zic4	~37	Nuclei of granular neurons, weaker on Purkinje cell nuclei	PCD	SCLC	Zinc finger protein found in cerebellum
mGluR1	~140	Purkinje cell cytoplasm, climbing fibre	PCD	Hodgkin's lymphoma	mGluR1
C. Antibodies that occur with or without cancer					
VGCC	64	Presynaptic neuromuscular junction	LEMS, PCD	SCLC	64-kDa P/Q voltage-gated calcium channel, acetylcholine release
VGKC	VGKC	Peripheral nerve	LE, neuromyotonia	SCLC, thymoma	Voltage-gated potassium channel
Ach R	Receptor	Postsynaptic neuromuscular junction	MG	Thymoma	ACh receptor

AchR, acetylcholine receptor; ANNA, antineuronal nuclear antibody; BE, brainstem encephalomyelitis; LE, limbic encephalomyelitis; LEMS, Lambert–Eaton myasthenic syndrome; MG, myasthenia gravis; mGluR1, metabotropic glutamate receptor type 1; OM= opsoclonus/myclonus; PCA, Purkinje cell cytoplasm antibody; PCD, paraneoplastic cerebellar degeneration; PEM, paraneoplastic encephalomyelitis; PND, paraneoplastic neurological disorder; SCLC, small-cell lung carcinoma; SN, sensory neuropathy; SPS, stiff person syndrome; VGCC, voltage-gated calcium channel; VGKC, voltage-gated potassium channel.

[??] No common band has been identified by western blot analysis.

TABLE 9.2 Detection frequency of PNA from 120 000 patients suspected of paraneoplastic neurological syndrome

PNA	Frequency (%)
ANNA-1	0.4
CRMP-5/CV-2	0.4
PCA-1	0.2
PCA-2	0.1
Amphiphysin	0.06
ANNA-2	0.02
ANNA-3	0.001
PCA-Tr (Tr)	0.002

TABLE 9.3 Classic and nonclassic neurological disorders associated with cancer

	Classic—strong cancer link	Nonclassic—weak cancer link
Central nervous system	Encephalomyelitis Limbic encephalitis Subacute cerebellar degeneration Opsoclonus–myoclonus	Brainstem encephalitis Stiff person syndrome Paraneoplastic visual syndromes Motor neuron syndromes
Peripheral nervous system	Subacute sensory neuronopathy	Acute sensorimotor neuropathy Chronic sensorimotor neuropathy Subacute autonomic neuropathy Paraneoplastic peripheral nerve vasculitis
Neuromuscular junction and muscle	Lambert–Eaton myasthenic syndrome Dermatomyositis	Myasthenia gravis Neuromyotonia Acute necrotizing myopathy Cachectic myopathy

Clinically, PNS can be defined as 'definite' or 'possible', based on combined evidence arising from neurological examination (classical or nonclassical syndrome), the involvement of cancer, and the presence of well-characterized PNA (Graus *et al.* 2004). The criteria for the definitive or possible diagnosis of PNS are shown in Table 9.4 later in the chapter. When present in a patient, the rare neurological illnesses of the classical syndrome imply a very high index of clinical suspicion of PNS diagnosis. A brief description of these conditions follows, together with antibodies associated with such conditions as LEMS, **myasthenia gravis**, **neuromyotonia**, and other relevant disorders.

Myasthenia gravis
Weakness and rapid fatigue of voluntary muscles.

Neuromyotonia
Abnormal nerve impulses from peripheral motor neurons causing twitching, stiffness, cramps, and slowed movement.

Key Point

Autoimmune neurological syndromes may or may not be associated with an underlying cancer.

SELF-CHECK 9.1

What is meant by a classical neurological syndrome?

Signs and symptoms of paraneoplastic syndromes

Limbic encephalitis

Inflammation of the brain leading to memory loss, drowsiness, confusion, disorientation, and seizures.

Encephalomyelitis

Inflammation of both brain (encephalitis) and spinal cord (myelitis).

Cerebellar degeneration

Damage to the cerebellum, with loss of muscle control and balance.

The most common signs and symptoms of PNS include difficulty in walking, maintaining balance, swallowing, loss of muscle tone and fine motor coordination, slurred speech, memory loss, vision problems, dizziness, sleep disturbances, dementia, seizures, numbness, and tingling in the limbs.

Key Point

The common neuroimmunological syndromes associated with well-recognized antibodies are myasthenia gravis, LEMS, limbic encephalitis, encephalomyelitis, and cerebellar degeneration.

SELF-CHECK 9.2

Define paraneoplastic neurological syndrome (PNS).

Paraneoplastic encephalomyelitis (PEM)

Encephalomyelitis (EM) is a generalized term used for inflammation of brain and spinal cord. In about 10% of patients, EM is paraneoplastic, where multiple areas of the brain are affected by neuronal loss and inflammatory infiltrates. The term paraneoplastic encephalomyelitis (PEM) alone provides limited information on the main clinical picture and therefore should not be used in isolation, especially if a single predominant area of the central nervous system is affected (Graus *et al.* 2004). Depending on the predominant area of central nervous system involvement, patients may be classified in different ways, which are discussed below. Some 9% of PEM patients have limbic encephalitis (affecting the hippocampus and limbic system), 10.5% have subacute cerebellar degeneration, 6% have brainstem encephalitis, and some have autonomic neuropathy. Fifty-four per cent of patients have dorsal root ganglia involvement causing subacute sensory neuronopathy. The spectrum of neurological symptoms can vary from numbness to respiratory failure (Graus *et al.* 2001). In 30% of cases, a single abnormality may manifest clinically.

Paraneoplastic cerebellar degeneration (PCD)

Paraneoplastic cerebellar degeneration (PCD), the most commonly occurring PNS, is a disorder of the cerebellum and occurs at a frequency of 37% in patients with PNA. The cerebellum consists of white and grey matter; the latter is subdivided into molecular and granular layers (containing densely packed granular cells). The Purkinje cells, which can be easily identified by their large size and location at the border of the granular layer facing the molecular layer, make up a mere 0.3% of the human cerebellum. Figure 9.1 shows the location of the cerebellum and Figure 9.2 its cellular structure.

Post-mortem studies on subjects with PCD reveal an almost complete absence of cerebellar Purkinje cells, an observation that might explain the reason behind the rapid onset of symptoms (from weeks to a few months). Functionally, the cerebellum is responsible for sensory

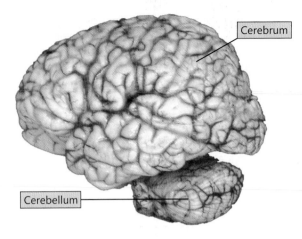

FIGURE 9.1

Human brain showing the location of cerebellum (Latin: 'little brain'), which is located in the inferior posterior region of the head and is made up of two hemispheres.

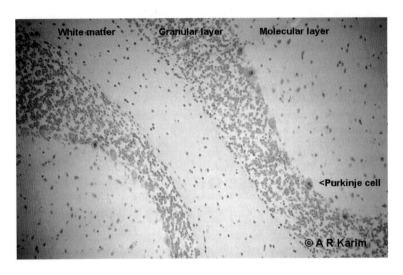

FIGURE 9.2

Haematoxylin- and eosin-stained section of primate cerebellum showing the white matter and the granular and molecular layers. Large Purkinje cells are located at the border of the granular and the molecular layer.

(information) perception, coordination, and motor control. Lack of coordination is known as ataxia; 50% of cerebellar ataxia is of paraneoplastic origin.

Clinically, the characteristic signs of cerebellar involvement are obvious: the patient walks with a wide-legged, unsteady, lurching gait and jerky limb movements. These acute symptoms are accompanied by nausea, vomiting, dizziness, and uncoordinated movement, which usually progress to a severe stage where simple tasks like walking, sitting, and eating cannot be performed without assistance. Patients may also suffer from inability to communicate verbally (due to slow and slurry speech) and/or in written form (owing to nystagmus and double vision, coupled with unsteady hands).

Paraneoplastic limbic encephalitis (PLE)

Paraneoplastic limbic encephalitis (PLE) is attributed to a disturbance in the limbic system (located at the base of the brain) and presents as changes in the individual's personality, rapid loss of short-term memory, drowsiness, confusion, disorientation, depression, irritability, and seizures (Gultekin *et al.* 2000, Dalmau and Bataller 2006). In 64% of cases, MRI findings show brain abnormalities. These symptoms are not confined solely to PLE but can also occur in association with other ailments such as brain metastases, toxic therapy, or herpes infection, thus complicating diagnosis. The onset of the symptoms can be acute or subacute and may accompany SCLC (40%), testicular germ-cell tumours (20%), breast cancer (8%), Hodgkin's disease, and thymoma. PLE can also exist without cancer (nonparaneoplastic origin).

Opsoclonus–myoclonus (OM)

Opsoclonus–myoclonus (OM)
Rapid, irregular eye movements (opsoclonus) coupled with quick, involuntary muscle jerks (myoclonus).

Opsoclonus–myoclonus (OM), also known as Kinsbourne's or 'dancing eyes–dancing feet' syndrome, is defined by the presence of rapid, irregular eye movements (opsoclonus) in either vertical or horizontal direction coupled with quick, involuntary muscle jerks (myoclonus) of the limbs and trunk. Symptoms of cerebellar dysfunction are also frequent with this disorder (Rossinol *et al.* 2008). Paraneoplastic OM (POM) is seen in 50% of children with neuroblastoma and about 20% of adults with OM have underlying malignancy of lung (SCLC), breast, or gynaecological origin. In some adults, POM can occur in conjunction with SCLC but without a related antibody. Reports of other neoplasms exist in the literature.

Stiff person syndrome (SPS)

Stiff person syndrome (SPS)
Progressive, severe muscle stiffness or rigidity, mainly in spine and legs.

Stiff person syndrome (SPS) is considered as a central nervous system syndrome and belongs to the nonclassical category of cancer. It is included here for the sake of completeness, and will not be mentioned later in the chapter. SPS is due to a malfunction of the fastigial nucleus in the cerebellum, whose function is concerned with antigravity muscle groups and other synergies involved with standing and walking. The fastigial nucleus contains excitatory axons and the likely candidate for neurotransmitter in these neurons is glutamate and/or aspartate.

Cross reference
You can find a fuller account of stiff person syndrome in the review by Meinck *et al.* (2002).

SPS is a rare form of autoimmune neurological disorder featuring symmetrical progressive and severe muscle stiffness or rigidity, mainly in the spine, and intense painful muscle spasms that may be triggered by sensory stimuli. Muscle rigidity can vary during the day and may reduce in intensity with sleep. Muscle spasm, which may be accompanied by intense pain, can immobilize the limbs so that walking becomes slow and difficult. Severe spasms have been known to inflict femoral fractures or abdominal hernia. In about 20% of cases, a paraneoplastic variation of SPS can also exists in patients with breast, colon, or lung cancer, Hodgkin's disease, and thymoma.

Paraneoplastic sensory neuronopathy (PSN)

Neuropathy
Disorder of peripheral nervous system involving motor, sensory, and/or autonomic nerves.

The term neuronopathy was coined to describe neurological syndromes arising from damage to the neurons of the peripheral nervous system observed in patients with tumours of lung origin, usually SCLC (70–80%), but it can also be identified with neoplasms of ovary, breast, or Hodgkin's disease (Graus *et al.* 2001). Approximately 20% of neuronopathies are of paraneoplastic origin. The main clinical complaints are subacute numbness and paraesthesia (pins and needles), which can be asymmetrical and patchy, usually starting with the upper limbs and rapidly progressing to a state where the patient becomes wheelchair- or bed-bound with the disability. The **neuropathy** is often painful (shooting, burning sensations) and when large sensory fibres are involved, sensory ataxia (unsteadiness due to reduced sensation) is also present. Sensory loss can affect the face, chest, and abdomen. Patients may also present with gastrointestinal pseudo-obstruction (constipation and vomiting), due to the involvement of the neurons of the myenteric plexus.

Myasthenia gravis (MG)

Myasthenia gravis (MG) is an autoimmune disorder of the peripheral nervous system affecting neuromuscular junctions (NMJ) and occurs at an approximate rate of 0.02% (1/5000). Clinically, it can be referred to either as ocular MG, where only the eyelids and extraocular muscles are affected with weakness, or generalized MG, in which subnormal muscle strength can be observed in other muscles. The weakness is variable, painless, and can fluctuate from day to day and is typically fatiguable (i.e. aggravated by exercise or activity).

Ocular MG leads to abrupt onset of weakness/fatiguability of the eyelids or eye movement. Ptosis (drooping of the eyelid) is usually bilateral, but asymmetrical ptosis is generally made worse with up-gaze; consequently, patients may have difficulties with reading and watching television.

The generalized form of MG can affect a variety of muscles, leading to unstable or waddling gait, weakness in the arms, hands, fingers, legs, and neck, difficulty in swallowing, shortness of breath, and impaired speech. Many patients may appear to be depressed, because they have an expressionless face resulting from fatigued facial muscles (Juel *et al.* 2007).

Lambert–Eaton myasthenic syndrome (LEMS)

This is another disorder of the neuromuscular junction, affecting different muscles from those involved in myasthenia gravis (respiratory, ocular, or bulbar muscles that control swallowing, breathing, and speech). In LEMS, trunk and leg muscles are involved. In over 90% of patients, muscle weakness starts in the legs proximally and then spreads to other muscles, resulting in fatigue and difficulty in swallowing (Vedeler *et al.* 2006). Autonomic symptoms are frequent features of LEMS, such as dry eyes and mouth, blurred vision, impotence, constipation, sweating, and orthostatic hypotension (Vincent 2008).

LEMS can be divided into two types, one associated with cancer (paraneoplastic LEMS) and the other not. Both types are indistinguishable in terms of clinical expression or electrophysiology (the test used to confirm LEMS). The disorder is paraneoplastic in about 60% of patients with LEMS, usually caused by SCLC. LEMS can also exist in conjunction with other PNS.

Neuromyotonia (NMT)

Neuromyotonia (NMT), also know as undulating myokymia or Isaac's syndrome and often described as peripheral nerve hyperexcitability (PNH), is an autoimmune disorder commonly found to impact the limbs and trunk. NMT is manifested as spontaneous and continuous muscle fibre hyperactivity of peripheral motor neurons, causing muscle stiffness, twitching (myokymia), painful cramps, and slowed movement. Muscle cramps in NMT are indistinguishable from other normal cramps, but the hyperactivity of muscle continues even during sleep. One of the autonomic complaints frequently experienced by these patients is excessive sweating. However, NMT is not a fatal condition but can also exist with thymoma (20%) and on occasions may coexist with central nervous system symptoms.

Paraneoplastic NMT has been reported with SCLC, thymoma, and Hodgkin's disease, predating the cancer by up to 4 years.

9.3 Malignancies commonly associated with PNS

PNS can be related to almost any type of malignant cancer with the exception of brain tumours, but only a handful are commonly occurring, such as SCLC, ovarian, breast, testicular, and Hodgkin's disease. Pathologically, PNS-associated cancers resemble any other cancer except for being small in size and infiltrated by immune mediators such as lymphocytes and plasma cells. The fundamental role of the immune system in the control of growth and metastasis is supported by literature reports: in rare cases, there has been spontaneous remission of cancer in patients harbouring PNAs and in 20% of PNS cases, the cancer is never found even at post-mortem examination. In most cases, the cancer can be detected up to 24 months after diagnosis of PNS. It is believed that the longer the cancer is undetectable, the less likely it will appear in the future.

Detection of cancer in patients harbouring PNAs should be carried out using a high-resolution whole-body ^{18}F-deoxyglucose positron emission tomography (FDG-PET) scan, especially when the CT scan is negative. In case the cancer cannot be found, a 6-month review of the patient is advisable in order to search for a possible underlying malignancy, especially in patients with a high risk of developing cancer (e.g. smokers). Monitoring should continue for up to 4 years (Vedeler *et al.* 2006).

9.4 Paraneoplastic neurological antibodies (PNA)

Paraneoplastic neurological antibodies (PNA) are perhaps the most important early diagnostic markers of PNS, which is thought to be immune-mediated in the absence of nonmetastatic complications of cancer and other specific aetiology such as vascular, infectious, metabolic, or treatment-related causes. Typically, the symptoms frequently precede the detection of the associated tumour by up to 2 years (Gultekin *et al.* 2000).

A relationship between neurological disorder and systemic tumours has been known for decades, with immunological involvement first being hypothesized in the early 1950s by

Russell Brain *et al.* (1951). The involvement of the immune system against cancer has been the subject of debate for many years. Over this period, evidence has accumulated from various models supporting the concept of natural immunity to cancer. For example, it is well known that there is a higher risk of cancer developing in patients who are immunocompromised, irrespective of whether the immunodeficiency is primary or caused by HIV infection or immunosuppressive therapy for organ transplantation (Grulich *et al.* 2007, Swann and Smyth 2007). This concept is further supported by the observation that in immunodeficient mouse models there is an increased incidence of cancers. Human disorders like PNS also provide additional valuable circumstantial evidence for immune system involvement.

Pathological post-mortem studies on brains with paraneoplastic cerebellar degeneration (PCD) have demonstrated a general loss of neurons in the affected areas of the central nervous system together with infiltration by B cells, CD4$^+$ T-helper cells, and cytotoxic CD8$^+$ T cells. Immune-mediated processes such as intrathecal IgG (oligoclonal bands) were also evident in the cerebrospinal fluid of patients with PNS. A conclusive breakthrough in this field came in the 1980s when evidence for immunological involvement in neurological disorders due to systemic neoplasm was provided by Posner and colleagues (Graus *et al.* 1985). These workers found specific ANNA1 (Hu) antibodies in the serum of a patient with PNS and SCLC. These antibodies were shown to bind not only to the patient's tumour but also to neuronal cells of the central nervous system. This discovery provided concrete scientific support for the autoimmune basis of paraneoplastic neurological disorders. The commonly accepted hypothesis for the pathogenesis of PNS is as follows:

Cross reference
See section 9.3 on malignancies commonly associated with PNS.

- The immunological response is initially triggered by brain antigens expressed by the tumour (also known as onconeuronal antigens), seemingly in an attempt to eradicate the cancer.

- Consequently, the antigen-specific cytotoxic T and B cells gain access to both the tumour and the brain tissue, thereby targeting cells that are expressing onconeuronal proteins. Such an autoimmune response against neuronal antigens is thought to be responsible for neuronal destruction and hence the clinical condition.

The symptoms exhibited are dependent on the area of the brain affected. Despite the important role of immunological factors in the pathogenesis of PNS, the direct pathogenic role of these antibodies (with the exception of a few) has yet to be proven. The immune attack is directed against intracellular (cytoplasmic or nuclear) antigens which have an important role in neuronal development and function. These groups of antibodies are probably an epiphenomenon or a marker for autoimmune disease processes, rather than directly involved in causing neuronal damage. For this reason, patients do not respond to any treatment that relies on diminishing the levels of these antibodies. Conversely, epitopes exposed on the extracellular surface can be accessible to autoantibody attack, thus characterizing them both as pathogenic and as diagnostically important disease-specific biomarkers. Consequently, treatment with immunomodulation therapy in patients harbouring such antibodies has seen greater success.

In the past two decades the list of anti-neuronal antibody specificities identified in patients with PNS has expanded steadily. With this expansion, the first consensus was initiated that aimed to provide clear guidelines for detection and classification of paraneoplastic antineuronal specific antibodies (Moll *et al.* 1995) for greater uniformity in laboratory screening of PNAs. Previously, detecting PNA suffered from variability due to nonstandard procedures, leading to difficulties in inter-laboratory comparison.

Despite these positive developments, a degree of confusion remains; not only can single antibody specificity be found associated with more than one neurological disorder, but individual syndromes can be associated with different antibody specificities. A further compounding factor is that less than 50% of patients with PNS will harbour PNAs and in 30% more than one PNA is likely to be detected (Pittock *et al.* 2004). For this reason screening is preferable to testing for specific PNA. It is also important to bear in mind that PNA can be found in up to 16% of cancer patients who are neurologically asymptomatic, while up to 11% of subjects with PNA and neurological symptoms may not have a detectable neoplasm. In view of these issues, further standardization of diagnostic criteria and classification of PNS became necessary. This challenge was addressed by a study supported by the European Union to define standards for the diagnosis and classification of PNS.

Cross reference

These guidelines (Graus *et al.* 2004) are referred to in the section on the use of PNAs in diagnosis.

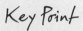

PNAs are not always tumour- or syndrome-specific, but there are well-recognized associations. Hence screening for a broad range of antibodies (e.g. using indirect immunofluorescence with primate cerebellar sections) may be preferable in neurological syndromes that are not so well defined.

Autoantigens

There are a multitude of antigens which are recognized by their respective PNA. The degree of their characterization varies significantly; no doubt a number also remain to be identified. The heterogeneity in both function and cellular location compounds the characterization of the antigens. Despite this, in most cases the antigens responsible for PNS have been identified and the respective genes have been cloned and sequenced. One must bear in mind that it is not necessarily the case that all tumours of a particular type express the antigens. The majority of the antigens are exclusive to the nervous system, an immunologically privileged site. There are one or two exceptions where the antigens have also been identified in individual organs. A number of the antigens are expressed by neuronal cells of both the peripheral and central nervous system, but some are specific to the central nervous system and a proportion are particular to the Purkinje cells of the cerebellum. These onconeuronal antigens responsible for PNS have since been identified and the genes involved cloned to produce recombinant proteins for both testing and research purposes.

PNA detection in the laboratory

'Neuro-oncoantigens' found in the cerebellar tissue are in their native environment, with structure and epitopes preserved. This provides an ideal environment for visualizing the antigen–antibody interaction, both specific and novel. The only drawback is co-localization of other non-neuronal antigens, which may exhibit reactivities similar to those of specific antibodies. To overcome this, it is desirable to confirm any positive reaction with an alternative method, e.g. western blotting, recombinant proteins, ELISA, or competitive assay.

Indirect immunofluorescence

Cross reference

Full details of the methodology are given elsewhere (Karim *et al.* 2005); it is based on the guidelines published by Moll et al. (1995).

In our hands the method of choice of screening for PNA is by indirect immunofluorescence (IIF) using primate cerebellar cryosections as this is rapid, reliable, and reproducible, and is used by 90% of laboratories that provide this service. Although rodent cerebellar sections can suffice and are frequently used, monkey tissues are preferable for reasons of antigenic similarity.

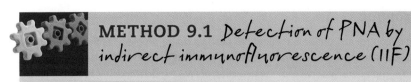

METHOD 9.1 *Detection of PNA by indirect immunofluorescence (IIF)*

- Frozen sections of monkey cerebellum are incubated with test sera at a dilution of 1/50 to allow specific antibody–antigen binding to take place.
- Unbound immunoglobulins are removed by a wash step.
- The bound human immunoglobulins (IgG class) are visualized using sheep anti-human IgG (monkey absorbed) conjugated to fluorescein.

All positive sera are subjected to alternative methods of confirmation of reactivity for the reasons mentioned. There are exceptions to this rule and these will be dealt with under the appropriate antibody section.

Confirmation of reactivity

Various test kits are available commercially that provide a qualitative assay for human IgG antibodies to highly purified antigens as coated parallel lines on strips. In addition to the usually six characterized onconeuronal antigens on a strip, there is also a control band to indicate the correct performance of the incubation step.

Western blots

Commercial preparations of western blots containing separated extract of primate cerebellum with additional recombinant proteins of the most common antigens and control bands are also available. In addition to verifying the specificity of PNA, these blots are very useful for determining the molecular size of novel antigens. A sample is considered positive only when it binds to a specific antigen of the relevant molecular weight and this is consistent with cerebellar pattern.

Key Point

If the screening tests for PNA are positive, further specific tests should be performed using immunoreactive strips or western blots.

Quality assurance

There exists a UK Neuroimmunology Discussion Group (NIDG) made up of members from laboratories around the country. The NIDG sends out patient samples once or twice a year and then meets to discuss and evaluate the outcome. The NIDG has also undertaken a survey to examine methodologies related to the screening and detection of PNA. In addition to improving consistency, it has facilitated sample exchange and sharing of experience.

At the time of writing no external quality control scheme was available, although discussions had taken place between the NIDG and the UK National External Quality Assurance Service (UKNEQAS) to set up a pilot scheme, rather like the NEQAS scheme that is in operation for the acetylcholine receptor antibody.

Internal controls

Internal quality control for routine screening has posed a major problem, as there are limited stocks available to share. For this reason the screening service is limited to a few centres that provide a full and comprehensive service for the detection of PNA. Understandably, these being rare antibodies, most centres guard their positives very jealously, thus limiting the supply of controls.

SELF-CHECK 9.3

What is the rationale for confirming antibody reactivity with an alternative methodology?

Role of PNA in diagnosis of PNS

The recommended guidelines for the use of PNAs to complement diagnosis can be divided into three categories:

1. Well-characterized antibodies that are strongly associated with both the neoplasm and a well-defined neurological disorder (Figure 9.3).

2. Partially characterized antibodies, which have an unidentified target antigen; the experience with this class of antibodies is often confined to one laboratory and/or reported in only a few patients (Figure 9.4)

3. Antibodies that occur with a specific disorder but do not differentiate between PNS and non-PNS cases (Figure 9.5).

Below we describe three scenarios where the combination of clinical and paraclinical tests can be utilized to diagnose PNS, with particular emphasis on the involvement of PNA (Graus *et al.* 2004).

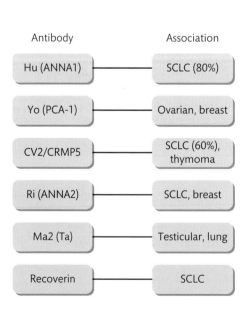

FIGURE 9.3
Defined PNAs and their commonly associated malignancies. SCLC, small-cell lung cancer.

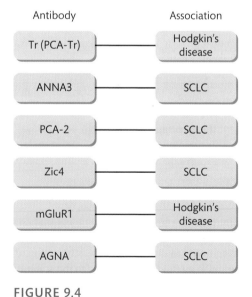

FIGURE 9.4
Partially defined PNAs that have been reported in a limited number of patients and often by a single group of workers. SCLC, small-cell lung cancer.

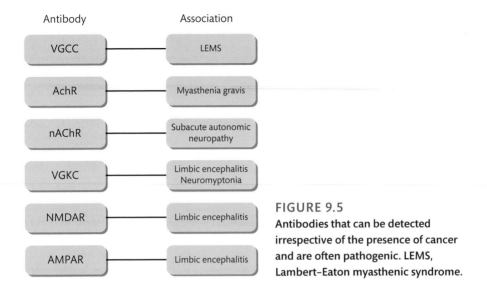

FIGURE 9.5
Antibodies that can be detected irrespective of the presence of cancer and are often pathogenic. LEMS, Lambert–Eaton myasthenic syndrome.

Looking at Table 9.4a, we see that PNAs can assist in 'a definitive' diagnosis of PNS if:

- the patient has a neurological disorder, does not have cancer, but is harbouring a well-characterized antibody
- the patient with nonclassical PNS is harbouring any PNA and develops a cancer within 5 years of diagnosis of the neurological disorder.

Looking at Table 9.4b, we see that a 'probable' diagnosis of PNS can be made if:

- a patient has a neurological disorder, does not have cancer, but is harbouring a partially characterized antibody.

The downside is that the guidelines do not address the issue of consensus on nomenclature for naming these antibody specificities, so most of the antibodies still have two names. One naming system uses two letters from the name of the original patients in whom the respective antibodies were identified; the other, which should have superseded the former, is based on the nature or cellular location of the antigen recognized.

TABLE 9.4 Diagnosis of PNS

Syndrome	Antibody	Cancer
A. Diagnosis of 'definite PNS' using a combination of clinical syndrome and the presence of PNA		
Neurological syndrome	Characterized	No
Nonclassic[a]	Any PNA	Develops within 5 years
B. Diagnosis of 'possible PNS' using the presence of partially characterized PNA and clinical syndrome		
Neurological syndrome	Partially characterized	No

[a] A nonclassic neurological syndrome is one that is loosely associated with cancer.

9.5 **Well-characterized antibodies**

The well-characterized antibodies have a recognizable immunocytochemical pattern resulting from reaction with a known recombinant protein (onconeuronal antigens) and are widely associated with malignancy and a well-defined neurological syndrome (Graus *et al.* 2004). The most efficient way to diagnose PNS is to identify one of the PNA in this category as they have a high specificity (>90%) for PNS. Anti-neuronal antibodies belonging to this category include (in descending order of occurrence):

ANNA-1 (Hu) > PCA-1 (Yo) > CRMP-5/CV-2 > (ANNA-2, Ri) > Ma2 (Ta) > amphiphysin.

These will now be described briefly.

Anti-neuronal nuclear antibody type 1 (ANNA-1, Hu)

ANNA-1, also known as Hu antibody, is the most commonly occurring and widely investigated PNA. The antigen associated with this antibody is HuD (Shams'ili *et al.* 2003), which consists of a family of neuronal nuclear proteins (HuD, HuC/ple21, Hel-N1, Hel-N2) that differ by alternative splicing of their mRNAs. It is an intranuclear RNA-binding antigen with three

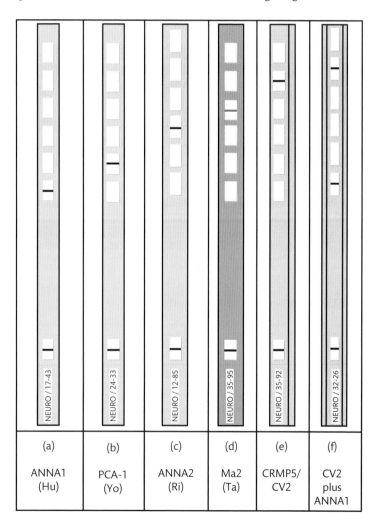

FIGURE 9.6

Strip coated with specific paraneoplastic antigens from the top down: amphiphysin, CRMP-5/CV-2, Ma2, ANNA-2, PCA-1, and ANNA-1, incubated with serum to confirm specificity against ANNA-1 (a); PCA-1 (b); ANNA-2 (c); Ma2 (d); and CRMP-5/CV-2 (e); an example of specificity of ANNA-1 coexisting with CRMP-5/CV-2 antibodies (f).

RNA recognition motifs. The expression of this antigen is normally restricted to the central and peripheral neurons and is thought to regulate the cell cycle, specifically in early neuronal development and maintenance. In addition to its expression in neuronal tissue, HuD is also expressed in the patient's own tumour and in SCLC of other patients, neuroblastomas, sarcomas, and prostate carcinomas (Dalmau and Posner 1999). However, the precise function of the protein both in its native location and in tumours is unknown.

ANNA-1 is usually present both in the cerebrospinal fluid and in serum in high titres, but low titres have also been found. However, any correlation between the antibody titre and the severity of the symptoms is uncertain. ANNA-1 antibody reacts with neuronal proteins of molecular weight 35–40 kDa (Figure 9.6a) and when tested immunocytochemically on primate cerebellar cryosections the staining is particularly prominent in the Purkinje cells (Figure 9.7c). ANNA-1 stains the nuclei of both central and peripheral system neurons (Figure 9.7a, b) with weak staining of the cytoplasm, and is absent in the nuclei of glial, endothelial, and non-neuronal cells. During detection and identification, it is important to differentiate it from other anti-nuclear antibodies, as these can have a similar distribution pattern to ANNA-1 (Karim et al. 2005).

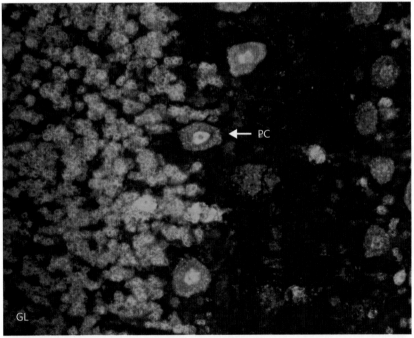

(a) ANNAI on cerebellum

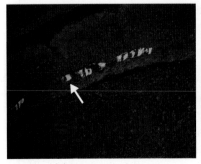

(b) Myenteric plexus

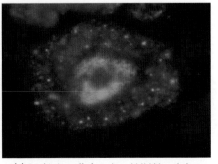

(c) Purkinje cell showing ANNAI staining

FIGURE 9.7
ANNA-1 antibody reactivity on primate cerebellum showing in (a): nuclear and cytoplasmic staining of all central (granular layer (GL) and Purkinje cells (PC)); and in (b) peripheral neurons (of the stomach (arrow)). The predominantly nuclear staining of the Purkinje cell (PC) is more clearly visible at the higher magnification (c).

In a series of 200 patients, the occurrence of ANNA-1 antibodies was more common in males and had a median age of onset around 62 years. In patients with PEM and ANNA-1 antibody, more than 85% had lung cancer (of which 77% were SCLC). The predominant neurological disorders were sensory neuronopathy (54%), cerebellar ataxia (10%), and limbic encephalitis (9%). Low titres of anti-ANNA-1 are found in 16% of SCLC patients who do not have neurological symptoms (Graus *et al*. 2001).

The prognosis for patients harbouring this antibody is very poor, with no improvement of neurological function after treatment of the cancer, but the symptoms are stabilized and further progression limited. Death occurs from PEM (60%) and tumour-related complications (40%).

Other ANNA-1-associated tumours include neuroblastoma, prostate tumours, rhabdosarcoma, seminoma, and adenocarcinoma of the gallbladder. The tumour may only become clinically apparent many months after the onset of the neurological conditions.

Purkinje cell antibody 1 (PCA-1, Yo)

PCA-1 antibody recognizes three types of Yo proteins, also known as cerebellar degeneration-related proteins: CDR34, CDR62 (CDR1), and CDR62 (CDR2), which are 34-, 52-, and 62-kDa proteins, respectively (Dalmau and Posner 1999). These antigens are the second most common onconeuronal antigens to have been reported and are highly expressed in the cerebellar Purkinje cell cytoplasm, testis, and some neuroectodermal cell lineages. CDR2 onconeuronal antigens are also expressed in tumours (such as ovarian and breast cancers) of patients with the PCA-1 antibody.

CDR1 is a polypeptide of 223 amino acids containing 34 tandem repeats of 6 amino acids and a leucine zipper motif (Giometto *et al*. 1999). The polypeptide CDR2 has 510 amino acid residues with a leucine zipper domain. This is the major epitope for the antibody. The antigen is expressed in the cerebellum, brainstem, intestinal mucosa, SCLC, squamous-cell lung cancer, and secondary tumours of adenocarcinoma of the colon. CDR2, an intracellular antigen, binds to myc and can be expressed in cancers found in neurologically normal individuals (Roberts and Darnell 2004).

PCA-1 is a polyclonal complement-fixing antibody, restricted to the IgG1 subclass, which to date has not been found to coexist with any other PNA. On cerebellar cryosections, coarse granular staining in the cytoplasm of Purkinje cell neurones with sparing of the nucleus is observed (Figure 9.8) (Karim *et al*. 2007). Immunoelectron microscopy has shown the antibody binds to ribosomes, the granular endoplasmic reticulum and the Golgi complex vesicles of Purkinje cells. These antibodies only recognize the tumour of the patient harbouring the antibody. Western blot analysis usually shows bands at 34, 52, and 62 kDa. Injection of the antibody into mice has not shed any light on its function, except that it does not cause disease or disrupt the blood–brain barrier. Figure 9.6b shows an example of blot-confirming antigen recognized by anti-PCA1 antibody.

This antibody is more frequently detected in women (60–65 years of age); very few cases have been reported in men. Patients suffer from cerebellar ataxia leading to rapid and progressive deterioration of speech, nystagmus, impaired coordination, and ataxic gait, leaving them severely incapacitated within 3 months of diagnosis. Death occurs from the debilitating neurological condition in 30% and from tumour progression in over 50% of the patients.

The incidence of PCD is about 40% in PCA-1 patients and 80% of these are likely to be associated with treatable gynaecological, breast, or ovarian malignancies. On treatment, however,

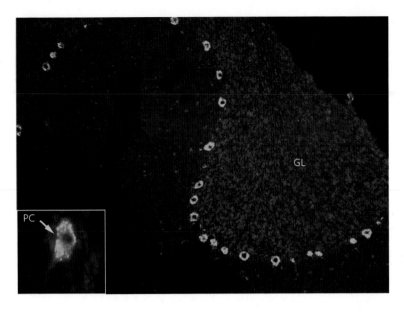

FIGURE 9.8
PCA-1 (Yo) staining on cerebellum can give an appearance of a 'pearl necklace' around the granular layer (GL) and is characterized by coarse speckling in the cytoplasm of Purkinje cells (PC, see insert).

there is no improvement in the neurological function and most patients remain neurologically disabled.

CRMP-5/CV-2

The molecular target of CRMP-5/CV-2 antibodies involves a family of proteins known as collapsin response-mediator brain proteins (molecular mass of 62–66 kDa), consisting of five cytosolic phosphoproteins (CRMP-1, CRMP-2, CRMP-3, CRMP-4, and CRMP-5). The dominant antigen is CRMP-5 and its specificity rests predominantly in the N-terminal epitopes; it exists as a tetramer in the adult brain and the gene responsible is located on human chromosome 2. CRMP-5 has a relatively low sequence homology with the other four members of the CRMP family but is expressed in the developing nervous system in a similar distribution pattern to that of CRMP-2.

In the adult rat, the immunocytochemical distribution of anti-CRMP-5/CV-2 antibody is restricted to the cytoplasm and processes of a subpopulation of oligodendrocytes in the white matter (Honnorat *et al.* 1996), where it recognizes a neuronal cytoplasmic antigen known as CRMP-5 (Yu *et al.* 2001).

Figure 9.9 shows the staining of anti-CRMP-5/CV-2. This type of staining is distinct from anti-ANNA-1 staining, which is confined to the neuronal nuclei, and when tested on cerebellar extract, a protein of molecular size 62–66 kDa is recognized. The anti-CRMP-5/CV-2 can coexist with other PNA such as ANNA-1 or anti-amphiphysin antibody. Figure 9.6e shows anti-CRMP-5/CV-2 alone, and you can see it coexisting with ANNA-1 in Figure 9.6f.

In the clinical setting, patients with this PNA tend to be male (70%), with an average age of about 62 years. This antibody is associated with peripheral neuropathy (47%), autonomic neuropathy (31%), cerebellar ataxia (26%), subacute dementia (25%), and disorders of the neuromuscular junction (12%). Patients with this antibody most frequently have SCLC (77%) and thymoma (6%). Other malignancies have been reported with CRMP-5/CV-2 reactivity. The mean survival time for the patients with SCLC and CRMP-5/CV-2 antibody is more than twice that of patients with the same tumour and similar symptoms but different PNA.

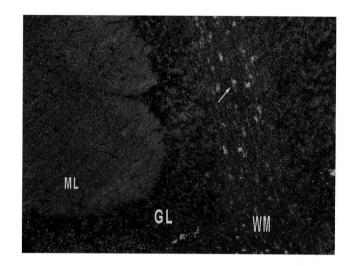

FIGURE 9.9

Anti-CRMP-5/CV-2 antibody is found localized in a subpopulation of oligodendrocytes in the cerebellar white matter (WM) with intense fine granular staining in the molecular layer (ML). GL, granular layer.

Antineuronal nuclear antibody type 2 (ANNA-2, Ri)

ANNA-2 antigens, also known as Ri, are highly conserved neuron-specific RNA-binding proteins encoded by the *Nova-1* and *Nova-2* genes. Nova-1 contains three RNA recognition motifs, which are homologous to the KH motifs of the hnRNP K protein. The third KH motif of Nova-1 is a target for the anti-ANNA-2 antibody; binding of the autoantibody results in inhibition of Nova-1 binding to RNA. An extensive study by Graus *et al.* (1993) revealed that all the areas of the central nervous system tested harboured the ANNA-2 antigen, with the exception of the gasserian ganglion, dorsal root, sympathetic ganglia, and the myenteric plexus. All nonneuronal tissue lacked the ANNA-2 antigen except for the pituitary gland.

ANNA-2 is a rare antibody and reacts with the target antigen in the nuclei and to a lesser extent in the cytoplasm of neurons of the central nervous system, with an immunocytochemical pattern resembling that of anti-ANNA-1. In contrast to ANNA-1, ANNA-2 does not react with the peripheral nervous system such as the myenteric neuron. On western blots of cerebellar extract, anti-ANNA2 IgG recognizes two bands with relative molecular weight 55 and 80 kDa. Anti-ANNA-2 antibody specificity can be confirmed by the recombinant protein; look at Figure 9.6c to see this. It is important to note that ANNA-2 can coexist with various other PNA such as ANNA-1, CRMP-5/CV-2, ANNA-3, and VGCC.

Clinically, the mean age of onset is around 65 years and 71% of the patients are smokers, presenting with a broad range of neurological signs and symptoms. Adult patients mostly harbour ANNA-2 antibody (Pittock *et al.* 2003) with neurological disorders affecting the brainstem (71%), cerebellum (50%), and peripheral nerves (25%). The predominant clinical features are ataxia and ocular movement disorders (opsoclonus–myoclonus). Opsoclonus can exist alone or with myoclonus, hence it is described as either paraneoplastic opsoclonus ataxia or paraneoplastic opsoclonus myoclonus ataxia. A higher incidence of this antibody is seen in women (ratio of 2:1) and underlying malignancy of breast carcinoma or SCLC is found in 75% of cases. Less frequent cases of ovarian, fallopian tube, bladder, and cervix cancer have been reported. The presence of antibodies has been reported in some cases of ovarian carcinomas without manifesting PNS. The detection of anti-ANNA-2 antibodies should prompt a careful search for an underlying tumour, especially breast cancer or SCLC. Occasionally a tumour may not be found, although the presence of an occult tumour cannot be ruled out, and this makes close follow-up advisable. Disability is severe: within a month of onset of neurological symptoms, 32% of patients are usually confined to a wheelchair (Pittock *et al.* 2003).

Ma2 (Ta)

The three Ma antigens were identified by probing cDNA libraries with patient sera; all three share significant sequence homology. Dalmau and Posner (1999) reported two onconeuronal proteins (Ma1 and Ma2, also known as Ma and Ta, respectively) associated with PNS. Like other paraneoplastic antigens, they are expressed in both tumours and immunoprivileged sites (neuronal tissue and testis). The distribution of Ma1 mRNA is highly restricted to the brain and testis. Ma1 is encoded on chromosome 14 and is a peptide of 330 amino acids and molecular weight 37 kDa, whereas Ma2 is encoded on chromosome 8, has a predicted molecular weight of 40 kDa (Figure 9.6d) and is expressed in the brain only (Rosenfeld *et al.* 2001). Ma2 displays a unique epitope(s) in that it is recognized by all patients' sera studied. The existence of a new family member, Ma3, has been reported in the literature (Rosenfeld *et al.* 2001). The gene for Ma3 is located on chromosome X and its mRNA is expressed in brain, testis, and several systemic tissues (kidney and trachea). The function of the Ma proteins is currently unknown (Dalmau and Posner 1999).

The predominant member of the Ma family is Ma2, an IgG polyclonal antibody found in the serum and cerebrospinal fluid of patients with paraneoplastic disorder, that reacts with nucleoli, but less so with the nucleus and cytoplasm of central nervous system neurones (Figure 9.10). There is no reactivity against glial cells. Ma1 reacts with both the brain and testicular germ cells, and Ma3 antibody reacts with systemic tissue as well.

In over 50% of patients with Ma reactivity, both Ma1 and Ma2 antibodies were present together and no evidence is available for the coexistence of any other PNA. Anti-Ma2 patients tend to be predominantly male (median age 23 years) with symptoms of short-term memory loss, seizures, confusion, excessive daytime sleepiness (32%), eye movement abnormalities (92%), and vertical gaze paralysis (60%), all of which develop from dysfunction of limbic, brainstem, or diencephalic system alone or in combination. Ataxia can be found in 38% of the Ma

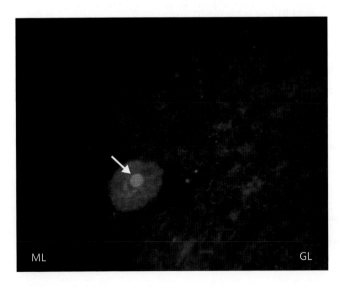

FIGURE 9.10

The nucleolus (arrow) of the Purkinje cell is predominantly stained with anti-Ma2 antibody. GL, granular layer; ML, molecular layer.

patients. Ma2-associated encephalitis is different from the classical PLE or brainstem encephalitis. Germ-cell tumours of the testis are found in 53% of such patients (Dalmau *et al.* 2004).

Immunity to Ma antigens appears unique, in that 50% of the patients with testicular cancer who respond well to treatment achieve complete remission of the tumour with accompanying improvement or stabilization in neurological deficit. As yet the reason for this is unclear.

In a study by Rosenfeld *et al.* (2001), Ma1 and Ma3 specificities were more common in older patients, who tended to develop a wider range of cerebellar symptoms with more intense dysfunction; a high proportion (82%) have non-germ-cell neoplasms, including lung (large-cell), parotid, breast, and colon.

CASE STUDY 9.1 *Ma antibody associated with mesothelioma*

SM was a 62-year-old man with a history of right-sided pleural effusion. He smoked 20 cigarettes a day, then changed habit to daily pipe smoking. He complained of double vision.

Neurological examination

Mostly normal except for:

- broad-based ataxic gait veering to both sides
- nystagmus on lateral gaze
- significant wasting of quadriceps
- no weakness or sensory symptoms

Laboratory and other investigations

All biochemical and immunological parameters were normal except for:

- iron, which was low
- immunoglobulin (IgG was 24.91 and IgA was 5.01 g/L)
- raised complement C3 (2.07)
- paraneoplastic neurological screen was positive for Ma2 antibody (look at Figure 9.10, which exemplifies the distribution seen on the cerebellum)
- Ma2 reactivity was confirmed on recombinant blot (look at the example given in Figure 9.6d)
- MRI of the head and spinal cord were normal
- pleural biopsy showed mesothelioma

Outcome

One year later, patient died.

Post-mortem examination

Tumour metastasized to lymph node with mediastinum, chest wall, right adrenal gland, and liver.

Of the three Ma antibodies (Ma1, Ma2, and Ma3), Ma2 antibody is more commonly identified and usually found in association with testicular tumour in younger men who frequently have limbic encephalitis but can be associated with other cancer in older patients. This is a rare antibody and about 50 cases have been reported around the world.

The case described in Case study 9.1 illustrates that although antibodies may have been initially described with one type of tumour and neurological syndrome (testicular cancer and limbic encephalitis), they may frequently be identified in other types of tumours and neurological signs (mesothelioma and cerebellar degeneration).

Amphiphysin

Amphiphysin, with its two isoforms, I and II, is a neuronal protein that is highly concentrated in the synaptic vesicles and has a molecular weight of 128 kDa. It plays a role in clathrin-mediated endocytosis and forms a dimer that binds to dynamin and synaptojanin through C-terminal Src-homoglogous (SH3) domains. It has been proposed to have a role in intracellular signalling and is essential for synaptic vesicle recycling in neurons. Amphiphysin is also expressed in certain types of endocrine cells (e.g. adrenal and pituitary), retina, and spermatocytes.

Anti-amphiphysin antibody is found in paraneoplastic stiff person syndrome (SPS) with malignancies of breast and lung (SCLC), as well as in patients with encephalomyelitis or sensory neuropathy, especially when the cancer involved is SCLC.

Serum positive for this antibody reacts with the neuropil of human and rodent frontal cortex, hippocampus, cerebellum, and spinal cord. In the cerebellum, there is intense, diffuse staining of the neuropil in cerebellar cortical molecular layer and intense granular staining in the periphery of perikarya and the granular cell layer, but little or no immunoreactivity in the Purkinje cell cytoplasm (Figure 9.11), nor any other neuronal cell body. This characteristic staining can easily be confused with anti-mitochondrial or anti-glutamic acid decarboxylase (GAD). In 74% of the patients, amphiphysin can coexist with other PNAs such as ANNA-1, CRMP-5/CV-2, and PCA-2, thus complicating the identification; therefore the specificity of the antibody may need to be confirmed by other methodologies, such as western blotting, which should reveal a protein of molecular size of around 128 kDa.

Neurological disorders accompanying amphiphysin reactivity are diverse; this may be due to the pathology associated with the presence other PNAs. The onset of symptoms is subacute, occurs around the age of 64 years, and leads to 40% of patients being confined to a wheelchair within 6 months. Symptoms include sensory neuropathy, encephalopathy, myelopathy (spinal cord involvements), cerebellar syndrome, and paraneoplastic SPS. With this antibody, paraneoplastic SPS is more common in women (39%) than men (12%).

A malignant neoplasm is found in 79% of the patients, the most common being SCLC and breast tumour. Other less frequent cancers, e.g. non-SCLC lung cancer and melanoma, have also been reported. Pittock et al. (2005) found that treatment had no significant effect on survival rate in patients with cancer.

Cross reference

A selection of typical and atypical immunofluorescence patterns seen on cerebellum can be found on the University of Birmingham clinical immunology website, http://www.ii.bham.ac.uk/clinicalimmunology/Neuroimmunology/

Key Point

Certain PNAs have well-characterized antigens, with Hu (ANNA1), Yo (PCA1), and CRMP-5/CV-2 antibodies being the most commonly detected.

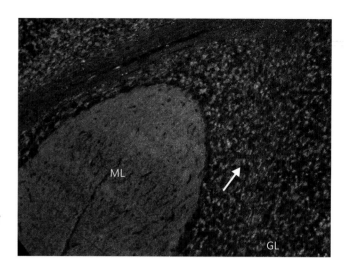

FIGURE 9.11
On cerebellum amphiphysin antibody reacts intensely with the neuropils in the granular layer (GL) but not with the granular cells, which are visible as seen as 'black holes' (arrow). The molecular layer (ML) is often uniformly stained.

9.6 Partially characterized antibodies

The partially characterized PNA lack clearly identified target antigen and are often reported by either a single group of investigators and/or in a few patients. The most frequent of the PNAs are:

PCA-Tr (Tr) > ANNA-3 > PCA2 > Zic4 > mGluR1.

PCA-Tr (Tr)

Tr antigen is found in the cytoplasm of central neurons, and to date no common bands have been identified on western blots, but it is widely expressed in the developing rodent brain. Abolition of the anti-Tr immunoreactivity by preincubation of the tissue with pepsin suggests that the antigen is a protein. The inability to detect common proteins on western blots may not be due to a low concentration of the antigen but to the antibody being directed against conformational epitopes which may have become modified during preparation (Graus *et al.* 1997).

IgG1 and IgG3 are the major subclasses of anti-Tr antibody found in the serum and cerebrospinal fluid of patient with Hodgkin's disease. In about 7% of patients, this antibody is only found in the cerebrospinal fluid. Immunohistochemically, the staining pattern on the cerebellum resembles PCA-1 distribution. The fine speckled staining of the cytoplasm and proximal dendrites of Purkinje cells is, however, distinct from that of PCA-1 (Yo) (Figure 9.12). The identification of anti-Tr reactivity is strictly based on immunocytochemical criteria where the Purkinje cell cytoplasmic staining is combined with a characteristic punctuate (dots) staining in the molecular layer of the cerebellum (not seen with PCA-1 antibody), and is suggestive of immunoreactivity against dendritic spines of the Purkinje cells. The immunoreactivity is confined to central neurons and the antibody rarely stains the neoplasm. The specificity of the antibody cannot be confirmed due to unavailability of antigen/recombinant protein.

In the clinical setting anti-Tr reactivity is found predominantly in men, with mean age of onset around 61 years, and there is a tight correlation between acute onset of symptoms, usually PCD and Hodgkin's disease (Bernal *et al.* 2003). Clinical improvements are seen in 14% of

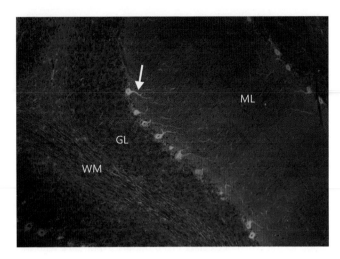

FIGURE 9.12

The Purkinje cell body and its dendrites (arrow) react with anti-PCA-Tr antibody. This fine-speckled (uniform) staining is distinct from that of the coarse speckles seen with PCA-1 (Yo). GL, granular layer; ML, molecular layer; WM, white matter.

younger patients after treatment of the disease and the antibodies are known to disappear spontaneously and also after successful treatment for Hodgkin's disease.

Anti-ANNA-3 antibody

This antibody is very rare, being described in only 11 patients with PNS, the majority of whom are afflicted with SCLC (Chan *et al.* 2001). Immunocytochemically, the staining of the cerebellum is distinct from that of ANNA-1 and ANNA-2, and the nucleoli are spared in all three. ANNA-3 staining is specifically nuclear. Purkinje cell nuclei are most prominently stained with much lower reactivity in the nuclei of molecular layer neurons. No staining is seen in the neurons of the granular layer or in the cytoplasm of other cerebellar neurons. Its unique reactivity is not only confined to the central nervous system antigen (molecular size 170 kDa) but also extends to the nuclei of the kidney podocytes (but not the cytoplasm). ANNA-3 has been reported to coexist with other PNAs (anti- CRMP-5/CV-2 (20%) and ANNA-1).

The precise function of the antibody is unclear, and the theory is that it can have an effective antitumour response through the activation of CD4+ helper T lymphocytes.

Because of the rarity of ANNA-3, information on its prognostic utility is quite limited. In addition to SCLC, it has been found in patients with adenocarcinoma, and it appears to be a specific marker for tobacco-related airway cancer.

The onset of symptoms in the adult is around 64 years, with approximately equal frequency in both genders. Like other PNA, ANNA-3 symptoms are also acute and diverse, usually multifocal and may include cerebellar ataxia, sensorimotor neuropathies, myelopathy, and brainstem and limbic encephalopathy.

Anti-Purkinje cell antibody type 2 (PCA-2)

Experience with this antibody is also limited and confined to only 10 patients. PCA-2 reacts in reticular fashion with cerebellar Purkinje cell cytoplasm and dendritic processes, together with the cytoplasm of dentate nucleus neurons (Vernino *et al.* 2000). In contrast to PCA-1 and

PCA-Tr, additional reactivity can be found in the nerves innervating the renal arterioles. The molecular size of both the tumour and cerebellar antigen is approximately 270 kDa.

PCA-2 can coexist with other neuronal autoantibodies, e.g. voltage-gated calcium channels, CRMP/CV-2, or acetylcholine receptor antibodies, and its function and pathological role is yet to be determined.

The onset of neurological symptoms is subacute and occurs predominantly in females (~2:1) around the age of 60 years. The underlying neoplasm is SCLC in 80% of patients who are mostly smokers and the presenting symptoms are limbic encephalitis (50%), cerebellar ataxia (30%), autonomic neuropathy (10%), and motor or sensory neuropathy (10%).

Anti-Zic4 antibody

Zic4 antibody is another addition to the panel of existing PNAs but the experience with this antibody is confined to one laboratory (Bataller *et al.* 2004). It has been identified in both the serum and the cerebrospinal fluid of patients with paraneoplastic neurological disorder and neoplasm of the lung (SCLC, 92%).

Zic proteins are thought to have an important role in the development of the nervous system. Mutations of Zic genes have been linked to cerebellar malformation, spina bifida, and/or sensorimotor gait.

Zic4 antibody can be screened on the brain, showing binding predominantly to the neuronal nuclei of the cerebellar granular layer and with less intense staining in other neurons, including Purkinje cells and brainstem. Detection of Zic4 may be complicated by its frequent coexistence with other onconeuronal antibodies (ANNA-1, ANNA-2, or CRMP-5/CV-2). On cerebellar western blots, Zic4 recognizes many proteins including a 37-kDa band, which is considered to be the Zic4 antigen. For definitive identification, confirmation by recombinant Zic4 should be utilized.

The onset of symptoms in Zic4 patients occurs at around 66 years. Only 18% of patients have Zic4 antibodies alone and these developed cerebellar syndrome (88% of males), increasing to 52% in the presence of coexisting SCLC-related PNAs (ANNA-1 and/or CRMP-5). As a result, 82% of these patients develop additional symptoms, including paraneoplastic encephalomyelitis. Paraneoplastic disorder was absent in 16% of the patients, despite harbouring a SCLC and Zic4 antibody.

Anti-metabotropic glutamate receptor 1 (mGluR1)

The antibody directed against metabotropic glutamate neurotransmitter receptors is believed to modulate excitatory synaptic transmission in the central nervous system and is thought to have a role in neural plasticity, learning, and memory function. Anti-mGLuR1 associated with paraneoplastic cerebellar ataxia recognizes a membrane neurotransmitter receptor of molecular weight 140 kDa, located on the dendritic spines of the Purkinje cell. Ataxia can be induced by blocking the mGluR1 receptor with anti-mGluR1 antibodies.

Anti-mGluR1 antibodies are IgG class that bind to the Purkinje cell bodies and dendritic spines, the latter staining appearing as intense punctate staining in the molecular layer.

These antibodies are found in Hodgkin's disease-associated cerebellar ataxia, often occurring during remission of the disease. The published data is reported in just two patients with anti-mGluR1 antibodies and PCD. Both subjects were female and after treatment one showed clinical improvement coupled with diminished serum antibodies, while the other was bedridden and showed no improvement in the ataxia despite being in complete remission (Sillevis Smitt *et al.* 2000).

Anti-glial nuclear antibody (AGNA)

Recently, a new antibody directed against the Bergmann glia of the Purkinje cell layer of cerebellum has been described in patients with PNS (usually LEMS) associated with SCLC (Graus *et al.* 2005). Screening for the candidate antigen using a fetal brain library showed the target to be SOX-1 protein (Sabater *et al.* 2008). SOX (Sry-like high-mobility group box) proteins are DNA-binding transcriptional factors with more than 20 proteins identified. SOX-1 and SOX-2 have an important role in neurogenesis and are both thought to be targets for AGNA, with higher positivity seen against SOX-1. Immunohistochemistry or immunofluorescence using rat cerebellum shows characteristic staining of the nuclei of Bergmann glia, which is a very useful screening tool. Currently, checking antibody specificity against SOX-1 or SOX-2 are performed mainly on a research basis in selected laboratories.

Key Point

More and more new antibodies and their clinical associations are being recognized.

9.7 **Antibodies with or without cancer**

The remainder of the chapter will deliberate on some syndromes in which the immune attack is directed against surface antigens, i.e. where the autoantibodies are believed to be pathogenic. This group of antibodies includes disorders which may also be of nonparaneoplastic or paraneoplastic origin (cancer-associated) and involves the peripheral nervous system (chiefly, neuromuscular transmission).

Neuromuscular transmission

Messages are transmitted by the brain to the muscles as electric signals (nerve impulses), which arrive at the junction of the nerve terminal and the muscle (neuromuscular junction, NMJ) and are converted into chemical signals for transmission across the gap (synaptic gap). At the NMJ, there are several transmembrane proteins vulnerable to antibody-mediated autoimmune attack. Of interest are four proteins, two of which are located on the presynaptic motor nerve terminal: the voltage-gated calcium channels (VGCC) and the voltage-gated potassium channels (VGKC). The other two are the acetylcholine receptor and the muscle-specific kinase (MuSK), which are present on the postjunctional folds of the muscle. Briefly, the electrical impulse opens the VGCC to allow influx of extracellular calcium into the nerve terminal. The increase in intracellular calcium triggers the release of a neurotransmitter (acetylcholine, ACh) into the synaptic gap, activating the muscle membrane and prompting the opening of the sodium and potassium channels. The movement of the ions that follows creates an electrochemical gradient across the plasma membrane (more sodium moves in than potassium out), producing a local depolarization of the motor endplate, known as an endplate potential, which spreads across the surface of the muscle fibres, thus initiating muscle contraction.

Transmembrane targets

These four transmembrane proteins located at the NMJ have been direct targets for autoimmune attack by pathogenic autoantibodies causing peripheral nervous system disorders. They include antibodies to P/Q-type VGCC in patients with LEMS, muscle acetylcholine receptor (AChR) or MuSK in patients with MG, VGKC in some patients with peripheral nerve hyperexcitability (neuromyotonia), and ganglionic acetylcholine receptor in some patients with autonomic neuropathy.

Voltage-gated calcium channel (VGCC) antibody

VGCC is a transmembrane protein, a pore-forming moiety that is exposed to the surface, divided into at least five categories (L, N, P/Q, R, and T) based on electrophysiological and pharmacological properties of its α_1 subunit. The P/Q type VGCC is highly expressed in the cerebellum and is sensitive to conotoxin, a neurotoxin from the marine cone snail. The P/Q-type channels are the most frequent targets in autoimmune LEMS and the associated antibodies (anti-VGCC) have been shown to reduce acetylcholine release when injected into animals. It is this process that is involved in the pathology of LEMS.

Anti-(P/Q)-VGCC antibody is associated with LEMS, most commonly in patients with SCLC (60%), although less common cancers have also been reported. There is a very high correlation between anti-VGCC antibody and LEMS (91%). LEMS is a disorder of neuromuscular transmission characterized by weakness of proximal muscle, depressed tendon reflexes, post-tetanic potentiation, and autonomic changes (Vedeler *et al.* 2006). Initially, the aetiology resembles MG, although the course of the two diseases is distinct.

In the paraneoplastic form, almost all patients with LEMS and SCLC have VGCC antibody usually against type P/Q channels. They also develop neurological signs and symptoms indicative of cerebellar involvement, together with clinical features of LEMS.

METHOD 9.2 Anti-VGCC and anti-VGKC measured by radioimmunoassay

Measuring antibodies to VGCC

Immunoprecipitation is a quantitative method that uses antigen–antibody reaction complexes to identify proteins that react specifically with an antibody in mixtures of proteins.

Briefly, a radiolabelled synthetic peptide, ω-conotoxin MVIIC (which has a high affinity for the P/Q subunit), is used to label the solubilized P/Q type VGCC extracted from cerebellum. This indirectly radiolabelled P/Q-VGCC is incubated with the test serum and will form a complex with the anti-VGCC IgG. The radioactivity in the precipitated complex is proportional to the concentration of the antibody.

Measuring antibodies to VGKC

Essentially the principal is the same as VGCC except that the protein extract comes from the cerebral cortex and the high-affinity radioligand is α-dendrotoxin. This assay measures antibodies to VGKC subtypes KV1.1, 1.2, and 1.6.

Voltage-gated potassium channel (VGKC) antibody

VGKC is also a transmembrane protein. Its α subunit forms the actual channels specific for potassium movement and has a crucial role in returning the depolarized cell to a resting state. VGKC belongs to the Shaker (drosophila-carrying mutant gene for VGKC) family of potassium channels. The three important isotypes of the α subunit (KV1.1, KV1.2, and KV1.6) present in both the central nervous system and the peripheral nervous system have very high affinity for the neurotoxin (α-dendrotoxin) found in the venom of the green mamba snake. It is this property of the α subunit that is utilized for measuring anti-VGKC antibodies.

Anti-VGKC antibodies were originally tested on rat cerebellum, where they stained molecular layer but not Purkinje cells. Reactivity was also found in the neurons of the hippocampus. A variety of antibodies can coexist with VGKC antibody, both neuronal (24%) and non-neuronal (49%), including anti-GAD65 (16%) and VGCC (10%) Routinely, these antibodies are measured using radioimmunoassay and have been detected in the serum of patients with neuromyotonia. Neuromyotonia is the most common form of peripheral nerve hyperexcitability, caused by autoantibodies to VGKC, resulting in an increase in the release of acetylcholine into the synaptic cleft and thus prolonging the action potential.

The onset of symptoms is either acute or subacute, affecting both genders with equal frequencies, and occurs at a median age of 65 years. Broad spectra of other neurological symptoms and neoplasms have been reported with VGKC autoimmunity. The neurological complications are multifocal, with a majority (75%) associated with cerebral cortex involvement (cognitive impairment in 71%, seizures in 58%, and hallucinations in 10%). Additional symptoms of coexisting autoimmunity can also be observed, such as diabetes mellitus (VGKC and anti-GAD65) and MG (VGKC and acetylcholine receptor antibody).

A neoplasm is found in 47% of the patients with anti-VGKC antibody, of whom the majority are smokers (Tan *et al* 2008). A variety of carcinomas are concurrently found with VGKC antibody including SCLC (7%), thymoma (6%), prostate adenocarcinoma (6%), and adenoma (7%).

Acetylcholine receptor (AChR) antibody

The acetylcholine receptor (AChR), an integral transmembrane protein, is classified according to its pharmacological property of relative affinity and sensitivity to nicotine and muscarine. Depending on the pharmacological response to these drugs, the receptors can be designated as either nicotinic or muscarinic. Antibody against the nictonic receptor causes the loss of receptor function and/or receptor density and leads to MG. When injected into an animal model these high-affinity antibodies tend to produce many of the symptoms seen with MG and are therefore considered to have a pathogenic role.

Approximately 15% of MG patients are seronegative for antibody but harbour instead antibodies to MuSK, which is found in and is required for the development of the NMJ. This antibody is present in about 70% AChR-seronegative patients (5–8% of all generalized MG patients). MuSK antibodies tend to be of the IgG4 subclass and do not cause complement-mediated loss of AChR, so it is not clear how the weakness is caused.

The AChR antibodies are IgG1 and IgG3 with high specificity, and confirm clinical suspicion of MG. Anti-AChR antibodies can be measured by either radioimmunoprecipitation assay or commercially available nonisotopic ELISA utilizing high-affinity α-bungarotoxin (snake venom from the banded krait *Bungarus multicinctus*). Recently, a new immunocytofluorescence assay has been developed to detect low affinity AChR antibodies in approximately 50% of previously 'seronegative' patients (5% of total MG) (Leite *et al.* 2008).

MG is a rare disorder but occurs in a bimodal distribution affecting predominantly young (less than 40 years) women (F:M ratio is 7:3) or older men (Juel *et al.* 2007). Anti-AChR antibodies are found in 80% of patients with generalized MG and 55% of those affected with ocular MG. Approximately 10% of the patients with MG have tumour of the thymus gland (Vincent 2008), which upon resection leads to clinical improvement.

NMDAR antibodies

Anti-*N*-methyl-D-aspartate receptor (NMDAR) antibodies have been recently described in patients with limbic encephalitis with prominent psychiatric presentation, with involuntary movements, autonomic symptoms, and respiratory depression (Dalmau *et al.* 2008). This syndrome has been initially described exclusively in young women with ovarian teratoma, but the spectrum is expanding, with non-neoplastic cases and men being increasingly described. Antibodies react to cell surface of nonpermeabilized hippocampal neurons. Immunocytofluorescence using HEK293 cells expressing the NR1/NR2B heteromers has been used in some centres as a diagnostic assay.

AMPAR antibodies

Antibodies to AMPAR (α-amino-3-hydroxy-5-methyl-4-isoxazolepropionic acid receptor), a glutamate receptor, have been described in a few patients with VGKC-negative limbic encephalitis, most whom had an underlying malignancy. Antibodies reacting against neuronal cell surface antigens were found to be reacting against the GluR1 and GluR2 subunits of AMPAR by immunoprecipitation. As in the NMDAR assay, HEK293 cells expressing GluR1/GluR2 receptors have been used for diagnostic testing of these antibodies in the sera or CSF (Lai *et al.* 2009). These antibodies are thought to reduce the GluR2-AMPAR clustering at the synapse, thereby causing the neurological syndrome. Presence of this antibody should lead to a hunt for any underlying neoplasm, most commonly lung, breast, or thymus.

9.8 Treatment of paraneoplastic syndromes

Treatment and management of PNS is tailored to individual needs as determined by clinical and paraclinical investigations confirming subtypes of PNS, presence or absence of tumour, detection and type of PNA. These factors will determine the course of the disease, which varies from patient to patient. PNS is considered as an autoimmune disorder; therefore it is only logical to consider immunomodulatory therapies such as steroids, plasma exchange, or intravenous immunoglobulin (IVIG), for these patients. Such intervention has been of little or no value in some subtypes of PNS, e.g. PLE, SSN, and PCD, where there has been irreversible neurological damage. Generally, early detection and treatment of the underlying tumour is by far the best current approach for stabilizing neurological symptoms and curtailing further permanent neurological damage. Symptomatic therapy should be provided in an attempt to improve the patient's quality of life.

Immunotherapy has been beneficial in patients with functional abnormalities, such as MG, LEMS, and PNH, where improvement has been seen, and may be of some benefit to children with POM but not adults. These recommendations were made by the European Federation of Neurological Society (EFNS) task force (Vedeler *et al.* 2006).

9.9 **Miscellaneous antibodies**

Glutamic acid decarboxylase (GAD)

GAD enzyme converts glutamic acid to γ-aminobutyric acid (GABA), an inhibitory neurotransmitter in the brain and a putative paracrine hormone found in pancreatic islet cells. GAD exists as two isoforms (65 and 67 kDa), which share 64% sequence homology and are expressed in the central nervous system, pancreatic islet cells, testis, oviduct, and ovary. GAD65 is a membrane-anchored protein responsible for vesicular GABA production. GAD67, on the other hand, is a cytoplasmic protein involved in the formation of cytoplasmic GABA. In the pancreas, GAD65 (found in β cells) is 200 times more abundant than GAD67 (α cells). Naturally, there are two anti-GAD antibodies, one involved in type 1 diabetes (GAD65) and the other associated with stiff person syndrome (GAD67).

Immunocytochemical detection of GAD67 antibodies utilizing cerebellum produces a characteristic staining pattern revealing peripheral GABA-ergic nerve terminals of the cerebellar glomeruli, which you can see in Figure 9.13a. GAD65 is best visualized on the pancreas, where it stains β cells (Figure 9.13b). These antibodies can also be detected by other methods (blot, ELISA, and radioimmunoassay).

Cross reference

Read Chapter 7 for more information on autoimmune type 1 diabetes.

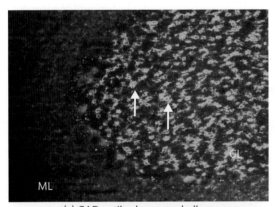

(a) GAD antibody on cerebellum

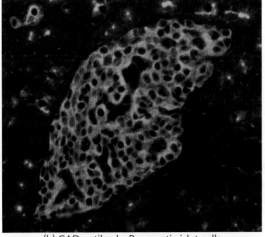

(b) GAD antibody: Pancreatic islet cells

FIGURE 9.13

Anti-GAD antibody showing reactivity in the granular layer (GL) of the cerebellum (a). Note the staining of the γ-aminobutyric acid nerve terminals (arrows), which is of a similar distribution to amphiphysin. Unlike amphiphysin there is no staining of the molecular layer (ML) with GAD antibody. Primate pancreas can express antigens for the GAD antibody in the cytoplasm of the β cells (b).

Very high titres of GAD antibody are usually found in patients with neurological disorders (82%, including SPS (36%), cerebellar ataxia (28%), and other CNS disorders (18%)). Interestingly, few cases of epilepsy in association with GAD antibodies exist. Patients with SPS and ataxia were predominantly women (over 86%) with a mean age of about 60 years, and half of them developed diabetes (Saiz *et al.* 2008). In a few cases, SPS and ataxia can coexist. Most patients have no underlying malignancy.

Four cases of paraneoplastic origin harbouring GAD antibodies have been reported without diabetes in men with a mean age of 67 years but with classical syndrome of LE, PEM, and PCD (Saiz *et al.* 2008). All four patients had underlying malignancy of the lung (SCLC and non-SCLC), pancreas, and thymus.

Anti-ganglioside antibodies (AGA)

Anti-ganglioside antibodies (AGA) are markers of immune-mediated neuropathies, and their target antigens (gangliosides) are located in the myelin sheath. Gangliosides share a common epitope and are compounds composed of a glycosphingolipid consisting of a hydrophobic ceramide and a hydrophilic oligosaccharide chain with one or more *N*-acetylneuraminic acid (sialiac acid) residues linked to the sugar chain. They are found widely distributed throughout the cell membrane, with the two hydrocarbon chains of the ceramide moiety embedded in the plasma membrane and the oligosaccharide on the extracellular surface. Gangliosides are abundant in the myelin sheath (Schwann cells of peripheral nervous system) and oligodendrocytes of the central nervous system. The fact that the onset often occurs after infections with *Campylobacter jejeuni*, cytomegalovirus, Epstein–Barr virus, *Mycoplasma pneumoniae*, or *Haemophilus influenzae* suggests that the pathogenesis may be due to antibodies against microbial ganglioside-like structures that may cross-react with gangliosides in the myelin sheath and induce inflammatory processes, thereby causing demyelination.

Measurements of clinically relevant AGAs (usually IgG and IgM) are widely available in many centres and include GM1, GM2, GD1a, GD1b, and GQ1b. See Table 9.5 for a detailed list. This range of antigens will capture almost all neuropathy-related antibodies. AGA are routinely measured by ELISA or screened by immunodot/line blots assay. In the latter case, quantification relies on visual examination of the colour of the dots or line, followed by classifying the reaction as negative, weak positive, or positive. With some commercial dot blots, a scanner and software is provided to assist with the interpretation, thus removing operator bias.

In the clinical setting, neuropathies (pain, numbness, paraesthesia, or weakness in the limbs) associated with AGA comprise acute inflammatory demyelinating polyneuropathy (AIDP), which can be subdivided into Guillain–Barré syndrome (GBS), acute motor axonal neuropathy (AMAN), and Miller–Fisher syndrome (MFS) (Figure 9.14).

GBS was first described in 1916 in two soldiers, as a potentially fatal disorder with rapidly progressive paralysis. GBS is an acute, predominantly motor, neuropathy that may be precipitated by infection and follows a monophasic course. GBS occurs at a frequency of 1 to 2 per 100 000 with a slight male predominance, and in a third of the patients AGA can also be found. Several clinical subtypes of GBS can exist:

- In **acute motor axonal neuropathy (AMAN)**, neurological deficit is entirely confined to motor neurons, often leading to respiratory failure but with normal sensation. The disease may be seasonal (summer epidemics), due to outbreaks of bacterial enteritis contaminating water supplies.

TABLE 9.5 Neuropathies associated with anti-ganglioside antibodies and their cross-reactions with other ganglioside due to shared epitopes. These antibodies are often associated with neuropathies but not always detected

Neuropathies	Class	Ganglioside	Other antigens with shared epitope
Acute motor axonal neuropathy (GBS)	IgG	GM1	GD1b
Multifocal motor neuropathy	IgM	GM1	
Chronic inflammatory demyelinating polyneuropathy	IgM	GM2	–
Acute motor neuropathy	IgM	GD1a	GM1, GM2, GT1a, GT1b
Acute ataxic sensory neuropathy	IgG	GD1b	GT1b, GQ1b
Chronic ataxic sensory neuropathy	IgM		
Miller–Fisher syndrome	IgG	GQ1b	GT1a, GD1b

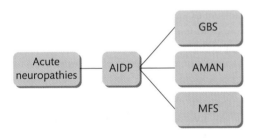

FIGURE 9.14

Antiganglioside antibodies can be associated with acute inflammatory demyelinating polyneuropathy (AIDP), which can be subdivided into Guillain–Barré syndrome (GBS), acute motor axonal neuropathy (AMAN), and Miller–Fisher syndrome (MFS).

- **Acute motor sensory axonal neuropathy (AMSAN)**, a subtype of AMAN where both the motor and sensory fibres involved cause severe axonal damage. Like AMAN, it is likely due to an autoimmune response against the axoplasm of peripheral nerves. Recovery is slow and often incomplete. AIDP, AMAN, and AMSAN usually affect all four limbs and can involve cranial nerves and respiration.

- **Miller–Fisher syndrome (MFS)** is a rare variant of GBS and was described in 1956 as an acute triad of ophthalmoplegia (paralysis of the extraocular muscles due to cranial nerve involvement), ataxia, and areflexia (absence of reflexes).

Treatment of GBS consists of good intensive care, recognizing respiratory failure and providing respiratory support as and when required. Plasma exchange and IVIG have proved equally effective.

Myelin-associated glycoprotein (MAG) antibodies

MAG, a glycoprotein component of myelin of both the central nervous system and the peripheral nervous system, has a similar epitope to that found on other glycolipids such as

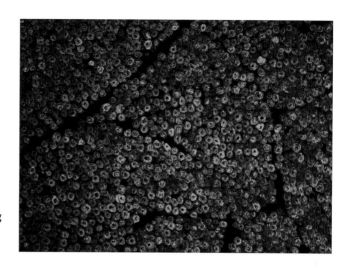

FIGURE 9.15
Transverse section of primate sciatic nerve axons showing staining of the inner and outer myelin sheath with IgM anti-myelin-associated glycoprotein antibody.

sulphated glucuronyl lactosaminyl paragloboside and sulphated 3-glucuronyl paragloboside. This glycoprotein, an integral membrane protein of molecular size 100 kDa, can be found in oligodendrocytes and Schwann cells. It is located in the periaxonal region of the myelin and may function in cell interactions and myelination.

High titres of anti-MAG antibodies are found in 50% patients with IgM paraproteinaemic demyelinating neuropathy. The IgM antibodies are considered to be responsible for demyelination seen in neuropathy. This type of IgM paraproteinaemia can be associated with Waldenstrom's macroglobulinaemia and multiple myeloma. Anti-MAG paraproteins show cross-reactivity with gangliosides, such as GD1b, GT1b, GQ1b, and sulphatides. These antibodies tend to be IgMκ, and can be detected by immunofluorescence using peripheral nerve (Figure 9.15) or quantified by ELISA.

Cross reference

For further information on anti-MAG antibodies the reader is referred to a recent article by the European Federation of Neurological Societies (2006).

Clinically, the syndrome associated with MAG antibody is chronic senorimotor demyelinating neuropathy, often with tremor. Anti-MAG (IgM) antibodies are considered as pathogenic and therapeutic strategy is directed at reducing circulating antibodies by plasma exchange, inhibition by intravenous immunoglobulin infusion, or reduction of synthesis by steroid administration.

Aquaporin 4 (AQP4) or NMO antibody

Neuromyelitis optica (NMO), also known as Devic's disease, is an immune-mediated inflammatory demyelinating disorder affecting the optic nerve and spinal cord. In the initial stages of the disease, NMO resembles multiple sclerosis (MS) and since neither disorder has had a specific marker until recently, 30% of patients with NMO may be misdiagnosed as having MS. It is important to distinguish NMO from MS as the outcome of NMO is worse and the treatment of each condition is also different. With the recent discovery of a specific antibody marker, NMO-IgG, the issue has become less problematic.

The antigen for the anti-NMO antibody is a water channel protein known as aquaporin 4 (AQP4), found in both central nervous system and other tissue. It is an integral protein of the plasma membrane and is the predominant water channel in the central nervous system, with a pathological role in brain oedema.

Anti-AQP4 recognizes antigens present in the distal tubules of renal medulla and the basolateral membranes of epithelial cells in the deep gastric mucosa. In central nervous system tissue,

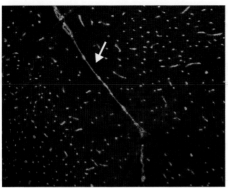

(a) Molecular layer: juxtaposed pial membrane and microvessels

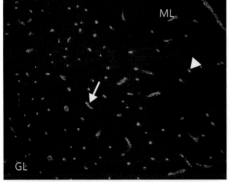

(b) Granular layer: microvessels

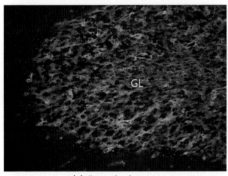

(c) Granular layer

FIGURE 9.16

Aquaporin 4 antibodies (AQP4) bind to the juxtaposed pial membrane of the cerebellum producing linear staining (a, arrow). The red colour in (b) is ethidium bromide staining the nucleus of the granular layer (GL) cells interlaced with microvessels (arrow) expressing the AQP4. Arrow head shows microvessels in the molecular layer (ML). Often the AQP4 sera can also be associated with other intense staining in the granular layer (c).

AQP4 binds predominantly to the juxtaposed pial membrane of the cerebellar cortex, producing a characteristic linear staining and also the microvessels of the white matter, the molecular, and granular layers (Figure 9.16).

AQP4 is found in 73% of patients with clinical NMO and in 46% of patients at high risk of developing NMO. Women with a median age of 41 years are predominantly affected (> 5:1). Clinical features of bilateral optic neuritis are present in 67% of patients, with 71% suffering from severe attack-related weakness. Within 5 years, there is loss of vision in at least one eye or an inability to walk independently. In 84% of the patients the brain MRI is different from that in MS. Immunological studies of the cerebrospinal fluid show that these patients do not usually have oligoclonal bands or abnormal levels of IgG.

Cross reference
For further information on anti-AQP4, the reader is referred to an article by Lennon *et al.* (2004).

Unlike MS patients, NMO patients derive benefit from plasmapheresis and immunosuppression, whereas in MS immunomodulation is currently the treatment of choice.

AQP4 is a welcome addition to the range of disease-specific markers and discriminates NMO from other optic neuritis, or myelitis, with high sensitivity (73%) and specificity (91%). With such specificity and sensitivity, the patient can benefit from early diagnosis and treatment. Furthermore, this can also provide valuable information on monitoring treatment and disease progression.

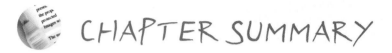

CHAPTER SUMMARY

- The immune-mediated processes involved in curtailment of a neoplasm are diverse and complex and have devastating effects on the nervous system.

- The discovery of highly specific anti-neuronal antibodies (an early diagnostic marker of PNS) may provide an invaluable adjunct for diagnosing PNS and alerting clinicians to search for an underlying tumour.

- Often, the specificity of the antibody can predict the likely location of the cancer.

- The association of these antibodies with rapidly deteriorating and devastating neurological symptoms that frequently lead to morbidity and mortality necessitates an early and rapid diagnosis followed by prompt treatment.

- There is then a greater chance of stabilizing the condition and preventing further neuronal cell death and permanent disability.

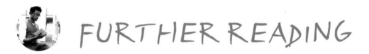

FURTHER READING

- European Federation of Neurological Societies/Peripheral Nerve Society (2006) Guideline on management of paraproteinemic demyelinating neuropathies. Report of a joint task force of the European Federation of Neurological Societies and the Peripheral Nerve Society. *J Peripher Nerv Syst*, **11**, 9–19.

- Karim AR, Hughes RC, Winer JB, Williams AC, Bradwell AR (2005). Paraneoplastic neurological antibodies: a laboratory experience. *Ann N Y Acad Sci*, **1050**, 274–285.

- Lennon VA, Wingerchuk DM, Kryzer TJ, *et al*. (2004) A serum autoantibody marker of neuromyelitis optica: distinction from multiple sclerosis. *Lancet*, **364**, 2106–2112.

- Meinck HM, Thompson PD (2002) Stiff man syndrome and related conditions. *Mov Disord*, **17**, 853–866.

- Moll JWB, Antoine JC, Brashear HR, *et al*. (1995) Guidelines on the detection of paraneoplastic anti-neuronal-specific antibodies: Report from the Workshop to the Fourth Meeting of the International Society of Neuro-Immunology on paraneoplastic neurological disease, held October 22–23, 1994, in Rotterdam, The Netherlands. *Neurology*, **45**, 1937–41.

ACKNOWLEDGEMENTS

I would like to express my gratitude to Dr J Winer (consultant neurologist), for comments and suggestion on the clinical section and Dr A Detta (principal research scientist) for critical review of the manuscript; both at Neuroscience Centre, University Hospitals of Birmingham NHS Foundation Trust.

 # DISCUSSION QUESTIONS

9.1   What evidence is there for the autoimmune basis of PNS?

9.2   Explain how a remote neoplasm can cause neurological deficit.

9.3   Explain how well-characterized paraneoplastic neurological antibodies can be used in the clinical setting.

9.4   What are the likely outcomes in patients with PNS?

Answers to these questions are provided in the book's Online Resource Centre; visit www. oxfordtextbooks.co.uk/orc/ahmed/

10

Flow cytometry and primary immunodeficiency

Learning Objectives

After studying this chapter you should be able to:

- describe a number of well-defined immunodeficiencies
- explain the clinical features of these immunodeficiencies
- outline the expected findings by flow cytometer
- discuss the limitations of flow cytometry in the diagnosis of immunodeficiency and other techniques available
- describe the current treatment options

Introduction

Our knowledge of the immune system has increased greatly over the past decade. The discovery of many new types of primary immunodeficiency and the study of these has played a huge part in unravelling the complexities of the immune system. This process is ongoing and it is difficult to keep up to date in this fast-moving field. Techniques for measuring the immune system and its function are relatively crude. Flow cytometry has proved to be a very useful tool for detecting abnormalities in the cells of the immune system. This chapter introduces some of the better-described primary immunodeficiencies in which flow cytometry plays a role in their diagnosis.

A healthy immune system has three main functions:

- to protect the body from infection and damage from foreign pathogens
- to protect against abnormalities of self that occur in malignancy
- to maintain tolerance of self, which depends on an intact immune system.

Immunodeficiency refers to defects in the immune system resulting in gaps in the body's defence against pathogens. This presents with recurrent, uncommonly severe or unusual

Immunodeficiency

Defects in the immune system resulting in gaps in the body's defence against pathogens.

TABLE 10.1 Examples of types of infections and associations with particular immunodeficiencies

Site of infection/clinical presentation	Type of infection	Possible immunodeficiency
Upper airways, sinus/chest, and ear infections	Bacterial infections: pneumococcus, *Staph aureus*/streptococci, and meningococcus	B-cell/antibody defects
Severe pneumonias, gut infections leading to diarrhoea, and failure to thrive. Unusual opportunistic infections	Viruses (CMV, VZV, adenovirus, molluscum contagiosum), fungi (candida, *Pneumocystis jirovecii*), and cryptosporidium	T-cell deficiencies
Recurrent pyogenic infections. Abscesses of skin and internal organs. Granulomatous	Bacterial infections: *Staph. aureus*, burkholderia. Invasive fungal infection, aspergillus	Neutrophil defect
Recurrent infections with the same type of pathogen	Neisseria	Complement
Invasive pneumococcal infection	*Streptococcus pneumoniae* or pneumococcus	IRAK4

infections. The type and site of infection will depend on which part of the immune system is defective. In many immunodeficiencies, autoimmunity and malignancy can also be seen. Primary immunodeficiency is present at birth and is caused by genetic mutations, which can be inherited, or that occur spontaneously. Other causes of immunodeficiency include side effects from therapeutic treatments such as certain drugs and radiation therapy.

Depending on severity, primary immunodeficiencies can present in the first few weeks of life, as in severe combined immunodeficiency (SCID), or they can manifest much later, presenting in adulthood, as in combined variable immunodeficiency (CVID). Immunodeficiency should be suspected if a patient has either recurrent or persistent infections, severe infections requiring hospital treatment, or unusual or so-called 'opportunist' infections not normally seen in the healthy population. Being involved in the investigation of a possible immunodeficiency is a chance to play detective. Factors such as type, site of infection, and age of onset all provide important clues. Knowledge of how the immune system deals with different types of pathogens will allow investigations to be targeted appropriately. For example, phagocytic cells clear extracellular pathogens, such as encapsulated bacteria. They do this by targeting organisms that have first been opsonized (coated) with complement and specific antibodies. To investigate a patient suffering from recurrent bacterial infections, it may be necessary to investigate the presence and function of the phagocytes, the specific antibodies, complement components, and the ability to opsonize the bacteria.

It is not within the scope of this book to give a complete list of primary immunodeficiencies. This chapter is an introduction to some well-described immunodeficiencies for which flow cytometry is useful in the diagnosis (Table 10.1). This is by no means a comprehensive list, and other texts should to be referred to.

10.1 **Lymphocyte subsets**

The availability of **monoclonal antibodies** has greatly increased our ability to study and define the cells of the immune system. When monoclonal antibodies started to be produced in increasing numbers an international nomenclature system was adopted. **Clusters of differentiation (CD)** numbers were allocated to define the specificities of the various clones. Antibodies specific for structures on the surface of cells can be used to define cell types, as in lymphocyte subsets, the stage of maturation, as in leukaemia typing, and also the status of the mature cell, i.e. naive or activated.

All cells in peripheral blood are derived from haematopoietic pluripotent stem cells, which are found in the bone marrow. White blood cells all play a role in the immune system and can be

Cross reference

Secondary or acquired immunodeficiency is caused by external factors such as viral infection; the classic example is HIV. This is discussed in Chapter 11.

Monoclonal antibodies

Antibodies produced from a single clone of cells, consisting of identical molecules.

Clusters of differentiation (CD)

Cell surface molecules on lymphocytes that are recognized by monoclonal antibodies to allow identification of the cell by flow cytometry.

Cross reference

You can read in more detail about white blood cells in the *Haematology* book of this series.

identified by light microscopy using differences in their size, shape of nucleus, and the presence or absence of granules in the cytoplasm.

There are three main populations of white blood cells found in peripheral blood:

- Neutrophils, eosinophils, and basophils have multiple or bilobed nucleus and granules in their cytoplasm and are collectively known as **granulocytes**.
- Monocytes and the smaller lymphocytes generally have a clear cytoplasm and a large single nucleus and are referred to collectively as **mononuclear cells**.
- **Lymphocytes** can be further broken down into three different subsets—T cells, B cells, and NK cells—which all appear similar when viewed by light microscopy. T cells can be further defined as helper T cells or cytotoxic T cells.

The identification and quantitation of the basic lymphocyte subsets by flow cytometry is an essential part of the diagnosis of many immunodeficiencies. Absent, decreased, or even increased populations of the various lymphocyte subsets can be useful in the diagnosis and monitoring of immunodeficiency.

By using a flow cytometer the size (forward scatter) and granularity (side scatter) of a cell can be determined, enabling differentiation of the white blood cells, but in addition the amount of fluorescence associated with the cell can also be detected. By using monoclonal antibodies conjugated to a fluorescent molecule and specific to different structures on the surface of lymphocytes, the various subsets can be identified. Different combinations of antibodies against various specificities can be combined. Antibodies are generally conjugated to a fluorescent molecule; if not, additional staining steps are required. If the antibodies are conjugated to different fluorochromes they can be used simultaneously, as flow cytometers have a number of detectors, to which light from different parts of the spectrum can be directed.

Granulocytes

White blood cells filled with granules some of which contain enzymes which enable digestion of microorganisms and production of inflammatory responses. Include neutrophils, eosinophils, and basophils.

Mononuclear cells

White blood cells with only one nucleus; includes monocytes and lymphocytes.

Lymphocytes

A type of white blood cell of which there are three subtypes: B cells, which give rise to humoral immunity, T cells, which give rise to cellular immunity, and Natural killer cells.

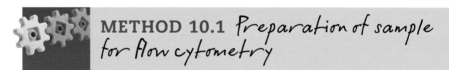

METHOD 10.1 *Preparation of sample for flow cytometry*

- To stain a sample, antibodies are mixed with whole blood and allowed to bind, usually at room temperature for 15 minutes (the time and temperature at which incubations should be carried out may differ—manufacturers' data sheets should always be referred to).

- A lysing solution (there are many commercial varieties available) is added to remove the red blood cells; again incubation times may vary.

- The sample may now require washing in phosphate-buffered saline to remove unbound antibodies and red cell debris.

- If the presence of a fluorescent antibody, and not cell size and granularity, is to be used to identify populations of cells, the sample may not require washing in phosphate-buffered saline to remove unbound antibodies and red cell debris. This will depend on local protocols and manufacturers' recommendations.

A number of tubes containing different antibody combinations may be required to identify all the populations of interest. This is generally referred to as a panel. The basic panel should enable a pure lymphocyte gate to be set (CD45 versus side scatter) and all major lymphocyte subsets to be identified. This can be seen in Figure 10.1. The inclusion of beads of known concentration into the tube will enable absolute counts to be calculated. This is now standard

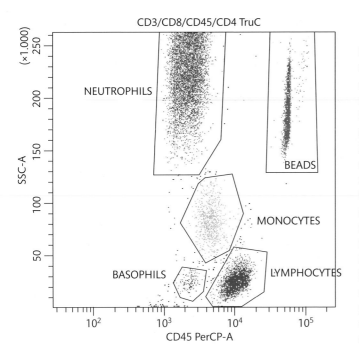

FIGURE 10.1

CD45 versus side-scatter lymphocyte gating. The plot shows an example of normal whole blood stained with an antibody to CD45, a pan white cell marker that is found at a higher density on lymphocytes than granulocytes. Red blood cells have been removed by lysis and the remaining cells run through a flow cytometer. The x-axis shows the amount of CD45 (the more CD45 antigen on the surface of the cell, the more fluorescent conjugated anti-CD45 antibody will bind and the greater the fluorescent signal detected by the flow cytometer). The y-axis denotes the amount of light the cells side scattered when they passed in front of the laser, and relates to the granules in a cell's cytoplasm. Neutrophils have a large number of granules in their cytoplasm and so have a high side-scatter signal. By plotting CD45 expression against granularity, four distinct populations appear. Beads are incorporated into the tube to enable an absolute count to be calculated.

practice in most clinical immunology laboratories. It allows an accurate measurement of the number of cells present in the sample using a single platform. Lymphocyte subsets are now routinely reported as both an absolute count (cells/µL) and as a percentage.

When constructing a panel for the first time it is essential to be aware of which markers are lineage-specific (e.g. CD3 is only expressed on T cells) and which are expressed on more than one cell type (e.g. CD4 is expressed on both helper T cells and monocytes). Table 10.2 shows which antibodies are used in the basic lymphocyte subset panel and which cell populations they can identify.

It is also important to consider the amount of antigen present on the cell. **Fluorochromes** differ in strength. For example, the number of molecules of phycoerythrin (PE) that need to be present on a cell before they can be seen above background is much less than for a weaker fluorochrome such as fluorescein isothiocyanate (FITC). The brightest fluorochrome should ideally be chosen for the weakest antigen.

> **Fluorochrome**
> A fluorescent chemical that emits a specific colour when illuminated by light.

SELF-CHECK 10.1

What antibodies would you use to identify cytotoxic T cells?

TABLE 10.2 Antibodies used in basic lymphocyte subset panel

Antibody specificity	Population identified in peripheral blood
CD3	T cells
CD19	B cells
CD16+CD56	NK cells (CD3 negative), CD16 also on neutrophils. CD56 is also on a subpopulation of T cells
CD4	Helper T cells (CD3+), also monocytes
CD8	Cytotoxic T cells (CD3+), also some NK cells
CD45	Panleukocyte marker
HLA-DR	B cells, monocytes, activated T cells

METHOD 10.2 *Quality assurance in flow cytometry*

Settings

It is important to ensure that the flow cytometer is correctly set up. It is possible to place a population anywhere on a plot by decreasing or increasing the power to a detector. Detectors are normally set using negative populations. There is also the problem of spectral overlap between the emission spectra of the various fluorescent molecules used. This will result in the signal being measured in more than one detector requiring that 'compensation' be applied to correct for this.

Instrument quality control

Various types of beads are used extensively to enable software to automatically set up suitable settings, including compensation, as well as to ensure that the flow cytometer is working optimally.

Samples

Cells are fairly labile and the age of samples and how they are stored can affect results. This may vary for different assays, but in general testing within 24 hours is preferable. Clots in samples will affect results, and adequate mixing of whole blood samples is essential if accurate absolute counts are required.

Once samples have been processed and stained they should be acquired on the flow cytometer as soon as possible or kept at 4 °C in the dark; this varies depending on the technique. Fluorochromes are sensitive to bright light.

Isotype controls

Each monoclonal antibody should bind only to its specific antigen. Structures on the surface of a cell may bind to the protein or fluorochrome. Antibodies with a specificity that should not be present in the assay can be used to determine any nonspecific binding. These antibodies should be of the same isotype (i.e. IgG1) and conjugated to the same fluorochrome as the primary antibody. Ideally, the isotype control should also be from the same manufacturer, as different companies use different protein levels.

There is some debate as to when isotype controls should be used. Where distinct stained and unstained populations are expected to be present, isotype controls are considered to be unnecessary. However, if weak staining is expected the use of an isotype control can be useful to set the cut-off between positive and negative. The behaviour of an isotype control cannot always be assumed to be exactly the same as the antibody of interest. Assays that require stimulation or other manipulation of the sample before staining may increase nonspecific staining by up-regulation of various receptors, and isotype controls may be helpful.

Lymphocyte subsets

The percentages of T, B, and NK cells found in a lymphocyte gate when added together, the so-called 'lymphosum', should be 100% ± 5%.

Where multiple tubes are set up in a panel on the same patient, any antigens measured more than once should be reproducible between tubes. Percentages would be expected to be within 3% and absolute counts within 10%.

CD4+ and CD8+ T cells when added together should be close to the CD3+ total.

Stabilized whole blood controls are available with target values, although these can be quite generous. These are whole-process controls, but as antibodies are used they can work out to be very expensive. There is no real consensus as to how often these should be run.

When measuring absolute counts using reference bead populations, accurate pipetting is critical. Processes should be in place to monitor the accuracy of pipettes and any automated sample preparation instruments used.

It can be useful to check lymphocyte counts against those obtained from a full blood count, as this will pick up any sample-specific pipetting errors such as small clots in the sample.

The next three sections of this chapter describe the three main types of lymphocytes. Knowledge of how cells develop, their functions, and interactions with other cells is critical to understanding the underlying defects that cause immunodeficiency. Possible causes of abnormal findings in the measurement of these different types of lymphocytes are also discussed.

Important factors in the interpretation of lymphocyte subsets

It is essential to interpret lymphocyte subset results in the context of age-related ranges. Children have much higher levels of lymphocytes than adults. What is a normal T cell result for an adult may be profoundly low for an infant.

When cells of a particular lymphocyte subset are absent, it is important to exclude the use of any treatments as being the cause. The use of monoclonal antibodies is becoming more common. Some, such as rituximab (anti-CD20 used in autoimmune diseases such as rheumatoid arthritis) target B cells. Other cytotoxic and immunosuppressive therapies can result in the depletion of various lymphocyte subsets.

Previous knowledge of the immune system, structure, and function is assumed in order to aid the understanding of this section. There are a number of good immunology texts that will support the following sections.

Cross reference

Suitable immunology textbooks include Janeway CA *et al.* (2001), Male *et al.* (2006), and Goldsby *et al.* (2003).

10.2 **T cells**

Development

T cells, like all cells found in peripheral blood, are derived from pluripotent haematopoietic stem cells, initially from fetal liver and subsequently from bone marrow. T cells differ from other blood cells in that they mature in the thymus. Stem cells seed the thymus, where they are provided with growth factors such as interleukin (IL)-7 and cell–cell interactions essential for development. Progenitor T cells first appear in the cortex of the thymus and do not express CD4 or CD8, and are therefore referred to as double negative (DN).

To fulfil their function, T and B cells require an immensely diverse repertoire of receptors enabling them to recognize all potential pathogens. Each mature T or B cell will have a unique receptor. Diversity is generated by DNA rearrangement of a relatively small set of germ-line genes: variable (V), joining (J), and in T-cell receptor (TCR) β and δ chains only, diversity (D)–VDJ. For example, when you throw one dice, you have the possibility of throwing six possible numbers. If you have two dice, this increases to 36. In TCR generation you have three dice (the V, D, and J genes). Although there is a relatively small number of each of these genes, by breaking them, resorting them randomly, and then rejoining them, a large number of different receptors can be generated. In addition, where these different segments join, nucleotides can be added or removed, increasing the diversity even more. This process is an adaptation of the normal DNA repair mechanisms, which exist to maintain the integrity of DNA when accidental damage from factors such as ionizing radiation occurs.

During this process several proteins have been shown to play a role. The products of the recombination-activating genes (RAG-1 and RAG-2) are important in initiating the break, but are not part of normal DNA repair. Other important factors such as Artemis, cernunnos, and DNA ligase IV also have a critical role in normal DNA repair.

Mature TCRs consist of two chains, either α and β or γ and δ. Some DN cells will remain DN and rearrange and express a γδ receptor. The majority of T cells rearrange the TCRβ chain first, which is then expressed on the surface as a pre-TCR complex in association with the CD3 molecule. If the gene rearrangement is unproductive this receptor will not be formed and the cell

Major histocompatibility complex

A group of genes that code for cell-surface histocompatibility antigens and are the principal determinants of tissue type and transplant compatibility.

Positive selection

The survival of a T cell through the TCR binding to MHC with weak affinity, ensuring T cells can recognize antigen in the context of self.

Negative selection

T-cell recognition of self-antigen in the thymus resulting in deletion by apoptosis.

Endocytosis

The process by which a cell ingests material with the formation of vesicles. Includes phagocytosis and pinocytosis.

will die from apoptosis. The TCR α chain gene rearrangement now occurs; cells express both CD4 and CD8, and are termed double positive (DP).

The likelihood of these rearrangements resulting in receptors recognizing self is high, so a process of selection now occurs during which more than 95% of thymocytes are eliminated. The survival of the T cell depends on interactions through the TCR. To survive, the TCR needs to bind with weak affinity to the **major histocompatibility complex (MHC)** expressed by thymic epithelial cells. No recognition results in cell death. This is referred to as **positive selection** and ensures T cells will recognize foreign antigen only in the context of self-MHC.

Cells that recognize self-antigens and therefore bind with high affinity are deleted by apoptosis. This is called **negative selection**. Ubiquitous self-antigens are presented mainly by dendritic cells. The autoimmune regulator (*AIRE*) gene activated in thymic epithelial cells enables organ-specific antigens to be expressed, which might otherwise not be presented to the immature T cells. Cells with TCR-recognizing MHC class I become CD8⁺ and those recognizing MHC class II become CD4⁺ T cells.

Function

Because of this selection process, T cells will only react with antigens in the context of MHC. This enables T cells to recognize antigens that originate from inside the cell. These antigens can be synthesized from within the cell, as in a viral infection, or taken up by **endocytosis** as occurs in antigen-presenting cells (APCs) such as macrophages, dendritic cells, and B cells. The antigens are processed and presented by MHC molecules, the binding sites of which hold the antigenic peptides and can therefore determine which part of the antigen is presented to the T cell. This may explain why MHC haplotype can affect susceptibility or resistance to autoimmunity and infection.

APCs are found mainly in the secondary lymphoid organs. Here, helper CD4⁺ T cells interact with the APCs, which provide costimulatory signals necessary for naive T cell activation. Using chemical messages such as cytokines or direct cell–cell contact, the activated CD4⁺ T cell sends a message back to the presenting cell. Interaction with a CD4⁺ T cell enables B cells to switch from their default of making IgM to other isotypes such as IgG, and macrophages to activate and destroy intercellular and extracellular antigens.

Cytotoxic CD8⁺ T cells with help from CD4⁺ T cells can secrete molecules capable of killing cells infected with virus. It is important therefore that MHC class I is expressed on most nucleated cells in the body, as a viral infection may occur anywhere.

Absent T cells

Severe combined immunodeficiency (SCID)

Complete absence of T cells can be seen in SCID. Even if B cells are present, their function is severely impaired in the absence of help from CD4⁺ T cells.

SCID is very rare, with an incidence of approximately 1 in 500 000, and is more common in boys than girls. Infants present within the first few months of life with poor growth, failure to thrive, and often a persistent low lymphocyte count. They have recurrent infections, often in the respiratory tract and gut, are unable to clear viruses, and are susceptible to opportunistic infections such as candida and pneumocystis pneumonia (PCP).

The diagnosis of SCID is a paediatric emergency. It is essential that the child be referred immediately to a specialist centre with facilities to provide a clean environment (free from pathogens).

TABLE 10.3 SCID classifications

Phenotype	Defect in	Mechanism	Inheritance
T⁻B⁻NK⁻	ADA (adenosine deaminase)	Premature cell death due to purine metabolism defect	AR
	Reticular dysgenesis, also low monocytes and neutrophils. Platelets and red blood cells are normal	? Adenylate kinase 2—important for cell survival	AR
T⁻B⁺NK⁻	Cytokine receptors are composed of 3 chains, α, β, and γ. In X-linked SCID the common γ chain (cγc) of the receptors for the cytokines IL-2, 4, 7, 9, 15, and 21 is absent.	IL-7 is required for T-cell development and survival, IL-15 is required for NK cell development	XL
	Janus kinase 3 (JAK3)	Kinase associated with cγc	AR
T⁻B⁺NK↓	CD45 (TCRγδ⁺)	CD45 important for TCR signalling	AR
	PNP (purine nucleoside phosphorylase)	Premature cell death due to purine metabolism defect	AR
T⁻B⁺NK⁺	α Chain of the receptor for the cytokine IL-7	IL-7 required for T-cell survival	AR
	The T-cell receptor is held within the CD3 molecule which is made up of:		
T⁻B⁺NK⁺ T↓B⁺NK⁺	δ ,ε chains ζ and γ (CD3 expression reduced, γδ T cells present)	Pre-TCR and TCR signalling required for survival	AR
T⁻B⁻NK⁺	RAG-1/2	Defective VDJ recombination required for both TCR and BCR (Ig)	AR
	Artemis (sensitive to ionizing radiation)	Artemis involved in VDJ recombination and DNA repair	

AR, autosomal recessive; XL, X-linked.

Live vaccines must not be given, e.g bacillus Calmette–Guérin (BCG), as this is a weakened but live form of the bacteria that cause tuberculosis and can become disseminated in the absence of functioning T cells. Blood products should be irradiated, as immunocompetent cells in the blood may cause graft versus host disease (GVHD). Blood products should also be cytomegalovirus (CMV)-negative as this could cause a fatal infection in an immunocompromised recipient. The prognosis in SCID is significantly worsened by any acquired infections.

There are many types of SCID (Table 10.3), and the phenotype reflects the type of defect. Many are inherited in an autosomal recessive manner (requiring an abnormal gene to be acquired from both parents), and consanguinity of parents should increase the index of suspicion for SCID.

Most SCID is T-cell negative; however, 'leaky' forms of SCID occur where high T cell numbers can be seen. An example of this is Omenn's syndrome (Clinical Correlation 10.2).

Key Point

Live vaccines such as BCG should never be given to patients suspected of having a primary immunodeficiency.

Another potential source of T cells in SCID is maternal fetal engraftment (MFE). In a normal fetus, T cells (which are absent in SCID) would destroy any maternal cells crossing the placenta. In SCID this does not occur and maternal T cells can survive and expand in the fetus. The presence of maternal T cells is considered to be one of the diagnostic criteria for SCID.

CLINICAL CORRELATIONS 10.2

Omenn's syndrome

Omenn's syndrome has been described in patients with mutations in RAG-1/2, artemis, and other defects associated with SCID. Clinically, it presents with often severe erythroderma (a general exfoliating dermatitis involving most of the patient's skin), and hepatosplenomegaly. Eosinophils can be increased, as can serum IgE levels. T cells can be greatly increased but are oligoclonal, highly activated, and do not proliferate in response to the mitogen phytohaemagglutinin (PHA).

CASE STUDY 10.1 Omenn's syndrome

Baby L was born at term to nonconsanguineous parents. She presented at 1 week old with a facial rash initially thought to be eczema, but that quickly developed into erythroderma. At 2 weeks she was admitted to hospital with rapid breathing that required oxygen. It was noted that she had a very high eosinophil count. The chest and skin improved with steroids and intravenous antibiotics. She was readmitted at 6 weeks with worsening chest and skin and generalized lymphadenopathy.

- ■ Her lymphocyte subsets were measured (see Figure 10.2).
- ■ T-cell proliferation to PHA was absent.
- ■ A diagnosis of Omenn's syndrome was made.

Key Point

The presence of T cells does not exclude a diagnosis of SCID.

The goal of treatment for SCID is for T- and B-cell function to be restored; this can be achieved by haematopoietic stem cell transplantation (HSCT). Success rates are good, especially if an HLA-matched sibling donor is available and the diagnosis was made prior to the acquisition of infections. For a limited number of SCID patients, such as those with defects in adenosine deaminase (ADA) or common γ chain (cγc), insertion of a corrected gene into the patient's own haematopoietic stem cells has been used to affect a cure. This is referred to as gene therapy but is only practicable if the genetic defect is well defined and discrete numbers of cells are affected. Ideally, cells expressing the transgene need to be long-lived and have a selective advantage so that they can outgrow affected cells.

Patients with SCID caused by adenosine deaminase (ADA) deficiency are often profoundly lymphopenic, but other cells are also affected. Skeletal, hepatic, renal, lung, and neurological abnormalities are also seen, in addition to the recurrent infections and failure to thrive caused by lack of lymphocytes. Lack of ADA causes a build-up of purine metabolites, which affects rapidly dividing cells such as lymphocytes. The defective enzyme (ADA) can be replaced conjugated to polyethylene glycol (PEG), which prolongs the half-life of the ADA by preventing

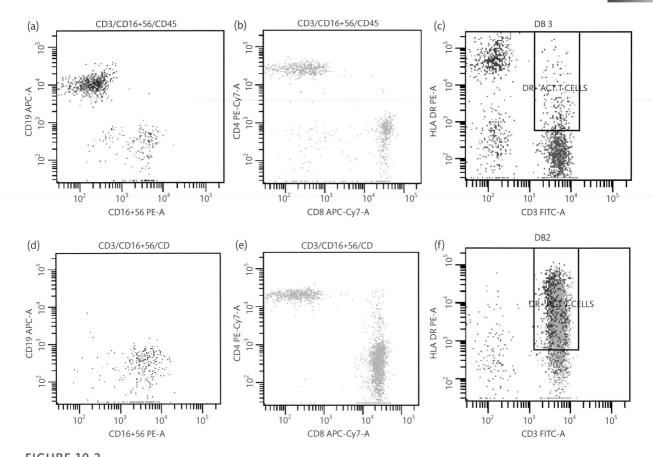

FIGURE 10.2

Omenn's syndrome. The top three plots show data from a normal child and the bottom three data for a patient with Omenn's. Plots (a) and (d) show data from CD3 positive lymphocytes. In (d) the B cell population is missing (CD19 positive). Plots (b) and (e) show CD3 positive lymphocytes; CD4 positive and CD8 positive T cells are present in both. Plots (c) and (f) show all lymphocytes. The percentage of T cells expressing HLA-DR in (f) is increased compared to the normal, and the HLA-DR positive, CD3 negative population (B cells) is missing.

it being excreted. This is often used only as a temporary measure to detoxify the metabolites, but does not usually enable lymphocyte numbers to recover.

Di George and CHARGE syndromes

Other conditions that can present with absent T cells include the Di George and CHARGE syndromes. Both, like most genetic diseases, have a broad spectrum, depending on multiple factors, including the specific mutation.

Di George syndrome is caused by a deletion in 22q11. This results in a number of defects including cardiac malformation, facial abnormalities, neonatal hypocalcaemia, and immunodeficiency. The immunodeficiency is caused by abnormalities in the thymus, which can lead to low T cell numbers; or, in the most severe form, the thymus may be absent. Unlike SCID there is no defect in the T cells, rather the absence of a thymus in which to develop. HSCT has been used to treat severe T-cell negative Di George, but with no thymus only peripheral expansion of the mature T cells given with the graft occurs. Recently, thymic transplants have been successful, and would now be the treatment of choice.

CHARGE syndromes consist of coloboma (abnormal eye development), heart defect, atresia choanae (closure of one or both nasal cavities), retarded growth and development, genital hypoplasia, and characteristic ear defects. It is due to mutations in *CHD7* and can result in severely reduced or absent T cells. There is some overlap with Di George syndrome, but the exact mechanism that causes complete absence of T cells is not yet known.

Low T cells

Low T cells can be seen in a number of immunodeficiencies. This can be further broken down into low CD4$^+$ T cells and low CD8$^+$ T cells. It is also important to take into consideration the ratio of CD4$^+$ T cells to CD8$^+$ T cells. A normal CD4:CD8 ratio is 1:5. Abnormal CD4:CD8 ratio may be an indication of maternal fetal engraftment (MFE), HIV infection, or leaky SCID. All of these will also have an increase in activation markers seen on the surface of the T cells.

Low CD4$^+$ T cells

When low CD4$^+$ T cells are seen, HIV should always be considered. In HIV the numbers of CD8$^+$ T cells are often increased, as are the percentages of T cells expressing activation markers such as HLA-DR.

Major histocompatibility complex (MHC) class II deficiency also results in low CD4$^+$ T cells. Class II is constitutively expressed on antigen-presenting cells such as B cells and monocytes. CD4$^+$ T cells only recognize antigen in the context of MHC class II and therefore cannot function normally. Measurements of T-cell proliferation in response to stimulation by mitogens such as PHA are normal, but responses to antigens are poor. Class II deficiency can be considered a form of SCID, and the presentation and treatment options are the same.

Low CD8$^+$ T cells

Very low numbers of CD8$^+$ T cells (often <50 cells/μL) are seen in ζ chain-associated protein (ZAP) 70 deficiency. ZAP 70 is a kinase associated with the ζ chain of the CD3 molecule and is essential for T-cell activation. Although T-cell proliferation to PHA is absent, normal proliferation can be achieved by bypassing the TCR/CD3 complex using phorbol myristate acetate (PMA) and ionomycin. PMA acts directly to activate protein kinase C (PKC), which is a key kinase downstream in the T-cell activation pathway of ZAP 70. Ionomycin is a calcium ionophore, which works in synergy with PKC. ZAP 70 can be considered a form of SCID and the treatment is the same.

Patients with absent or reduced expression of MHC class I (sometimes also class II), also referred to as bare lymphocyte syndrome, have reduced CD8$^+$ T cells. There is a wide spectrum of severity of disease; some present with severe infections within the first few months of life and others are completely asymptomatic.

Key Points

Absent T cells can lead to a straightforward diagnosis of SCID.

T cells, when present, should always be looked at closely, including CD4:CD8 ratio, numbers of cells, and the presence of activation markers. All of these are present in the basic panel described. Any abnormalities will provide clues as to what further investigations are required.

10.3 **B cells**

Development

Like T cells, B cells are also derived from pluripotent haematopoietic stem cells. Unlike T cells, B cells develop in the fetal liver before birth and in the bone marrow after birth.

Pro-B cells are the earliest cells committed to the B-cell lineage and express CD10 and CD19 on their surface. Surface immunoglobulin forms the receptor on a mature B cell, consisting of two light and two heavy chains associated with the Ig β and α subunits (these are responsible for intracellular signalling). The B-cell receptor undergoes the same process of VDJ recombination to generate a diverse repertoire as T cells. The immunoglobulin heavy chain (IgH) undergoes rearrangement first. RAG and terminal deoxynucleotidyl transferase (TdT) (involved in the addition of new nucleotides during the joining of the VDJ gene rearrangement) are highly expressed at this pro-B cell stage. Successful synthesis of the μ protein enables progression to pre-B cell. At this stage no light chains have been rearranged and so Igμ protein associates with surrogate light chains $λ_5$ and VpreB proteins. This, plus Igα and β, forms the pre-B cell receptor. This receptor appears to send a survival message once assembled—no binding of the receptor with a ligand is required. Various proteins are important in this signalling pathway including B-cell linker (BLNK) and Bruton's tyrosine kinase (Btk). This signal also inhibits IgH rearrangement of the other chromosome (allelic exclusion, when only one chromosome is used).

B cells have genes for two light chains, of which only one is required. The κ gene undergoes rearrangement first; if productive, this will inhibit rearrangement of the λ light chain. This is why there are more B cells expressing κ than λ on their surface. The light chain will then combine with μ protein to form IgM; this is expressed on the surface of the cell now called an immature B cell. B cells now also undergo a process of negative selection similar to T cells. Any immature B cells that are autoreactive have a chance of survival by undergoing a second gene rearrangement. If the receptor still reacts with self-antigens, the B cell is deleted. This process occurs independently of T cells. Mature B cells now exit the bone marrow, expressing IgM and IgD on their surface.

In the secondary lymphoid organs, B cells that recognize antigen and, with appropriate help from a CD4$^+$ T cell, will undergo **class switch recombination**, which leads to the production of antibody of various isotypes (ie IgG and IgA, rather than just IgM). A further process called **somatic hypermutation**, in which mutations are introduced into the variable region at a very high frequency, will further increase the affinity of the antibody.

Function

B cells recognize extracellular pathogens and, unlike T cells, recognize antigen in its native or only partly denatured state. To respond effectively to protein antigens, B cells require T cell help. Antigens with repeating segments such as polysaccharide and lipids can activate the B cells independently of T cells. Blood-borne antigens will come into contact with B cells mainly in the spleen. Antigens entering through skin and other epithelial surfaces contact B cells in draining lymph nodes where mature B cells migrate. B cells found in mucosal lymphoid tissue will come into contact with inhaled or ingested antigens and tend to produce IgA.

The main function of a B cell is the production of antibody. The B-cell receptor is the immunoglobulin molecule expressed on its surface. B cells express MHC class II and act as APCs, presenting antigen to CD4$^+$ T cells from which they require signals to class switch.

Class switch recombination
The process by which a B cell upon recognition of antigen will switch the production of immunoglobulin from IgM alone to other isotypes, e.g. IgG and IgA.

Somatic hypermutation
The introduction of mutations into the variable region of an antibody, to increase the antibody affinity.

Absent B cells

Key Point

SCID should always be considered in an infant with no B cells (MFE, Omenn's). The T-cell subsets and activation markers should be looked at more closely to determine if the T cells appear normal.

X-linked agammaglobulinaemia (XLA)

XLA occurs in 1 in 100 000 to 1 in 200 000 of the population. It is caused by mutations in Btk. Btk is found downstream of the pre-B cell receptor, which is required for survival and maturation.

Affected boys present early, from 4–6 months, after maternal antibodies start to decrease. They present with recurrent bacterial infections, small tonsils (absent germinal centres in the lymph nodes), and low immunoglobulins of all isotypes. Unlike in T-cell defects, growth is usually normal. T cells will be normal in number and function and, although often completely absent, a small number of B cells may be present.

Treatment requires replacement of immunoglobulin with 3-weekly intravenous or subcutaneous injections. As with many immunodeficiencies, recurrent infections can lead to irreversible long-term organ damage. Prompt and aggressive treatment of any breakthrough infections is required.

Mutations causing immunodeficiency carried on the X chromosome have some unique characteristics that can be useful in diagnosis. Males only have one X chromosome, and females randomly inactivate one of their two. In mutations resulting in failure of a cell type to develop, such as X-linked cγc SCID, all maternal T cells will have the normal X chromosome—this is referred to as non-random X inactivation. In conditions where the mutation affects function and not development of a cell type, as in chronic granulomatous disease, the maternal cells will be about 50% normal and 50% will have the defect. In XLA, Btk is found in monocytes, platelets, and B cells but is only essential for B-cell development.

Cross reference

See section 10.9 for more information on chronic granulomatous disease. Figure 10.6 shows the maternal cells, displaying 50% normal and 50% defective cells.

SELF-CHECK 10.2

When staining for Btk presence in a carrier, what would you expect to find?

Autosomal recessive forms of agammaglobulinaemia can also occur, due to mutations in the μ, Igα, BLNK, or λ5 genes.

Low B cells

Common variable immunodeficiency (CVID)

CVID occurs in 1 in 25 000 to 1 in 66 000 of the population. It is clinically heterogeneous and can occur at any age, but often presents in the second or third decade with recurrent bacterial infections, hypogammaglobulinaemia (IgM can be normal) and impaired antibody responses. B cells are generally present but are often low in number. T-cell function, as determined by proliferation responses to the mitogen PHA, can be poor. Patients can develop chronic lung disease, and there is a strong association with inflammatory bowel disease. A subgroup develop granulomata and resemble sarcoidosis.

A diagnosis of CVID is made if:

- there is a failure to make specific antibody responses to antigen after exposure
- there is markedly reduced serum levels of IgG, IgA, and often IgM
- and for other causes if antibody deficiencies have been excluded.

Recently, CVID patients have been further classified on the bases of their B-cell phenotypes.

The diagnosis of CVID is made only when all other known causes have been eliminated; however, a number of genetic defects have now been identified in patients previously classified as having CVID or with decreased IgG and IgA and variable IgM deficiency.

Cross reference
See Wehr (2008) for more detail about the EURO class trial.

Defects in the inducible co-stimulator (ICOS) and B-cell activating factor (BAFF) can lead to reduced B-cell numbers. BAFF is one of the family of tumour necrosis factor cytokines; it is secreted by mainly myeloid cells in the bone marrow and lymphoid follicles and provides maturation and survival signals to the B cells. ICOS expression on T cells is induced after stimulation by the T-cell receptor and is essential for T–B cell interaction.

Defects in transmembrane activator, calcium-modulating, cyclophilin ligand interactor (TACI) and CD19, normally present with normal B-cell numbers. CD19 forms part of a B-cell co-receptor complex that includes a complement receptor that binds to C3d. When this complex is stimulated, the signalling pathways of the B-cell receptor are greatly enhanced. C3d is produced when complement is activated and can be found on microbes or antigen–antibody complexes. Although important in enhancing a B-cell response, CD19 is not essential for its development. CD19-deficient patients have normal B-cell numbers but low or undetectable CD19 on their surface.

Key Point

The percentages of T, B, and NK cells should account for 100% ± 5% of the lymphocytes. CD3 and CD19 expression can either be reduced or absent in some immunodeficiencies.

Treatment of CVID is very similar to that of XLA, with replacement of immunoglobulin with 3-weekly intravenous or subcutaneous injections.

10.4 Natural killer (NK) cells

Development and function

Natural killer (NK) cells are derived from pluripotent stem cells in the bone marrow. Unlike T and B cells, they do not have unique receptors. As well as killing target cells, NK cells also interact with other cells by secreting interferon-γ in response to interleukin (IL)-12 secreted by activated macrophages, enabling the macrophages to kill any ingested pathogens.

NK cells have two mechanisms for recognizing a target. They express CD16 on their surface, which is a low-affinity receptor for the Fc portion of IgG1 and IgG3. Pathogens coated in immunoglobulin will therefore be targeted. The second mechanism involves a balance between stimulatory and inhibitory signals. Cytotoxic T cells play an important role in killing virally infected cells, but rely on viral antigen being presented by MHC class I. However, virally infected or malignant cells can down-regulate MHC class I. NK cells express an activation receptor called NKG2D, the ligands for which are not expressed on normal cells but are up-regulated by stress or DNA damage and are often expressed on virally infected or tumour cells.

Inhibitory receptors on NK cells such as the killer cell Ig-receptor (KIR) recognize different alleles of the HLA-A, B, and C molecules, ensuring that normal cells expressing HLA will not be killed. Only virally infected cells that have down-regulated MHC class I would remove the NK cells inhibition.

Absent NK cells

Key Point

T$^-$B$^+$NK$^-$ SCID should always be considered in an infant with absent NK cells (MFE, Omenn's). The T-cell subsets and activation markers should be looked at more closely to determine if the T cells appear normal.

There is a specific NK cell deficiency, but this is very rare, with only a handful of cases reported. Clinical symptoms manifest in early childhood, with increased susceptibility to viral infections, especially herpesvirus (CMV), varicella zoster virus (VZV), and herpes simplex virus (HSV). Lymphoproliferative disease driven by Epstein–Barr virus (EBV) was reported in one of the cases.

The defect has not yet been identified, but studies of affected families have mapped the defect to the centromeric region of chromosome 8.

10.5 **Additional antibodies**

The next four sections describe additional antibodies that can be used in the diagnosis of primary immunodeficiency. These include some that are absent in resting cells of peripheral blood and require stimulation before they can be detected. Antibodies can also be used to measure proteins found inside the cell, which require the cell membrane to be permeablized.

There are a number of primary immunodeficiencies that would give normal results using the routine lymphocyte subset panel. Two examples are given of specific conditions which, if suspected, would require the setting up of additional antibodies. Also described is B-cell phenotyping, useful for the classification of CVID and diagnosis of other primary immunodeficiencies.

Autoimmune lymphoproliferative syndrome (ALPS)

Clinically, this condition presents with chronic, non-malignant lymphadenopathy ± hepatosplenomegaly, severe autoimmune cytopenias (e.g. haemolytic anaemia, thrombocytopenia, and neutropenia) and susceptibility to malignancy. It can present early in the first few years of life.

ALPS is caused by a defect in apoptosis. Four types are described:

- **Type 1a:** patients have a defect in Fas (tumour necrosis factor receptor superfamily member 6, TNFRSF6).
- **Type 1b:** patients have a defect in Fas ligand.

- **Type 2a:** patients have a defect in caspase 10.
- **Type 2b:** patients have a defect in caspase 8.

A useful diagnostic finding is the presence of increased numbers of TCRαβ double negative T cells. Small numbers of double negative T cells can be detected in normal samples, but these are generally TCRγδ. Increases in this population can be seen in viral infections. However, DN TCRαβ T cells are usually less than 1% of T cells. Antibodies against CD3, CD4, CD8, and TCRαβ would be required to detect this population. What is considered a significant level is variable, but some quote figures as low as 1% of T cells. As with any low-event group, when looking for these small populations, large numbers of events should be acquired.

HSCT has been used successfully to treat this condition.

Immune dysregulation, polyendocrinopathy, enteropathy, X-linked syndrome (IPEX)

Symptoms of IPEX often appear in early childhood as protracted diarrhoea, type 1 diabetes, thyroiditis, and haemolytic anaemia. There are often massive infiltrations of T cells into the skin (resembles eczema) and gut, and high levels of autoantibodies against thyroid and pancreatic cells.

Mutations in the Forkhead Box 3 (*FOXP3*) gene have been identified, leading to an absence of T regulatory cells (Tregs). Tregs are a small subset of CD4⁺ T cells; classically they have high CD25⁺ expression and have been shown to be critical for the maintenance of peripheral tolerance. Although activated T cells express CD25, the absence of CD25-bright T cells can be a useful screen. An example of Tregs can be seen in Figure 10.3.

HSCT has been used successfully to treat this condition.

Key Point

When diagnosing any immunodeficiency it is important to remember that there is usually a wide spectrum of presentations and laboratory findings. Absent protein expression may be diagnostic, but the presence of protein does not exclude the diagnosis, as it may be nonfunctioning. The detection of mutations in a gene is an important addition to diagnosis but is not always in itself diagnostic.

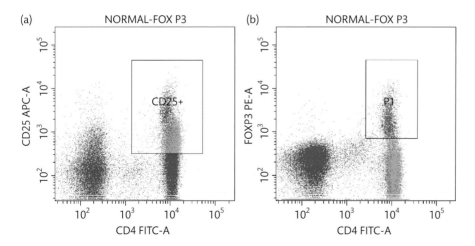

FIGURE 10.3
T regulatory cells. (a) and (b) show peripheral blood mononuclear cells first stained with anti-CD4 FITC and anti-CD25 APC antibodies, then permeabilized and stained with anti-FOXP3 PE. The FOXP3⁺ population denoted by the rectangle in (b) are seen as the purple population in the rectangle in (a). As shown, they are CD25 bright.

B-cell phenotype

On exiting the bone marrow, mature B cells are naive in that they have not encountered antigen. IgM and IgD are expressed on their surface and they will preferentially home to the secondary lymphoid organs. Upon binding to antigen, CD27 is expressed. B cells process antigen and present to CD4+ T cells. Recognition of the antigen by the CD4+ T cell results in up-regulation of CD40 ligand (CD154) on the surface of the T cells, which then binds to CD40 on the B cell, enabling the B cell to class switch from IgM to other isotypes. When this occurs, IgM and IgD are no longer expressed. Antibodies against CD27, IgM, and IgD can be used to determine the presence of naive, memory/activated, and class-switched B cells using flow cytometry.

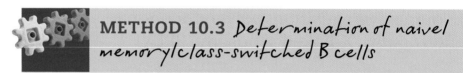

METHOD 10.3 *Determination of naive/ memory/class-switched B cells*

■ If whole blood is used, cells must be washed first to remove any IgM in the plasma. Antibodies will generally bind to free antigen first, rather than to bound antigen.

■ It is important to determine the number of events (usually cells) of a particular type to be acquired (i.e. data analysed) for each tube. A number of factors should be considered, including the number of events likely to be present in the stained sample/ tube and what percentage/numbers of various subsets are likely to be present.

■ Since low levels of class-switched B cells can be expected (1% is normal for infants), they should be treated as a rare event and suitable numbers (10 000) of B cells should ideally be acquired.

Absence of class-switched memory B cells is found in hyper IgM syndrome and a subset of CVID patients. Infants have high numbers of B cells compared to adults, the majority of which are naive; less than 1% of B cells are class switched in infants. Care needs to be taken to interpret B-cell phenotypes in the context of age. See Figure 10.4 for an example of B-cell phenotyping.

10.6 **Inducible antigens**

All of the antibodies described so far to identify lymphocyte subsets have been against structures present on the surface of resting peripheral blood lymphocytes. Some structures are only present for brief periods on the surface during activation, such as CD40 ligand. CD40 is constitutively expressed on B cells. Upon activation by antigen through the TCR/CD3 complex, CD4+ T cells will up-regulate CD40 ligand, which binds to CD40 on B cells, resulting in the ability to class switch (i.e. make immunoglobulin classes other than IgM). CD40 ligand is expressed relatively briefly. An example can be seen in Figure 10.5.

Activation markers such as HLA-DR take a couple of days to up-regulate and remain for a number of days, and are therefore readily detected on T cells in peripheral blood. HLA-DR expression on T cells is a useful marker, since it will be increased in viral infections but also in oligoclonal T cell populations such as those found in Ommen's syndrome.

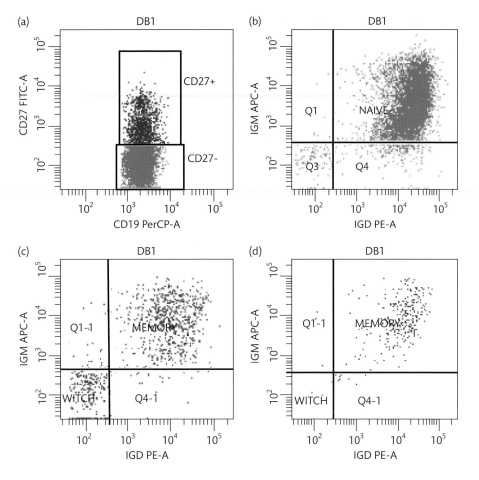

FIGURE 10.4

B-cell phenotyping. The figures above are of lysed whole blood stained with anti-CD19 PerCP, anti-CD27 FITC, anti-IgD PE, and anti-IgM APC: (a)–(c) A normal child gated (a) on B cells; (b) on CD27⁻ B cells; (c) on CD27⁺ B cells. Pink represents CD27⁻ and therefore naive; the majority of these cells still express IgD and IgM on their surface. Blue represents activated B cells, some of which have class switched and no longer express IgD or IgM (bottom left-hand quadrant). (d) CD27⁺ B cells from an infant with CD40-ligand deficiency; no class-switched B cells are present.

METHOD 10.4 *Detection of CD40 ligand (CD154)*

- ■ This can be carried out on whole blood or PBMCs.
- ■ T cells will require stimulation usually with PMA and ionomycin, for at least 4 hours. Antibodies against CD154 (CD40 ligand) can then be added, mixed, and incubated.
- ■ CD154 is only expressed on CD4⁺ T cells, so markers used should enable this population to be identified. Usually CD3 and CD4 would be required.
- ■ Unstimulated cells should be stained as a negative control.
- ■ CD69 behaves in a similar manner to CD154 but is expressed on all T cells upon activation. It should be included as a positive activation control.
- ■ Patients with CD40 ligand deficiency have complete absence of the ligand.
- ■ Not all CD4⁺ T cells can be induced to express CD154, but it should be detected on the majority. Carriers of CD4OL deficiency will have reduced numbers of CD4⁺ T cells expressing CD154.
- ■ Stimulation of T cells will cause down-regulation of CD3 and especially CD4.

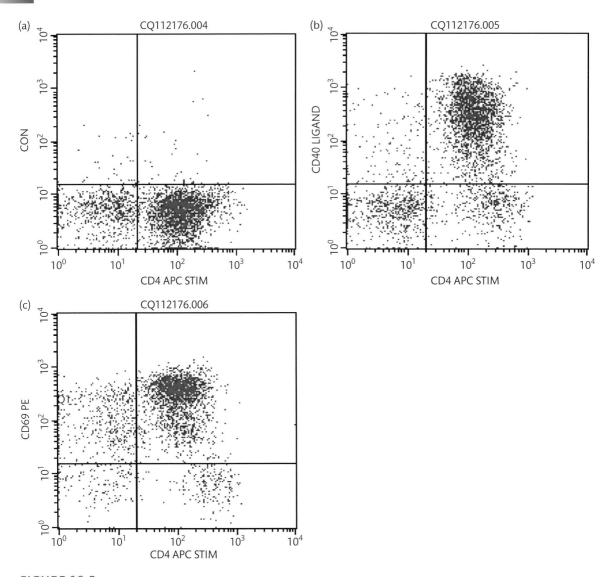

FIGURE 10.5

CD40 ligand assay. Peripheral blood mononuclear cells that have been stimulated with PMA and ionomycin for 4 hours at 37 °C and then stained with anti-CD3 and anti -CD4. All plots are gated on CD3+ expression. (a) Stained with the isotype control, which is negative; (b) stained with anti-CD40 ligand; shows the majority of CD4+ cells are positive; (c) stained with anti-CD69, which is positive for both CD4+ and CD4− cells.

Hyper IgM syndrome

This is a collective term for a group of disorders, which share a similar phenotype (Table 10.4). In the most severe forms, such as CD40 ligand deficiency, which present in infancy, patients have symptoms of a humoral defect, e.g. recurrent bacterial infection, but also of a T-cell defect such as pneumocystis pneumonia (PCP). They often have protracted diarrhoea due to *Cryptosporidium parvum* and liver disease, such as sclerosing cholangitis. Up to 50% of patients will also have neutropenia. IgM levels are normal or increased, but levels of all other isotypes are reduced. Defects in the class-switching of B cells are present and no class-switched

TABLE 10.4 Hyper IgM syndromes

Classification	Inheritance	Clinical symptoms
1. CD40 ligand (CD154)	XL	Recurrent bacterial infection, PCP, cryptosporidium, and neutropenia
2. AID (activation-induced-cytidine deaminase)	AR	No opportunistic infections, only bacterial. Lymphoid hyperplasia. Can present early in childhood but milder and can present later
3. CD40	AR	Similar to CD154: severe bacterial and opportunist infections
4. Unknown Defective class switch, normal SHM	AR	Similar to AID No opportunistic infections, only bacterial. Lymphoid hyperplasia
5. UNG	AR	Similar to AID No opportunistic infections, only bacterial. Lymphoid hyperplasia
6. NEMO(NFκB essential modulator)	AR	Ectodermal dysplasia (abnormal hair, teeth (pointed), sweat glands). Severe bacterial and atypical mycobacteria infections

AR, autosomal recessive; XL, X-linked.

memory B cells are detected. CD40 is expressed not only on B cells but also on monocytes/dendritic cells and myeloid progenitors. This may explain the abnormal cellular T-cell immune response, as monocytes and dendritic cell present antigen to CD4+ T cells. This cannot be corrected for by immunoglobulin substitution therapy.

Haematopoietic stem cell transplantation has been used successfully to treat the more severe forms. Milder forms are generally treated with immunoglobulin replacement therapy.

10.7 Intracellular staining

All staining described so far has been to structures on the cell surface. Intracellular proteins can also be detected by monoclonal antibodies if the cell is first fixed and the membrane is permeabilized. Many commercial reagents are now available. In the diagnosis of primary immunodeficiency there are many examples where this technique is useful.

METHOD 10.5 Intracellular staining

- To allow for the entry of an antibody inside a cell, the membrane needs first to be fixed and then permeabilized.

- It is not possible to determine if fluorescence detected by flow cytometry is intracellular or on the surface.

- Some permeabilization procedures can alter the expression of certain structures both on the surface and inside the cell.

- WASP and FOXP3 proteins, absent in Wiskott–Aldrich syndrome and IPEX respectively, can be determined by intracellular staining and flow cytometry.

- Cytokines produced by cells after appropriate stimulation can be blocked from exiting the cell. This enables then to be detected intracellularly while simultaneously staining surface structures to identify the producing cell.

- BrdU is a pyrimidine analogue and is incorporated in place of thymidine into the DNA of proliferating cells. Anti-BrdU antibodies can be used to enumerate the proliferation of T cells in response to mitogens.

10.8 **Functional assays**

The presence of a cell type does not always mean it can function normally. B-cell function can be determined in a number of ways, the simplest of which is to measure the immunoglobulins present. As previously described (see Methods 10.3) the presence of class-switched B cells can also be detected. Specific antibody response to immunization antigens is a good method for assessing humoral immunity. T-cell function is more diverse than that of B cells and therefore more difficult to measure.

Measuring T cell function

A basic function that can be measured is the T cell's ability to respond to stimulation, to become activated, and to proliferate. This is an essential requirement of T cells as part of the adaptive immune response.

In vivo T cells are stimulated by recognition of antigen in the context of MHC by the TCR with appropriate co-stimulatory signals. T cells can be activated *in vitro* by plant lectins such as PHA, antibodies such as anti-CD3, and antigens such as PPD (purified protein derivative –TB).

The most commonly used method is based on measuring the incorporation of tritiated thymidine into the DNA of proliferating cells. The major drawback of this method is the use of radioactive material. Other techniques that look at T-cell activation involving the use of flow cytometry include the expression of various activation markers, such as CD69, and the secretion of cytokines. Methods that are equivalent to thymidine uptake, i.e. those that actually measure T-cell proliferation, include the measurement of the number of T cells in S phase using DNA staining, and antibodies to BrdU. Both these methods require permeabilization of the cells.

Another method uses carboxyfluorescein diacetate succinimidyl ester (CSFE), which labels intracellular molecules with fluorescence. With each cycle of cell division, the fluorescence is halved. This does not require a permeabilization step and allows for surface staining to identify specific cell populations.

Measuring NK cell function

The function of NK cells can be tested by flow cytometry using a human leukaemia cell line K562 that does not express MHC class I.

 METHOD 10.6 NK cell killing assay

- A K562 cell line needs to be maintained.
- PBMCs are prepared from whole blood by density gradient.
- Monocytes are removed by incubation for 1 hour on a plastic surface, to which they adhere.
- K562 cells are stained with a fluorescent dye to ensure they are readily identified from the PBMCs.

- PBMCs (effector cells) are mixed with the K562 (target cells) at ratios of 100, 50, 25, and 12.5 to 1. These are gently centrifuged and incubated in a 37 °C 5% CO_2 incubator for 2 hours.

- K562 death is ascertained by staining with propidium iodide (PI), which is only taken up by dead cells.

- The percentage of dead (killed) K562 cells is determined by gating on K562 cells and measuring the number that have taken up PI.

- Background K562 death should be determined by adding PI to K562s not mixed with PBMCs.

- As with any functional assay, a normal control should always be tested alongside a patient sample.

- This assay can also be performed using a chromium release assay.

10.9 Neutrophil defects

This final section describes primary immunodeficiency due to neutrophil defects in which flow cytometry plays a role in diagnosis.

Neutrophil function

Neutrophils, like lymphocytes, are derived from haematopoietic pluripotent stem cells and develop in the bone marrow. They are short-lived and are initially released into the peripheral blood circulation. To function effectively they need to be able to exit the circulation and migrate to the site of infection. They do this by responding to chemotactic signals such as one of the complement components, C5a. To exit the blood vessels neutrophils need to adhere to the endothelium, which is facilitated by adhesion molecules present on both the neutrophils and endothelial cells. Neutrophils will then migrate to the site of infection. Receptors on their surface include those to many common components of pathogens such as lipopolysaccharide found in bacterial cell walls, as well as receptors to the Fc component of immunoglobulin and to complement. Pathogens coated in immunoglobulins and complement are said to be **opsonized** and are readily phagocytosed by neutrophils. Once the pathogen is in the phagosome, the activated neutrophil will undergo the respiratory burst during which highly toxic reactive oxygen species are produced. Granule proteases are released as a result of this, and these are primarily responsible for killing ingested bacteria.

Opsonization
The binding of complement and antibodies to the surface of a pathogen or foreign substance to aid phagocytosis.

There are many congenital neutrophil defects, but only two will be discussed here as flow cytometry plays a useful role in their diagnosis.

Leukocyte adhesion deficiency (LAD)

LAD is a very rare condition. In the severe form patients present very early with recurrent severe bacterial infections, especially on mucosal surfaces (perianal abscess). Those who survive into early childhood have severe periodontitis and gingivitis. They have poor wound healing with lack of pus, and one of the earliest signs is delayed separation of the umbilical cord. A leucocytosis is also present, as neutrophils are unable to leave the circulation.

In LAD 1 there is a defect in the synthesis of the common β chain (CD18) shared by three leukocyte integrins, LFA-1, Mac-1 (CR3), and p150.95 (CR4). These can be readily detected on the surface of neutrophils with appropriate antibodies. The severity of the disease relates to the degree of CD18 that is detectable; less than 1% of normal CD18 in severely affected children. LAD1 can be treated by HSCT.

LAD 2 presents in a very similar fashion to LAD 1 but with no delayed cord separation and also includes mental retardation and the Bombay or hh blood group. CD15 (Sialy-Lewis X) is absent. It is a much less severe condition than LAD 1, and infections are generally not life-threatening.

Chronic granulomatous disease (CGD)

This is one of the more severe neutrophil defects and affected children do not usually survive beyond early adulthood. There is a failure in intracellular killing, especially of catalase-positive organisms, such as staphylococci, as well as fungi such as *Aspergillus*. There is formation of granulomas especially in the liver, lungs, and gut.

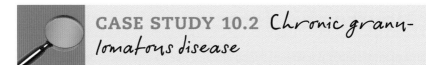

CASE STUDY 10.2 *Chronic granulomatous disease*

A 4-year-old boy presented with cervical lymphadenopathy. He had a biopsy taken of his right cervical lymph node, which showed caseous granuloma. He was started on intravenous antibiotics for high inflammatory markers and spiking temperature. He was also started on antitubercular medication, but the spike temperatures still continued. On transfer to a paediatric infectious disease unit it was noted that he had had a mild failure to thrive and previously had a perianal abscess, which needed to be incised and drained.

- Following abnormalities noticed on a chest radiograph, a CT scan was performed which showed a lung abscess. A biopsy from this grew *Burkholderia cepacia*.
- A neutrophil oxidative burst assay was performed on both his neutrophils and his mother's. Results are shown in Figure 10.6.
- A diagnosis of CGD was made.

The defect is in one of four components of NADPH oxidase that produces reactive oxygen intermediates (ROIs) important for the killing of phagocytosed pathogens. One of these components is coded for on the X chromosome, gp91phox. The other three components, p22phox, p67phox, and p47phox, are inherited in an autosomal recessive fashion.

Dihydrorhodamine is a dye that changes to a fluorescent form, rhodamine, when oxidized by H_2O_2 in the presence of a peroxidase. This can be used to detect the respiratory burst by flow cytometry (Figure 10.7).

(a)
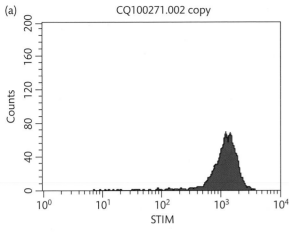

(b)
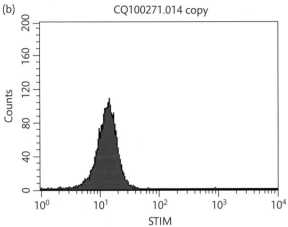

(c)
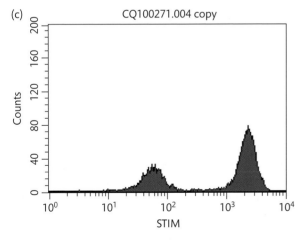

FIGURE 10.6
Dihydrorhodamine assay in chronic granulomatous disease.
(a) A normal DHR shift after stimulation of neutrophils with
PMA. The histogram shows data gated on neutrophils on the
basis of forward and side scatter; (b) a CGD patient with no shift
in DHR; (c) the mother of the CGD patient in (b); she has two
populations, demonstrating that she is a carrier.

FIGURE 10.7
Neutrophil oxidative mechanisms for the production of reactive oxygen species (ROS) during the oxidative burst process. H_2O_2, hydrogen peroxide; HOCl, hypochlorous acid; MPO, myeloperoxidase; O_2^-, superoxide; SOD, superoxide dismutase.

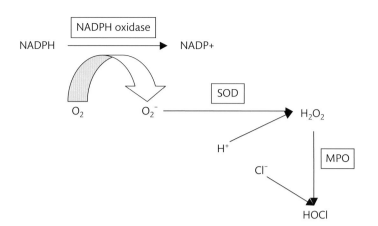

METHOD 10.7 *Neutrophil oxidative burst*

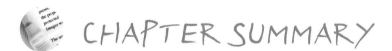

- Whole blood EDTA samples can be used for this assay.

- Red blood cells need to be lysed (not using commercial lysing agents, containing formaldehydes, which would kill the neutrophils).

- After washing, the leukocytes are incubated with dihydrorhodamine in a 37 °C water bath.

- Neutrophils are then stimulated using PMA.

- An unstimulated tube for each sample and a normal control should always be tested alongside each patient sample.

- Samples should be processed the same day the sample is taken, because of the short half-life of neutrophils.

- Myeloperoxidase (MPO) deficiency will affect this assay and should be excluded in an abnormal result.

CHAPTER SUMMARY

- Flow cytometry plays a role in the diagnosis of a number of primary immunodeficiencies.

- A basic panel of antibodies can be used to screen for certain diseases such as SCID.

- The presence of a cell type or protein does not exclude a functional defect.

- For many primary immunodeficiencies a more directed approach is required to ensure the correct test is carried out.

- A number of techniques are available, enabling intracellular proteins and cell function to be assessed.

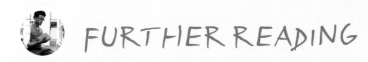

FURTHER READING

- Goldsby RA, Kindt TJ, Osborne BA, *et al.* (2003) *Kuby's Immunology*, 4th edition. W.H. Freeman, New York.

- Janeway CA, Travers P, Walport M, Shlomchik M (2001) *Immunobiology. The Immune System in Health and Disease, 5th edition*. Garland Science, New York.

- Male D, Brostoff J, Rith D, Roitt I (2006). *Immunology*, 7th edition. Mosby, St Louis.

- Wehr C, Kivioja T, Schmitt C, *et al.* (2008) The EUROclass trial: defining subgroups in common variable immunodeficiency. *Blood*, **111**, 77–85.

DISCUSSION QUESTIONS

10.1 Describe the functions of T cells.

10.2 Which primary immunodeficiencies would have absent B cells? How would you differentiate between them?

10.3 What are the clinical symptoms of autoimmune lymphoproliferative syndrome (ALPS)? What is the defect? What test could you do to help with diagnosis?

10.4 What would you expect to see in the mother carriers of the following conditions: X-linked SCID, XLA, CGD?

Answers to these questions are provided in the book's Online Resource Centre; visit www.oxfordtextbooks.co.uk/orc/ahmed/

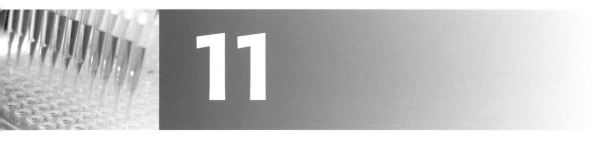

11

Human immunodeficiency virus (HIV)

Learning Objectives

After studying this chapter you should be able to:

- describe how HIV transmission occurs
- understand how HIV infects cells and replicates
- describe the clinical features of HIV disease
- outline the assays and techniques used to test for HIV infection
- describe how the disease is monitored
- outline the treatment regimens for HIV disease
- discuss how drug resistance may occur
- understand how HIV transmission and infection may be prevented

Introduction

Cross reference
See http://www.who.int/hiv.

The human immunodeficiency virus (HIV) affects over 33 million people worldwide and it is the most widespread cause of immunodeficiency. It is estimated that in the last three decades over 25 million people have died as a result of HIV infection (World Health Organization 2007).

11.1 The human immunodeficiency virus

HIV is a retrovirus, a member of the lentivirus family. It can be further subdivided into two types, HIV-1 and HIV-2. At a molecular level HIV-2 is more homologous with simian

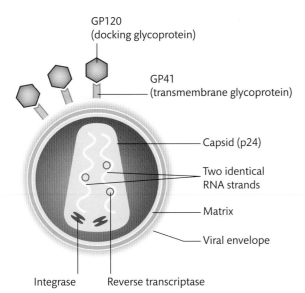

GP120
(docking glycoprotein)

GP41
(transmembrane glycoprotein)

Capsid (p24)

Two identical
RNA strands

Matrix

Viral envelope

Integrase   Reverse transcriptase

FIGURE 11.1
**Diagrammatic representation
of HIV virus.**

immunodeficiency virus (SIV), a virus which when introduced into macaque monkeys causes an acquired AIDS-like disease. HIV-1 has three main classes: M (major), O (outlying), and N (new). HIV-1 class M accounts for around 90% of HIV-1 infections and can be further subdivided into nine different clades (or subtypes) A, B, C, D, F, G, H, J, and K. As a result of continuous transmission, mutation, and recombination, the distinction between different clades has become blurred.

The HIV virus is around 20 nm in diameter and almost spherical (Figure 11.1). The plasma membrane is derived from the host plasma membrane which encloses a capsid. The capsid contains two copies of single-stranded RNA, which is tightly bound to the nucleocapsid proteins. Also enclosed within the capsid are the regulatory proteins Vif (virus infectivity factor), Vpr (viral protein U), Nef (negative regulatory factor), p7, and viral protease.

11.2 The life cycle of HIV

Knowledge of the HIV life cycle is necessary for the design of strategies to help prevent infection and disease progression. You can see the stages of the life cycle in Figure 11.2.

HIV-1 uses the CD4 receptor and a chemokine co-receptor, either CXCR4 or CCR5, to bind to and infect CD4+ cells. CXCR4 was the first HIV coreceptor to be discovered, and is considered the most important in HIV-1 infection of CD4T lymphocytes. Viruses utilizing CCR5 are macrophage-trophic and more important in the infection of macrophages. Viral HIV-1 strains differ in their ability to infect different cell populations and in their ability to utilize the different co-receptors. Mutations or deletions in the CCR5 co-receptor have been shown to render some individuals resistant to HIV-1 infection (Libert 1998, Quillent 1998).

Following cellular attachment, the virus fuses with the target cell membrane and enters the cell. The viral envelope is removed by enzymes normally present inside the cell, and the internal core exposed and broken down. Once the viral RNA is exposed, an enzyme attached to it, known as reverse transcriptase, begins to make a complementary single-strand DNA copy (cDNA) of the viral RNA and subsequently the same enzyme makes double-stranded DNA. This DNA is then integrated into the host T-cell DNA, where it may remain quiescent (latent infection), or be used as a template to make new viral particles. Multiple copies of mRNA are

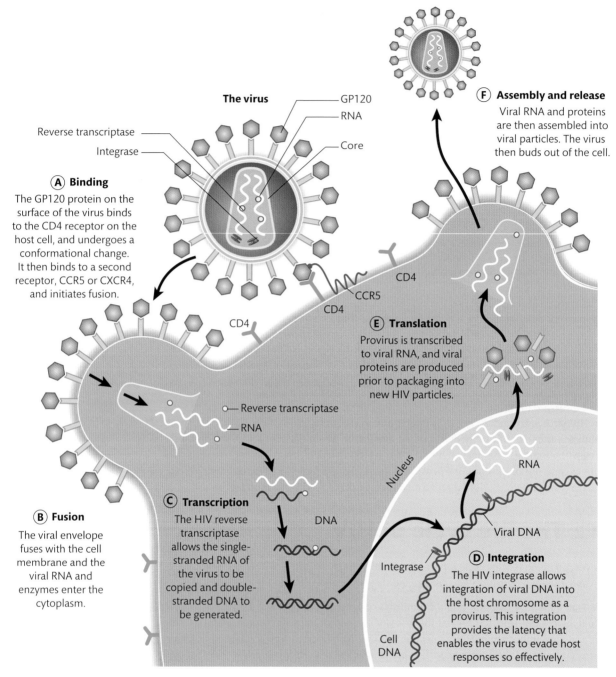

FIGURE 11.2
Schematic representation showing replication of HIV.

transcribed and the subsequent translation of mRNA results in the synthesis of viral polypeptides and proteases. RNA and structural proteins then gather at the host cell surface, where they are cleaved by polypeptides into functional HIV-1 proteins. The virus then buds from the cell's surface and infects further CD4 cells.

Viral RNA copies are integrated into the host genome in the form of proviral DNA. The detection of such integrated, replication-competent proviral DNA is an important diagnostic marker in the evaluation of HIV-1 infection of newborns born to HIV-1 seropositive women. It is clear that viral integration and viral reservoirs established early in infection serve as a major obstacle in eradication of HIV-1 infection. Several anatomical reservoirs may exist, including the lymphatic system, the male genitourinary tract, and the central nervous system. However, it is the presence of latently infected CD4 cells that provides a long-term reservoir of HIV-1 replication-competent cells. Proviral DNA can be used to evaluate viral infection in the absence of measurable amounts of the viral RNA in the plasma.

11.3 Transmission of HIV

Infection with HIV may occur following sexual contact with an HIV-positive individual, sharing of contaminated needles and/or syringes among drug users, or (very rarely) through transfusion of contaminated blood or blood products. This last cause is now extremely rare thanks to improved screening of donations and predonation questionnaires—individuals with high-risk behaviours such as drug addicts and/or those with a history of unsafe sexual practices are discouraged from giving blood.

Maternal–fetal transmission may affect up to 30% of pregnancies to HIV-positive women, though this has been reduced dramatically to less than 1% by successful antiretroviral therapy (ART) and delivery by caesarean section. A further 5–20% of babies born to HIV-positive women may be infected through breastfeeding, and consequently this is discouraged. Maternal–fetal transmission is still a serious problem in the developing world, because of poor education about disease transmission and prevention, poor or nonexistent access to ART, and taboos surrounding bottle-feeding. The advice is further confused by the observation that transmission occurs more readily in babies receiving mixed feeding (breast and bottle), and mothers are now advised to choose only one type of feeding.

Although health-care workers have been infected with HIV after needlestick injury and through blood entering an open wound or mucous membrane, this is extremely rare. Transmission by a health-care worker to a patient is also extremely rare, although a case has been described whereby six patients were infected by a dentist following dental treatment. There is no evidence to suggest transmission through mosquito bites or other insect or animal bites.

11.4 Effects of HIV on the immune system

CD4 is a specific receptor for HIV-1. By infecting the very cell required to mediate B-cell and cytotoxic cell responses, the body's ability to raise antibodies or kill virally infected cells is compromised. In response to HIV-1 infection, more T cells are produced, which mature to become T helper cells, but then also become targets for viral infection themselves, thus helping to provide a fresh reservoir of susceptible cells.

With time, infection with HIV results in a progressive decline in the number of CD4 T cells and reversal in the normal CD4:CD8 ratio, causing a severe, progressive immunodeficiency. In particular, HIV-1 infects CCR5$^+$CD4$^+$ T cells. Effector memory T cells (T_{EM}), which express CCR5 (CD4$^+$CD45RA$^-$, CD27$^-$, CCR5$^+$) are prime targets for HIV infection, comprising around 15% of the peripheral blood T cells and regenerated from naive and central memory T cells, and it is this population which is initially depleted in early HIV infection. The decrease in the CD4T cell count may be a result of a number of different mechanisms. These include killing of infected cells by the virus itself, by the development of pores in the cell membrane of infected cells as a result of viral budding; fusion of uninfected cells with infected cells; or apoptosis or programmed cell death of HIV-infected and uninfected 'bystander' cells.

Cells other than $CD4^+$ T cells, also expressing the CD4 antigen, are susceptible to HIV infection; these include monocytes/macrophages, follicular dendritic cells, microglial cells, and Langerhans cells, and may serve as a further reservoir for HIV infection and exacerbate the pathogenesis of the disease due to abnormal function. CD4 cells are necessary for the proper functioning of the immune system, through their interaction with antigen-presenting cells, B cells, cytotoxic T cells, and natural killer cells. Lack of T cell help may lead to a number of disorders, as described below.

The gut also serves as a large reservoir for HIV-infected CD4T cells. In acute infection, there is an enormous depletion in the number of GALT-associated CD4 cells. Since the majority of intestinal lymphocytes express CCR5, it is not surprising that lymphocyte depletion is most significant within this subset of T cells.

There is strong evidence that HIV infection is associated with severe damage to the B cell compartment. **Hypergammaglobulinaemia**, exhausted tissue-like CD21 low B cells, and polyclonal B cell activation are hallmarks of the extensive B cell dysregulation in HIV infection and may be reversed by ART. Memory B cells expressing CD27 may make up around 40% of the peripheral blood B cells; these cells can be further subdivided into IgM and class-switched memory B cells—a pool of antigen-specific B cells which can rapidly differentiate into antibody-secreting **Plasmoblasts** on restimulation. The IgM memory subset is extensively lost during acute HIV infection, and this effect is not reversed by ART. HIV infection results in progressive damage to the population of memory B cells ($CD19^+CD27^+$), resulting in impaired vaccination responses to common antigens like tetanus toxoid and associated with increased susceptibility to invasive bacterial disease.

Hypergamma-globulinaemia

An increase in serum immunoglobulins.

Plasmoblast

A precursor cell of the plasmocyte, which constitutes 1% of the nucleated white blood cells. Not commonly seen in the peripheral blood of normal people, but can be seen in chronic infections, granulomatous and allergic diseases, and plasma cell myeloma.

Seroconversion

The detection of antibodies in response to an antigen (infectious organism). In HIV infection, the conversion from an antibody-negative to an antibody-positive state can take from 1 week to several months.

Infectious mononucleosis

The disease caused by a severe infection of Epstein–Barr virus (EBV). Symptoms include extreme fatigue, fever, sore throat, swollen lymph nodes, and an increase of lymphocytes in the blood. Patients with weakened or suppressed immune systems are at risk of serious complications of infectious mononucleosis.

CLINICAL CORRELATIONS 11.1

Effects of depletion in CD4 cells

- Hypergammaglobulinaemia through lack of CD4 cell control of B-cell function
- Autoimmune disease such as rheumatological disorders, systemic lupus erythematosus (SLE), Graves' disease, idiopathic thrombocytopenic purpura (ITP), and antiphospholipid syndrome
- Increased infections—viral, fungal, and bacterial
- Dementia
- Inflammation and symptomatic bowel disease is common, and the gut has been proposed as a major site of HIV replication

---

11.5 Clinical features of HIV infection

Following infection with HIV-1, around 10% of individuals develop an acute illness called **seroconversion** illness. Seroconversion illness usually occurs 2–6 weeks after infection but may occur up to 3 months later. It resembles **infectious mononucleosis**; the symptoms may include fever, headache, sore throat, enlarged or swollen lymph nodes, malaise, and rash. Following infection, most individuals will remain asymptomatic for periods of between 2 and

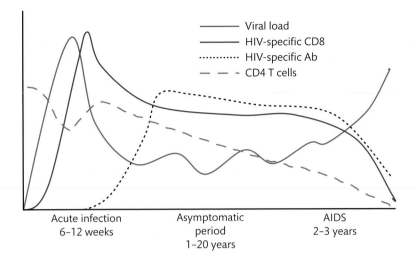

FIGURE 11.3

Effect of HIV disease progression on CD4 counts and viral load with time. Seroconversion illness is associated with a sharp increase in HIV-1 viral load and decrease in CD4 count. Following this, there is some regeneration of the immune system as seen by an increase in CD4 count to slightly subnormal levels and controlled viraemia. Over time, without treatment, the regenerative capacity of the immune system is lost, as seen by increase in viral load and steady decline in CD4 cell count.

15 years. The course of the disease varies considerably from individual to individual; in the absence of treatment, some individuals may rapidly progress to acquired immunodeficiency syndrome (AIDS) while others are termed long-term nonprogressors or 'elite controllers' and even after many years of infection remain asymptomatic with normal levels of CD4 cells, undetectable plasma HIV-1 viral load, and an absence of opportunistic infections. In the absence of ART, progressive damage to the immune system eventually leads to the development of symptoms and recurrent infections with other viruses, such as herpes zoster, and bacterial or fungal infections. These infections often involve the skin or mucous membranes, frequently in the buccal cavity. Skin disorders such as eczema or psoriasis may also be present, and the virus may affect the gastrointestinal tract, causing weight loss, diarrhoea, and appetite loss. Figure 11.3 shows the laboratory observations at different stages in the disease.

11.6 **Progression to AIDS**

Continued damage to the immune system eventually leads to the development of AIDS—this is the most advanced stage of HIV infection. The Center for Disease Control and Prevention's definition of AIDS includes all HIV-1 positive individuals with a CD4 count of less than 200 cells/μL, or less than 14% of the total lymphocyte count. This late stage of the disease is characterized by a collection of opportunistic infections which would not normally occur in individuals with a healthy immune system.

CLINICAL CORRELATIONS 11.2

Opportunistic infections frequently found in AIDS

- **Pneumocystis pneumonia***
- **Toxoplasmosis***
- **Tuberculosis***
- **Extreme weight loss and wasting* exacerbated by diarrhoea, which can be experienced in up to 90% of HIV patients worldwide**
- **Meningitis and other brain infections**
- **Fungal infections**

- **Syphilis**
- **Malignancies such as lymphoma*, cervical cancer, and Kaposi's sarcoma***

*AIDS-defining illnesses.

11.7 Laboratory diagnosis of HIV infection

HIV-1 antibody measurement

Antibodies to HIV usually appear 2–8 weeks (mean 22 days) after infection, with IgM antibodies usually preceding the appearance of IgG antibodies. The first antibodies to be detected are usually those directed to the p24 (core) antigen, followed by antibodies to gp41 (transmembrane) proteins.

Antibody screening alone may not identify HIV-infected individuals in the 'window period' prior to seroconversion, and hence diagnosis in the acute phase of infection can be improved by the measurement of p24 antigen, which usually precedes that of the antibody (mean 16 days after exposure). However, p24 antigen levels in serum decline shortly after seroconversion, so this antigen alone may only be present in approximately 70% of patients. The formation of p24 antigen–antibody complexes may account for the apparent decline in level of p24.

Enzyme-linked immunosorbent assays (ELISAs) are the most common way of identifying HIV infection, and many commercial HIV screening tests combine the testing of p24 antigen and anti-HIV antibodies to enhance assay sensitivity. ELISA plates may be coated with anti-p24 antibodies to identify the presence of p24 antigen, together with HIV-1 antigens, such as gp160, gp41, and/or peptides from HIV-2 envelope proteins, to identify antibodies with reactivity to both HIV-1 and HIV-2. The presence of HIV antigen or HIV-reactive antibody is determined by reactivity with an enzyme-conjugated anti-human antibody which, following the addition of a suitable substrate, will catalyse a colour reaction.

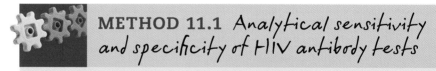

METHOD 11.1 Analytical sensitivity and specificity of HIV antibody tests

- **HIV ELISA tests have a high sensitivity (98.4–99.9%) and high specificity (99.3–100%).**
- **It is important to remember that false negatives may occur in the window period before seroconversion.**

Positive HIV tests are usually confirmed using a western blot or a line immunoassay. In line with immunoassays, different HIV-1 and HIV-2 antigens are coated at discrete locations on a test strip and the reactivity of the antibody to particular antigens is determined. For example, an HIV-1 positive sample may bind to gp120 and gp41 but not gp105 and gp36, while a sample positive for HIV-2 may react with gp105 and gp36, but not with gp120 and gp41.

Rapid screening tests or point-of-care testing using whole blood have a major role in the developing world, where access to laboratory equipment is limited. The three main rapid methods available are:

- **Particle agglutination:** HIV-1-positive whole blood is mixed with latex particles coated with specific HIV antigens; the antibody cross-links the latex particles, resulting in the visual agglutination of the particles.

- **Immunoconcentration:** HIV antigens are immobilized on a solid-phase column and blood samples applied to the column. These assays require sequential additions of washing buffers and detection substrate and are thus slightly more complex to perform. A positive sample is identified by antibody binding to the specific antigens and visualization is colorimetric. Some immunoconcentration assays allow for differentiation of HIV-1 from HIV-2.

- **Immunochromatography:** in this rapid assay, antigen and signal reagents are combined on a nitrocellulose strip. Samples applied to an absorbent pad move by capillary action along the strip and if antibody is present it will combine with the HIV antigen and signal reagents to produce a visual band at a defined position.

HIV-1 viral load measurement

HIV-1-infected patients are monitored through measurement of plasma HIV-1 viral load, which measures the degree of viraemia (the concentration of viral RNA in the plasma). The prognosis for patients is worse for those with a high HIV viral load. Although the HIV-1 viral load test is not usually recommended as a diagnostic test, it may well be positive before sero-conversion and hence when the HIV test such as those described above is negative.

ART may reduce the plasma viral load to levels below that of detection—routinely to a lower limit of detection of 40–50 copies HIV-1 RNA per mL.

There are two main methods for detecting viral RNA: reverse transcription-PCR (RT-PCR) reactions and the branched DNA (bDNA) assay.

The RT-PCR based methods involve on three main processes:

- isolation of RNA from the viral particle
- reverse transcription of the target RNA to generate complementary DNA (cDNA) using HIV-1-specific primers
- PCR amplification of the target cDNA and detection by fluorescent probe.

It is essential that the primer and detection probes are designed to bind to a highly conserved regions in the genome and thus are not affected by the mutations that occur frequently during viral replication/mutations.

Quantification is made possible by the addition of an internal standard of known copy number, with identical primer-binding region but reconfigured probe-binding region. The internal standard generates a DNA product of the same length as the target RNA, but by using two different detection probes with different emission spectra, the HIV DNA product can be discriminated from the internal standard—put simply, quantification is possible by comparing the fluorescent output from DNA amplification product and that of the internal standard.

Fairly recently, a new method for PCR quantification has been developed, called real-time or kinetic PCR. Real-time PCR enables the scientist to view the increase in DNA with sequential

PCR cycles. Essentially, there are three main types of real-time PCR methods, differing in the way the increase in PCR product is visualized; these utilize TaqMan probes, molecular beacons, and SYBR Green, respectively.

METHOD 11.2 *Real-time PCR probes*

- **TaqMan probes** consist of oligonucleotide probes labelled with two different types of fluorophore, a green reporter protein and a quencher fluorophore, which bind to specific regions in the target DNA. When the probe is intact, the fluorescence of the reporter probe is suppressed by the proximity of the quencher. With sequential cycles of PCR, the reporter and quencher dyes are separated and fluorescence from the reporter protein is released and can be quantified. Each cycle of PCR is represented by an increase in fluorescence intensity.

- **Molecular beacons** also consist of reporter and quencher dyes, but with this system the reporter dye is wrapped around into a hairpin-like configuration, bringing the reporter and quencher dye into close proximity, eliminating the reporter's ability to fluoresce. Unlike the TaqMan probe, the quencher and reporter dyes remain intact with each round of PCR. On binding to a complementary strand of DNA, however, the probe elongates, removing the reporter dye from the quenchers' influence, enabling a fluorescent signal to be released.

- **SYBR Green** is a dye which binds to all double-stranded DNA and can be used in real-time PCR methods. SYBR Green has no sequence specification, however, and therefore may lack specificity.

In contrast to RT-PCR methods, the branched DNA (bDNA) assay relies on signal amplification rather than amplification of DNA. In this method, synthetic DNA probes bind to HIV-1 RNA immobilized on the well of a microtitre plate. The HIV-1 virus is initially concentrated by high-speed centrifugation, then lysed to liberate the viral RNA. The RNA is then bound to the well of a microtitre plate, using HIV-1-specific capture probes. Sequential additions of further synthetic probes (DNA constructs) specific for the HIV-1 virus are added, which hybridize (i.e. bind) to the immobilized RNA. Quantification is made possible by adding an alkaline phosphatase and a substrate which releases a luminescent signal that is proportional to the amount of virus present and comparing the signal to that of the standard curve.

Some laboratories have developed in-house HIV-1 viral load assays, which are used routinely to determine HIV-1 viral load.

Sometimes viral loads may become positive after a series of previously undetectable results; this is referred to as a 'blip'. Blips may be due to the sensitivity of the assay at the lower detection limit or may suggest adherence problems, developing drug resistance, illness, or vaccination. Following a blip, it is usually recommended to repeat the viral load test as soon as possible. Repeated blips can be a sign of imminent failure of ART.

In addition to plasma, HIV-1 viral load can also be measured in other tissues such as the cerebrospinal fluid (CSF), seminal fluid, and breast milk. The detection of HIV-1 in the CSF may be linked with dementia, and CSF may serve as an important reservoir for HIV-1.

METHOD 11.3 *Analytical sensitivity of commonly used commercial HIV viral load assays*

Roche and Abbott real-time PCR

■ The concentration of HIV RNA within EDTA plasma can be detected to a lower limit of 40 copies/mL with a positivity rate exceeding 95%.

■ The dynamic range is 40–10×10^7 copies/mL.

Siemens Versant bDNA

■ The estimated limit of detection is 68 HIV-1 RNA copies/mL, with the upper one-sided 95% confidence limit of 73 HIV-1 RNA copies/mL

HIV-1 can also be detected in the seminal fluid of HIV-1-positive men. Many HIV-discordant couples (HIV-positive man and HIV-negative woman) may wish to conceive their own biological child, but unprotected sex will necessarily put mother and child at risk of infection. To reduce this risk, some couples chose artificial insemination using 'washed sperm'; this process can reduce the viral load to levels below the detection limit, commonly around 100 copies/mL, and significantly reduce the risk of infection.

Only a handful of laboratories also measure HIV-2 viral load and there is currently no commercially available HIV-2 viral load assay.

CD4 count measurement

HIV infection is characterized by a progressive depletion in CD4+ T cells and a decrease in the CD4:CD8 ratio. The CD4 count is a good prognostic marker for the development of AIDS. The likelihood of an individual progressing to AIDS in the absence of treatment increases with decreasing CD4 count. CD4 (and CD8) count can be measured by flow cytometry.

Lymphocytes may be gated by forward- and side-scatter characteristics, or a pan-leukocyte marker, such as CD45, and side-scatter characteristics, to distinguish them from other leukocytes such as granulocytes and monocytes. CD4+ and CD8+ T lymphocytes may then be stained with fluorescently labelled specific monoclonal antibodies. By using antibodies labelled with different fluorescent dyes and specific filters to detect each dye, multiple subpopulations of lymphocytes can then be analysed in a single tube and identified by their differing fluorescence emission profiles. While the percentage of CD4 and CD8 cells and the CD4:CD8 ratio is important, absolute counts are important prognostic indicators of disease progression. An absolute CD4 count can be obtained by adding to each tube a preparation containing a known number of fluorescent beads and comparing the number of cellular flow cytometric events with that in the bead preparation, or by analysing only those cells within a predefined volume. A CD4 count of between 200 and 500 indicates that some damage has already occurred to the immune system. Less than 200 cells/µL suggests progression to AIDS. Therefore, most laboratories now measure the absolute CD4 count. Future flow cytometric tests to monitor HIV infection and disease progression may address the expression of CD45RA

Cross reference

More information on measurement of CD4+ and CD8+ T cells by flow cytometry can be found in Chapter 10.

(a marker of naive T and B cells) and CD27 to differentiate between naive, memory, and effector memory T cells and the effect of HIV infection on these cell populations.

The effects of HIV infection on B cells may also be examined by flow cytometry, although currently measurement of B-cell dysregulation is more likely to be carried out in a research setting, rather than a routine diagnostic laboratory. Deficiencies in B-cell memory can be determined by the expression of CD19$^+$CD27$^+$IgD$^+$/IgD$^-$ cells and exhausted B-cell populations by the expression of CD19$^+$CD10$^-$CD27$^-$CD21^{low} cells. HIV-induced B-cell immune activation may be evidenced by the increased expression of B-cell activation markers CD70, CD71 (transferrin receptor; TFRC), CD80, and CD86.

Proviral DNA measurement

HIV-1 proviral DNA is integrated into the host genome. The identification of proviral DNA is a useful tool in the diagnosis of infection in neonates. Neonates born to HIV-positive mothers may have maternal antibodies in the circulation in the absence of HIV-1 infection, and therefore a positive HIV-1 antibody test may be misleading. Demonstration of proviral DNA in neonates provides evidence of HIV-1 infection and effective replication. It is a useful tool in the diagnosis of these infants, enabling prompt initiation of ART as needed.

ART may reduce the plasma HIV viral load to below the limit of detection, but does not completely eliminate infection or replication, as evidenced by positive proviral DNA. Proviral DNA can be measured in isolated peripheral blood mononuclear cells/cell lines (PBMCs) using RT-PCR.

11.8 Treatment regimens for HIV-1 infections

Presently, there are three main classes of drugs available for treatment and /or suppression of HIV infection:

- **Nucleoside reverse transcriptase inhibitors (NRTIs)** are analogues of DNA building blocks which must be phosphorylated by the body before they become active. During replication, the reverse transcription enzyme may insert NRTIs instead of natural DNA bases and terminate transcription; in this way, NRTIs prevent HIV from copying its genetic information and replicating. NRTI's include AZT (retrovir), which was the first ever anti-HIV drug. When first used on its own, AZT had serious side effects. Now it is used in much lower doses in combination with other drugs. Other NRTIs include lamivudine, abacavir, zidovudine, tenofovir, and stavudine.

- **Non-nucleoside reverse transcriptase inhibitors (NNRTIs)** have a similar mode of action to NRTIs. They include efavirenz, nevirapine, delaviridine, and etravirine.

- **Protease inhibitors (PIs)** prevent the virus from assembling correctly before leaving CD4 cells. They include saquinavir, nelfinavir, and ritonavir.

CLINICAL CORRELATION 11.3

HLA-B*57:01 and HIV

- Abacavir is associated with a severe hypersensitivity reaction in some HLA-B*57:01 individuals. Screening is now becoming increasingly common before deciding on a particular course of antiretoviral therapy.

■ **HLA-B*5701 is much more common in whites—the incidence is 5–8%, as compared with <1% in Asian or sub-Saharan African individuals.**

New classes of antiretroviral drug

The new classes of antiretroviral drugs include HIV fusion inhibitors and integrase inhibitors.

- **Fusion inhibitors** work by attaching themselves to proteins on the surface of T cells or proteins on the surface of HIV particles and prevent HIV binding to T cells and consequently from entering the cell. Currently there is only one fusion inhibitor approved by the U.S. Food and Drug Authority: enfuvirtide (Fuzeon, T-20). This drug targets the gp41 protein on the surface of HIV. Some experimental drugs target proteins on T cells: ibalizumab (TNX-355) targets the CD4 protein, and vicriviroc and maraviroc (Celsentri) target the CCR5 protein. These drugs are designed to prevent HIV infection of CD4 cells by blocking the receptors recognized by the virus.

- **Integrase inhibitors**, on the other hand, work by inhibiting integration of the viral DNA (after the action of the viral reverse transcriptase to convert RNA to DNA). There is apparently no functional equivalent of this enzyme in human cells.

Immune-based therapies

Other treatment options may include immune-based therapies using interleukin-2 (IL-2). This naturally occurring cytokine boosts CD4 production and hence strengthens the immune response. Clinical trials are under way investigating the long-term effect of IL-2 therapy.

Drug resistance

The HIV-1 virus shows great heterogeneity both phenotypically and genotypically. During HIV-1 replication, reverse transcriptase encoded by the virus makes a RNA:DNA hybrid from which a double-stranded DNA copy is generated. However, as the HIV-1 RT enzyme lacks 3′ activity, errors made during transcription cannot be repaired. As the virus replicates, variants may appear which can survive and replicate despite ART, i.e. the virus becomes 'resistant'. In patients taking ART, pre-existing drug-resistant strains of the virus confer a selective advantage, and assuming replicative fitness, they may rapidly predominate and become resistant to ART.

Two main techniques are available to identify drug-resistant strains of HIV-1: phenotypic resistance and genotypic resistance.

Phenotypic resistance

Phenotypic testing is a direct measure of drug resistance, whereby the patient's virus is cultured in the presence of antiretroviral drugs and the ability of the virus to replicate is measured. This procedure can be time-consuming, as the virus must be cultured *in vitro*. However, amplifying key portions of the genes within the patient's virus and inserting them into a laboratory strain of HIV deficient in those genes allows the production of a laboratory strain of HIV which is genetically identical to the patient's virus. The ability of the virus to grow in the presence of antiretroviral drugs is compared to that of a completely susceptible strain of the virus. One particular benefit of phenotypic testing is that combinations of drugs may be tested in combination or in parallel, and it mimics the situation *in vivo*.

Genotypic resistance

Genotypic resistance testing involves analysing the viral genotype to determine the arrangement of nucleotides in the virus' genome. When a mutation occurs in the virus which alters the coding for a particular amino acid, this may affect the viral susceptibility to ART.

There are two main types of resistance testing: sequencing assays and point mutation assays or LiPAs. Both methods look for mutations at specific locations within the protease and reverse transcriptase enzymes of the viral RNA. Sequencing involves determining the nucleotide order of the amplified RT-PCR product and hence the amino acids encoded for, whereas LiPAs identify only a limited selection of mutation-associated changes in the genome.

Differences detected in the viral genome are compared with those known to be associated with drug resistance. If a particular mutation is found in the reverse transcription enzyme, for example, this could mean that the virus is not susceptible to the antiretroviral drug targeting this part of the genome. This enables the clinician to prescribe only drugs to which the patient is susceptible. Mixed viral populations may also be detected, suggesting emerging resistance.

The commercial sequencing assays generally have integral software packages with which the patient's HIV viral sequence can be compared, which highlights the currently known resistance-associated mutations and the viral susceptibility or lack of/ resistance to particular antiretrovirals. Databases are also available on the internet, such as the Stanford University database, with which viral sequences can be compared to determine whether a certain mutation confers resistance to a particular antiretroviral. These databases are continually developing to keep up with novel observations regarding resistance. Future genotyping tests will need to remain up to date with the newly developed antiretrovirals and look for resistance to integrase inhibitors, etc.

CLINICAL CORRELATION 11.4

Testing guidelines for HIV resistance

The Current European Resistance Testing Guidelines, published in *AIDS* (2001;15:309–320) suggest testing in the following circumstances:

- **Treatment-naive patients**, especially if transmission is suspected from an antiretroviral 'experienced' individual.

- **Chronic infection,** especially where transmission rates are high, as evidenced by high viral loads.

- **Post-exposure**—if a sample from the index case is available, this may be tested, although ART may be initiated before obtaining an HIV-genotype.

- **Virological failure,** i.e. where the viral load is increasing despite ART.

- **Pregnancy**—if the mother has a detectable viral load.

- **Paediatrics**—in infants with detectable viraemia.

Cross reference

The 2009 update of the European HIV Drug Resistance Guidelines is available online at http://www.europeanaidsclinicalsociety.org/

Sequencing assays can also be used to determine the clade (or subtype) of infecting virus and this can be useful in determining the likely origin of that strain of virus.

Why is it so important to ensure that antiretroviral drugs are taken at regular intervals/consistently, and that missed doses are avoided?

HIV tropism measurement

As mentioned above, HIV-1 gains entry to $CD4^+$ cells by binding to the CD4 receptor and the co-receptors CXCR4 or CCR5. Some patients are infected with a strain of HIV-1 which preferentially uses either the CCR5 or CXCR4 receptor or a combination of both, and this is referred to as the virus's 'tropism'.

Assays are available to determine viral tropism. HIV particles constructed from the patient's envelope protein are cultured in the presence of cells expressing CXCR4 or CCR5. These viral constructs or vectors are also encoded with the gene for the bioluminescent molecule luciferase. On infecting a cell and replicating, the luciferase is released, and can be quantified.

A knowledge of viral trophism is important in identifying which patients may benefit from treatment with CCR5 antagonists.

CASE STUDY 11.1 *Grievous bodily harm*

A couple (A & B) in a long-term relationship attend two separate sexual health clinics for HIV tests in June 2004. Both state that the test results are negative for HIV.

Several months later, A attends the local hospital Emergency Department complaining of severe flu-like symptoms, night sweats, and an unusual skin rash. The symptoms are consistent with HIV seroconversion illness; A is tested again for HIV and found to be HIV-positive. A insists on having had no sexual relationships with anyone other than partner B.

When B had a second HIV test, it was also found to be positive. On reviewing the couple's HIV test results from June 2004 it was found that B had in fact tested HIV-positive on initial screening. It was suggested that B had lied to A about HIV status and was the source of A's seroconversion illness. B denied this. A then accused B of grievous bodily harm.

Questions

What blood tests would you perform to confirm HIV infection?

What other tests could you perform to confirm HIV infection?

Why might A's HIV antibody test be negative at the time of seroconversion?

What tests could you perform to determine the origin of A's HIV infection?

11.9 **Prevention of HIV transmission and infection**

From recent epidemiological data, it is clear that new diagnoses are not falling, and indeed new diagnoses in Europe now outnumber deaths from AIDS, meaning that the numbers of people living with HIV is increasing, with major implications for health care, economic growth, cost, and suffering.

Novel methods of preventing both infection and disease progression are therefore necessary. Behavioural changes including circumcision, microbicides, and prophylactic drugs and vaccines have all been considered.

Vaccines

Special challenges for a successful HIV vaccine are due to HIV integration, HIV variation, and its early harm to the immune system. These factors make the challenge of an HIV vaccine uniquely difficult compared to past successful vaccines.

Potential vaccines are being considered, developed and put into trial which

- reduce susceptibility to infection (prophylactic vaccines)
- slow disease progression (therapeutic vaccines)
- reduce infectivity and therefore make transmission less likely.

A prophylactic vaccine should offer sterilizing cross-protective immunity to all the different clades of virus that are circulating. It should be safe, effective, and cheap. Current vaccines in trials include some designed to induce humoral immunity (antibodies) only, some designed to induce HIV-specific cell-mediated responses alone, and some designed to produce both. Many small phase I trials have been performed or are being undertaken; only two large trials have been performed, and neither has shown the vaccine to be effective.

Few therapeutic vaccine trials (with or without other immunomodulatory therapy) have been carried out. Some hopeful, although relatively short-lived, responses have been observed, and it seems certain that such novel therapy will be most appropriate in individuals already receiving successful ART.

The possibility of modifying disease with a vaccine which, although not offering sterilizing immunity, may allow extra years of disease-free, ART-free life for the patient, and may also have an impact on the infectivity of the HIV-positive individual, is exciting. It has been predicted that the numbers of new infections averted in 15 years could range from 5.5 million to 28 million from the most modest scenario (30% efficacy and 20% coverage) to the most optimistic (70% efficacy and 40% coverage).

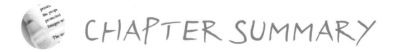 CHAPTER SUMMARY

- HIV-1 infection is the most common cause of immunodeficiency and continues to be a major problem throughout the world.

- As yet there is no cure, though disease progression can be slowed significantly by the use of ART.

- The ultimate goal is to eradicate the disease by production of a vaccine which protects against all the clades of virus and is realistic/practical for use in the developing world.

- Diagnosis relies on the detection of antibodies and/or viral proteins, usually by ELISA, although some rapid tests are available which can prove particularly useful in the developing world.

- Prognosis is generally worse for those individuals with high viral loads and low CD4 counts.

- Response to treatment is determined by monitoring CD4 count and viral load.

- Failure to control the adverse effects on the immune system, as seen by decreasing CD4 count and increasing viral load, may suggest treatment failure (developing resistance) or poor patient compliance; the former can be determined by genotypic and phenotypic resistance testing.

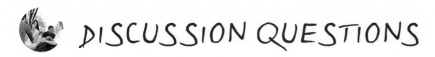

DISCUSSION QUESTIONS

11.1 How can you test for HIV?

11.2 Do the current methods for HIV also detect HIV-2?

11.3 What do you understand by the term 'seroconversion'?

11.4 What symptoms might you expect to see during seroconversion?

11.5 What do you understand by the term 'long-term nonprogressor'?

11.6 How can you monitor disease progression and/or therapy efficacy?

11.7 How can you determine why a treatment regimen is failing?

11.8 If no resistance mutations are detected, why else might ART be failing?

11.9 Why do you think there is no effective HIV-1 vaccine?

Answers to these questions are provided in the book's Online Resource Centre; visit www.oxfordtextbooks.co.uk/orc/ahmed/

References

Chapter 2

Beetham R (2000) Detection of Bence Jones protein in practice. *Ann Clin Biochem*, **37**, 563–570.

Brouet JC, *et al.* (1974) Biologic and clinical significance of cryoglobulins. A report of 86 cases. *Am J Med*, **57**, 775–788.

Dierlamm T, *et al.* (2002) IgM myeloma: A report of four cases. *Ann Hematol*, **81**, 136–139.

Ferri C, Zignego AL, Pileri SA (2002) Cryoglobulins. *J Clin Pathol*, **55**, 4–13.

Vladutiu AO (2000) Immunoglobulin D: Properties, measurement and clinical relevance. *Clin Diagn Lab Immunol*, **3**, 131–140.

Chapter 4

Agostoni A, Cicardi M (1992) Hereditary and acquired C1-inhibitor deficiency: Biological and clinical characteristics in 235 patients. *Medicine*, **71**, 206.

Bowden DW, Rising M, Akots G, *et al.* (1986) Homogeneous, liposome-based assay for total complement activity in serum. *Clin Chem*, **32**, 275.

Canova-Davis E, Redemann CT, Vollmer YP, Kung VT (1986) Use of a reversed-phase evaporation vesicle formulation for a homogeneous liposome immunoassay. *Clin Chem*, **32**, 1687.

Cicardi M, Beretta A, Colombo M, *et al.* (1996) Relevance of lymphoproliferative disorders and of anti-C1 inhibitor autoantibodies in acquired angio-oedema. *Clin Exp Immunol*, **106**, 475.

Colten HR, Rosen FS (1992) Complement deficiencies. *Annu Rev Immunol*, **10**, 809.

Daha MR, Fearon DT, Austen KF (1976) C3 nephritic factor (C3NeF): Stabilization of fluid phase and cell-bound alternative pathway convertase. *J Immunol*, **116**, 1.

Davis AE (1988) 3rd C1 inhibitor and hereditary angioneurotic edema. *Annu Rev Immunol*, **6**, 595.

Davis AE (1989) Hereditary and acquired deficiencies of C1 inhibitor. *Immunodeficiency Rev*, **1**, 207.

Davis AE, Aulak KS, Zahedi K, Bissler JJ, Harrison RA (1993a) C1 inhibitor. *Meth Enzymol*, **223**, 97.

Davis AE, Bissler JJ, Cicardi M (1993b) Mutations in the C1 inhibitor gene that result in hereditary angioneurotic edema. *Behring Inst Mitt*, **93**, 313.

Ebanks RO, Jaikaran AS, Carroll MC, *et al.* (1992) A single arginine to tryptophan interchange at beta-chain residue 458 of human complement component C4 accounts for the defect in classical pathway C5 convertase activity of allotype C4A6. Implications for the location of a C5 binding site in C4. *J Immunol*, **148**, 2803.

Egan LJ, Orren A, Doherty J, Wurzner R, McCarthy CF (1994) Hereditary deficiency of the seventh component of complement and recurrent meningococcal infection: Investigations in an Irish family using a novel haemolytic screening assay for complement activity and C7 M/N allotyping. *Epidemiol Infect*, **113**, 275.

Figueroa J, Andreoni J, Densen P (1993) Complement deficiency states and meningococcal disease. *Immunol Res*, **12**, 295.

Frank MM, Gelfand JA, Atkinson JP (1976) Hereditary angioedema: The clinical syndrome and its management. *Ann Intern Med*, **84**, 580.

Goldberg B, Lad P, Ghekierre L, Wolde-Tsadik G (1997) Comparison between assays for complement fragments and total hemolytic complement in the routine assessment of complement activation. *J Clin Ligand Assay*, **20**, 212.

Gotze O (1986) In Rother K, Till GO (eds) *The Complement System*, p. 154. Springer, Heidelberg.

Holmskov U, Malhotra R, Sim RB, Jensenius JC (1994) Collectins: Collagenous C-type lectins of the innate immune defense system. *Immunol Today*, **15**, 67.

Janatova J, Tack BF (1981) Fourth component of human complement: Studies of an amine-sensitive site comprised of a thiol component. *Biochemistry*, **20**, 2394.

Kozono H, Kinoshita T, Kim, YU, *et al.* (1990) Localization of the covalent C3b-binding site on C4b within the complement classical pathway C5 convertase, C4b2a3b. *J Biol Chem*, **265**, 14444.

Lachmann, PJ (1991) The control of homologous lysis. *Immunol Today*, **12**, 312.

Lachmann PJ, Hughes-Jones NC (1984) Initiation of complement activation. *Semin Immunopathol*, **7**, 143.

Lambris JD (1988) The multifunctional role of C-3, the third component of complement. *Immunol Today*, **9**, 387.

Law SK, Dodds AW (1990) C3, C4 and C5: The thioester site. *Biochem Soc Trans*, **18**, 1155.

Mandle R, Baron C, Roux E, *et al.* (1994) Acquired Cl inhibitor deficiency as a result of an autoantibody to the reactive center region of Cl inhibitor. *J Immunol*, **152**, 4680.

Morgan BP, Harris CL (1999) *Complement regulatory proteins*. Academic Press, London.

Morgan BP, Orren, A (1998) Vaccination against meningococcus in complement-deficient individuals. *Clin Exp Immunol*, **114**, 327.

Morgan BP, Walport MJ (1991) Complement deficiency and disease. *Immunol Today*, **12**, 301.

Reid KB (1986) Activation and control of the complement system. *Essays Biochem*, **22**, 27.

Reid KB, Day AJ (1989) Structure–function relationships of the complement components. *Immunol Today*, **10**, 177.

Reid KB, Turner MW (1994) Mammalian lectins in activation and clearance mechanisms involving the complement system. *Semin Immunopathol*, **15**, 307.

Schreiber RD, Muller-Eberhard HJ (1974) Fourth component of human complement: Description of a three polypeptide chain structure. *J Exp Med*, **140**, 1324.

Strife CF, Leahy AE, West CD (1989) Antibody to a cryptic solid phase C1q antigen in membranoproliferativenephritis. *Kidney Int*, **35**, 836.

Turner MW (1991) Deficiency of mannan binding protein—a new complement deficiency syndrome. *Clin Exp Immunol* **86** (Suppl 1), 53.

Waytes, AT, Rosen, FS and Frank, MM (1996) Treatment of hereditary angioedema with a vapor-heated C1 inhibitor concentrate. *N Engl J Med*, **334**, 1630.

Wener, MH, Uwatoko, S and Mannik, M (1989) Antibodies to the collagen-like region of C1q in sera of patients with autoimmune rheumatic diseases. *Arth Rheum*, **32**, 544.

Wisnieski JJ, Naff GB (1989) Serum IgG antibodies to C1q in hypocomplementemic urticarial vasculitis syndrome. *Arthritis Rheum*, **32**, 1119.

Wisnieski JJ, Baer AN, Christensen J, et al. (1995) Hypocomplementemic urticarial vasculitis syndrome. Clinical and serologic findings in 18 patients. *Medicine*, **74**, 24.

Wurzner R, Mollnes TE, Morgan BP (1997) In Johnstone AP, Turner MW (eds) *Immunochemistry 2*, p. 197. IRL Press, Oxford.

Yamamoto S, Kubotsu K, Kida M, et al. (1995) Automated homogeneous liposome-based assay system for total complement activity. *Clin Chem*, **41**, 586.

Zwirner J, Wittig A, Kremmer E, Gotze O (1998) A novel ELISA for the evaluation of the classical pathway of complement. *J Immunol Meth*, **211**, 183.

Chapter 5

Casciola-Rosen L, Nagaraju K, Plotz P, et al. (2005) Enhanced autoantigen expression in regenerating muscle cells in idiopathic inflammatory myopathy. *J Exp Med*, **201**, 591–601.

Nielen MM, van Schaardenburg D, Reesink HW, et al. (2004) Specific autoantibodies precede the symptoms of rheumatoid arthritis: A study of serial measurements in blood donors. *Arthritis Rheum*, **50**, 380–386.

Rantapää-Dahlqvist S, de Jong BA, Berglin E, et al. (2003) Antibodies against cyclic citrullinated peptide and IgA rheumatoid factor predict the development of rheumatoid arthritis. *Arthritis Rheum*, **48**, 2741–2749.

Stolt P, Bengtsson C, Nordmark B, et al. (2003) Quantification of the influence of cigarette smoking on rheumatoid arthritis: Results from a population based case-control study, using incident cases. *Ann Rheum Dis*, **62**, 835–841.

Suber TL, Casciola-Rosen L, Rosen A (2008) Mechanisms of disease: Autoantigens as clues to the pathogenesis of myositis. *Nat Clin Pract Rheumatol*, **4**(4), 201–209.

Chapter 6

Csernok E, et al. (2004) Evaluation of capture ELISA for the detection of antineutrophil cytoplasmic antibodies directed against proteinase 3 in Wegener's granulomatosis: First results from a multicentre study. *Rheumatology*, **43**, 174–180.

Esnault VLM (2002) Apoptosis: the central actor in the three hits that trigger antineutrophil cytoplasmic antibody related systemic vasculitic. *Nephrol Dial Transplant*, **17**, 1725–1728.

Holle J, et al. (2005) Variations in performance characteristics of commercial enzyme immunoassay kits for detection of antineutrophil cytoplasmic antibodies: What is the optimal cut off? *Ann Rheum Dis*, **64**, 1773–1779.

Popa ER, et al. (2002) *Staphylococcus aureus* and Wegener's granulomatosis. *Arthritis Res*, **4**, 77–79.

Popa ER, et al. (2003) Staphylococcal superantigens and T cell expansions in Wegener's granulomatosis. *Clin Exp Immunol*, **132**(3), 496–504.

Thomas R, et al. (2005) Wegener's granulomatosis presenting as multiple staphylococcal lung abscesses. *Respir Med Extra*, **1**, 43–46.

Chapter 8

Berg PA, Klein R (1986) Mitochondrial antigens and autoantibodies: From anti-M1 to anti-M9. *Klin Wochenschr*, **64**(19), 897–909.

Boberg K, Aadland E, Jahsen J, Raknerud N, Stiris M, Bell H (1998) Incidence and prevalence of primary biliary cirrhosis, primary sclerosing cholangitis and autoimmune hepatitis in a Norwegian population. *Scand J Gastroenterol*, **33**, 99–103.

Bogdanos DP, Baum H, Grasso A, et al. (2004) Microbial mimics are major targets of cross reactivity with human pyruvate dehydrogenase in primary biliary cirrhosis. *J Hepatol*, **40**, 31–39.

Bottazzo GF, Florin-Christensen A, Fairfax A, et al. (1976) Classification of smooth muscle antibodies detected by immunofluorescence. *J Clin Pathol*, **29**, 403–410.

Donaldson PT, Baragiotta A, Heneghan M, et al. (2006) HLA class II alleles, genotype and amino acids in primary biliary cirrhosis: A large scale study. *Hepatology*, **44**, 667–674.

Field JJ, Heathcote EJ (2003) Epidemiology of autoimmune liver disease. *J Gastroenterol Hepatol*, **18**, 1118–1128.

Gregorio GV, Davies ET, Mieli-Vergani G, Vergani D (1995) Significance of extractable nuclear antigens in childhood autoimmune liver disease. *Clin Exp Immunol*, **102**, 308–313.

Gregorio GV, Portmann B, Karani J, *et al.* (2001) Autoimmune hepatitis/sclerosing cholangitis overlap syndrome in childhood: A 16-year prospective study. *Hepatology*, **33**, 544–553.

Ingelman-Sundberg M, Daly AK, Oscarson M, Nebert DW (2000) Human cytochrome P450 (CYP) genes: Recommendations for nomenclature of alleles. *Pharmacogenet Genom*, **10**, 91–93.

Liu HY, Deng AM, Zhou Y, Yao DK, Xu DX, Zhong RQ (2006) Analysis of HLA alleles polymorphism in Chinese patients with primary biliary cirrhosis. *Hepatobiliary Pancreat Dis Int*, **5**, 129–132.

Manns M, Gerken G, Kyriatsoulis A, Staritz M, Meyer zum Büschenfelde KH (1987) Characterisation of a new subgroup of autoimmune chronic active hepatitis by autoantibodies against a soluble liver antigen. *Lancet* **i** (8528), 292–294.

Mieli-Vergani G, Vergani D (2008) Autoimmune paediatric liver disease. *World J Gastroenterol*, **14**, 3360–3367.

Muratori P, Muratori L, Ferrari R, *et al.* (2003) Characterization and clinical impact of anti-nuclear antibodies in primary biliary cirrhosis. *Am J Gastroenterol*, **98**, 431–437.

Rizzetto M, Swana G, Doniach D (1973) Microsomal antibodies in active chronic hepatitis and other disorders. *Clin Exp Immunol*, **15**, 331–344.

Stechemesser E, Klein R, Berg PA (1993) Characterisation and clinical relevance of liver-pancreas antibodies in autoimmune hepatitis. *Hepatology*, **18**, 1–9.

Vergani D, Alvarez F, Bianchi F, *et al.* (2004) Liver autoimmune serology: A consensus statement from the committee for autoimmune serology of the International Autoimmune Hepatitis Group. *J Hepatol*, **41**, 677–683.

Chapter 9

Bataller L, Wade DF, Graus F, *et al.* (2004) Antibodies to Zic4 in paraneoplastic neurologic disorders and small-cell lung cancer. *Neurology*, **62**, 778–782.

Bernal F, Shams'ili S, Rojas I, *et al.* (2003) Anti-Tr antibodies as markers of paraneoplastic cerebellar degeneration and Hodgkin's disease. *Neurology*, **60**, 230–234.

Brain WR, Daniel PM, Greenfield JG (1951) Subacute cortical cerebellar degeneration and its relation to carcinoma. *J Neurol Neurosurg Psychiat*, **14**, 59–75.

Chan KH, Vernino S, Lennon VA (2001) ANNA-3 anti-neuronal nuclear antibody: marker of lung cancer-related autoimmunity. *Ann Neurol*, **50**, 301–311.

Dalmau J, Bataller L (2006). Clinical and immunological diversity of limbic encephalitis: A model for paraneoplastic neurological disorder. *Hematol Oncol Clin North Am*, **20**, 1319–1335.

Dalmau JO, Posner JB (1999) Paraneoplastic syndromes. *Arch Neurol*, **56**, 405–408.

Dalmau J, Graus F, Villarejo A, *et al.* (2004) Clinical analysis of anti-Ma2-associated encephalitis. *Brain*, **127**, 1831–1844.

Dalmau J, Gleichman AJ, Hughes EG, *et al.* (2008) Anti-NMDA-receptor encephalitis: Case series and analysis of the effects of antibodies. *Lancet Neurol*, **7**, 1091–1098.

European Federation of Neurological Societies/Peripheral Nerve Society (2006) Guideline on management of paraproteinemic demyelinating neuropathies. Report of a joint task force of the European Federation of Neurological Societies and the Peripheral Nerve Society. *J Peripher Nerv Syst*, **11**, 9–19.

Giometto B, Taraloto B, Graus F (1999). Autoimmunity in paraneoplastic neurological syndromes. *Brain Pathol*, **9**, 261–273.

Graus F, Cordon-Cardo C, Posner JB (1985) Neuronal antinuclear antibody in sensory neuropathy from lung cancer. *Neurology*, **35**, 538–543.

Graus F, Rowe G, Fueyo J, Darnell RB, Dalmau, J (1993) The neuronal nuclear antigen recognized by the human anti-Ri autoantibody is expressed in central but not peripheral nervous system neurons. *Neurosci Lett*, **150**, 212–214.

Graus F, Dalmau J, Valldeoriola F, *et al.* (1997) Immunological characterization of a neuronal antibody (anti-Tr) associated with paraneoplastic cerebellar degeneration and Hodgkin's disease. *J Neuroimmunol*, **74**, 55–61.

Graus F, Keime-Guibert F, Rene R, *et al.* (2001) Anti-Hu-associated paraneoplastic encephalomyelitis: Analysis of 200 patients. *Brain*, **124**, 1138–1148.

Graus F, Delattre JY, Antoine JC, *et al.* (2004) Recommended diagnostic criteria for paraneoplastic neurological syndromes. *J Neurol Neurosurg Psychiat*, **75**, 1135–1140.

Graus F, Vincent A, Pozo-Rosich P, Sabater L, Saiz A, Lang B, Dalmau J (2005). Anti-glial nuclear antibody: Marker of lung cancer-related paraneoplastic neurological syndromes. *J Neuroimmunol.* **165**(1–2), 166–171.

Grulich AE, van Leeuwen MT, Falster MO, Vajdic CM (2007) Incidence of cancers in people with HIV/AIDS compared with immunosuppressed transplant recipients: A meta-analysis. *Lancet*, **370**, 59–67.

Gultekin AH, Rosenfeld MR, Voltz R, *et al.* (2000) Paraneoplastic limbic encephalitis: Neurological symptoms, immunological findings and tumour association in 50 patients. *Brain*, **23**, 1481–1494.

Honnorat J, Antoine JC, Derrington E, Aguera M, Belin MF (1996) Antibodies to a subpopulation of glial cells and a 66 kDa developmental protein in patients with paraneoplastic neurological syndromes. *J Neurol Neurosurg Psychiatry*, **61**, 270–278.

Juel VC, Massey JM (2007) Myasthenia gravis. *Orphanet J Rare Dis*, **2**, 44.

Karim AR, Hughes RC, Winer JB, Williams AC, Bradwell AR (2005) Paraneoplastic neurological antibodies: A laboratory experience. *Ann N Y Acad Sci*, **1050**, 274–285.

Karim AR, Hughes RG, El-Lahawi M, Bradwell AR (2007) Paraneoplastic neurological antibodies: Purkinje cell cytoplasm. In Shoenfeld Y, Gershwin E, Meroni PL (eds)

Textbook of Autoantibodies, 2nd edition, pp. 637–643. Elsevier, New York.

Lai M, Hughes EG, Peng X, *et al.* (2009) AMPA receptor antibodies in limbic encephalitis alter synaptic receptor location. *Ann Neurol*, **65**, 424–434.

Leite MI, Jacob S, Viegas S, Cossins J, Clover L, Morgan B Paul, Beeson D, Willcox N, and Vincent A (2008) IgGI antibodies to acetylcholine receptors in 'seronegative' myasthenia gravis. *Brain* 2008.

Lennon VA, Wingerchuk DM, Kryzer TJ, *et al.* (2004) A serum autoantibody marker of neuromyelitis optica: Distinction from multiple sclerosis. *Lancet*, **364**, 2106–2112.

Meinck HM, Thompson PD (2002) Stiff man syndrome and related conditions. *Mov Disord*, **17**, 853–866.

Moll JWB, Antoine JC, Brashear HR, *et al.* (1995) Guidelines on the detection of paraneoplastic anti-neuronal-specific antibodies: Report from the Workshop to the Fourth Meeting of the International Society of Neuro-Immunology on paraneoplastic neurological disease, held October 22–23, 1994, in Rotterdam, The Netherlands. *Neurology*, **45**, 1937–41.

Pittock SJ, Lucchinetti CF, Lennon VA (2003) Anti-neuronal nuclear autoantibody type 2: Paraneoplastic accompaniments. *Ann Neurol*, **53**, 580–587.

Pittock SJ, Kryzer TJ, Lennon VA (2004) Paraneoplastic antibodies coexist and predict cancer, not neurological syndrome. *Ann Neurol*, **56**, 609–610.

Pittock SJ, Lucchinetti CF, Parisi JE, *et al.* (2005) Amphiphysin autoimmunity: Paraneoplastic accompaniments. *Ann Neurol*, **58**, 96–107.

Rees JH (2004) Paraneoplastic syndromes: When to suspect, how to confirm, and how to manage. *J Neurol Neurosurg Psychiatry* **75** (suppl II), ii43–ii50.

Roberts WK, Darnell RB (2004) Neuroimmunology of the paraneoplastic neurological degenerations. *Curr Opin Immunol*, **6**, 616–622.

Rosenfeld MR, Eichen JG, Wade DF, Posner JB, Dalmau J (2001) Molecular and clinical diversity in paraneoplastic immunity to Ma proteins. *Ann Neurol*, **50**, 339–348.

Rossinol T, Graus F (2008) Paraneoplastic syndromes. In Shoenfeld Y, Cervera R, Gershwin ME (eds) *Diagnostic Criteria in Autoimmune Diseases*. Springer, New York.

Sabater L, Titulaer M, Saiz A, *et al.* (2008) SOX1 antibodies are markers of paraneoplastic Lambert–Eaton myasthenic syndrome. *Neurology*, **70**, 924–928.

Saiz A, Blanco Y, Sabater L, *et al.* (2008) Spectrum of neurological syndromes associated with glutamic acid decarboxylase antibodies: Diagnostic clues for this association. *Brain*, **131**, 2553–2563.

Shams'ili S, Grefkens J, de Leeuw B, *et al.* (2003) Paraneoplastic cerebellar degeneration associated with antineuronal antibodies: Analysis of 50 patients. *Brain*, **126**, 1409–1418.

Sillevis Smitt P, Kinoshita A, De Leeuw B, *et al.* (2000) Paraneoplastic cerebellar ataxia due to autoantibodies against a glutamate receptor. *N Engl J Med*, **342**, 21–27.

Swann JB, Smyth MJ (2007) Immune surveillance of tumours. *J Clin Invest*, **117**, 1137–1146.

Tan KM, Lennon VA, Klein CJ, Boeve BF, Pittock SJ (2008) Clinical spectrum of voltage-gated potassium channel autoimmunity. *Neurology*, **70**, 1883–1890.

Vedeler CA, Antoine JC, Giometto B, *et al.* (2006) Management of paraneoplastic neurological syndromes: Report of an EFNS Task Force. *Eur J Neurol*, **13**, 682–690.

Vernino S, Lennon VA (2000) New Purkinje cell antibody (PCA-2): Marker of lung cancer-related neurological autoimmunity. *Ann Neurol*, **47**, 297–305.

Vincent A (2008) Autoimmune disorders of the neuromuscular junction. *Neurol India*, **56**, 305–313.

Yu Z, Kryzer TJ, Griesmann K, *et al.* (2001) CRMP-5 neuronal autoantibody: Marker of lung cancer and thymoma-related autoimmunity. *Ann Neurol*, **49**, 146–154.

Chapter 11

Quillent C, Oberlin E, Braun J, *et al.* (1998) HIV-1-resistance phenotype conferred by combination of two separate inherited mutations of CCR5 gene. *Lancet*, **351**, 14–18.

Libert F, Cochaux P, Beckman G, *et al.* (1998) The deltaccr5 mutation conferring protection against HIV-1 in Caucasian populations has a single and recent origin in Northeastern Europe. *Hum Mol Genet*, **7**, 399–406.

Glossary

Adaptive immunity The immunity that is acquired following sensitization with antigens.

Aetiology The cause or origin of disease.

Alleles Variations of a single genetic locus.

Allergens Antigens that induce immune responses which cause allergy.

Allergy A hypersensitivity reaction initiated by immunological mechanisms.

Allotypes Allelic polymorphisms in a gene that can be determined using specific antibodies for the gene product.

Alternative pathway The complement pathway that provides a rapid, antibody-independent route for activation and amplification of complement on foreign surfaces.

Antibodies Antigen-specific proteins that are produced by B lymphocytes in response to exposure to the antigen.

Antibody excess The state in an antibody/antigen mixture where the concentration of antibody exceeds that of antigen.

Antigen excess The state in an antibody/antigen mixture where the concentration of antigen exceeds that of antibody.

Antigens Protein molecules recognized by the immune system as foreign and against which the immune system specifically reacts.

Antisera Antibodies that are targeted against a specific antigen. Often used to identify antigens in immunological assays such as ELISA or indirect immunofluorescence (IIF).

APECED Autoimmune polyendocrinopathy, candidiasis, ectodermal dystrophy.

Apoptosis Programmed cell death.

Atopy A genetic predisposition to produce prolonged IgE antibody responses to commonly occurring allergens.

Autoantigen A self-antigen that is the target of an immune response, such as in autoimmune disease.

Autoimmune disease (autoimmunity) Breakdown of tolerance, resulting in production of antibodies and/or T-cells directed against own cells and tissues.

Bence Jones proteins Monoclonal light chains found in the urine of patients with renal failure; named after the English physician Henry Bence Jones (1813–1873), who described some of their physicochemical properties in 1847.

Calcinosis The formation of tiny deposits of calcium in the skin.

Cationic Referring to a positively charged molecule.

Cell-mediated immunity (cellular immunity) Immune response mediated by cells such as T lymphocytes.

Cerebellar degeneration Damage to the cerebellum with loss of muscle control and balance.

Cholangiography Imaging of the biliary tract.

Cirrhosis Irreversible change in liver tissue that results in the degeneration of functioning liver cells and their replacement with fibrous connective tissue.

Citrullinated proteins Citrullination is the post-translational modification of arginine within a protein to citrulline by enzymes called PADs (peptidylarginine deiminases) to form citrullinated proteins.

Class switch recombination The process by which a B cell upon recognition of antigen will switch the production of immunoglobulin from IgM alone to other isotypes, e.g. IgG and IgA.

Classical pathway The complement pathway that is triggered by antibody bound to particulate antigen. Many other substances, including components of damaged cells, bacterial lipopolysaccharide, and nucleic acids can also trigger the classical pathway in an antibody-independent manner.

Clusters of differentiation (CD) Cell surface molecules on lymphocytes that are recognized by monoclonal antibodies to allow identification of the cell by flow cytometry.

Complement A group of blood proteins that enhance the immune response.

Complementarity determining region (CDR) A short amino acid sequence found in the variable region of an immunoglobulin.

Conjugate The term generally used to describe an immunoglobulin that has a marker attached, such as an immunofluorescent label or an enzyme. These immunoglobulins are used to label human antibodies in techniques such as indirect immunofluorescence or ELISA.

Continuing professional development (CPD) is a process of lifelong learning, which enables you to expand and fulfil your personal and professional potential, as well as meet the present and future needs of patients and deliver health outcomes and priorities. It assures that you meet the requisite knowledge and skills levels that relate to your evolving scope of professional practice (www.IBMS.org).

CREST syndrome A limited form of scleroderma, consisting of calcinosis (calcium deposits), Raynaud's phenomenon (a vascular defect), oesophangeal motility problems causing difficulty with swallowing, sclerodactyly (enlarged swollen fingers), and telangiectasia (a defect of surface blood vessels in the skin).

Crithidia lucilae A microorganism with a kinetoplast that contains only double stranded DNA. Commercial preparations of this organism are available for test purposes.

Cryoglobulin Abnormal immunoglobulins (IgG or IgM) that precipitate when serum is cooled.

Cytokines Proteins produced by cells of the immune system that act as regulatory proteins and intercellular mediators facilitating the immune response.

Densitometry The quantitative measurement of optical density.

Encephalomyelitis Inflammation of both brain (encephalitis) and spinal cord (myelitis).

Endocytosis The process by which a cell ingests material with the formation of vesicles. Includes phagocytosis and pinocytosis.

Enteropathy A disease of the intestinal tract.

Epiphenomenon A secondary symptom that appears during the course of a disease, secondary to the existing disease symptoms.

Epitope The region on an antigen that is recognizable by the immune system.

Fixative a compound (such as ethanol or formaldehyde) that preserves or stabilizes tissues and cells for microscopic study.

Fluorochrome A fluorescent chemical that emits a specific colour when illuminated by light.

Gastritis Inflammation of the stomach lining.

Genotype The genetic constitution of an organism.

Genotyping The process of defining the genotype of an individual using laboratory techniques such as DNA sequencing and PCR. This is useful in determining if an individual has disease-associated genes.

Glomerulonephritis (mPGN) Inflammation of the glomeruli of the kidney.

Grand round A conference in which clinicians/experts present the case studies of individual patients, or new topics in the field of medicine and use this as an educational tool for other staff members.

Granulocytes White blood cells filled with granules, some of which contain enzymes which enable digestion of microorganisms and production of inflammatory responses. Includes neutrophils, eosinophils, and basophils.

Granuloma A mass of immune cells (lymphocytes, macrophages) that accumulates at sites of inflammation, injury, or infection.

Haematemesis Vomiting blood.

Haematuria Blood in urine.

Haemolytic uraemic syndrome (HUS) A deficiency in factor H and factor I can lead to a susceptibility in HUS, which consists of the triad of thrombocytopenia, Coombs negative microangiopathic haemolytic anaemia, and acute renal failure.

Haemoptysis Coughing up blood.

Hapten A complex of a small molecule with a carrier, usually protein.

Hepatitis Inflammation of the hepatocytes in the liver.

Hereditary angioedema (HAE) Genetic mutations resulting in the absence of C1 esterase inhibitor in serum are found in approximately 85% of patients (type I). The remaining 15% of patients have normal or elevated serum concentrations, but the protein produced by one allele is dysfunctional (type II). This clinically results in angioedema.

Heterophile An antibody against an antigen from one species that also reacts against antigens from other species. Often seen in indirect immunofluorescence.

Human leukocyte antigen (HLA) A genetically determined series of markers (antigens) present on human white blood cells (leukocytes) and on tissues that are important in histocompatibility.

Humoral immunity Immune response mediated by B cells and antibodies.

Hypergammaglobulinaemia An increase in serum immunoglobulins.

Hypersensitivity The reaction that causes reproducible signs or symptoms, following exposure to a defined stimulus, in a susceptible individual.

Hyperthyroidism Excessive production of thyroid hormones caused by overactivity of the thyroid gland.

Hypoparathyroidism Underactivity of the parathyroid, the gland that controls calcium levels in both blood and bone.

Hypothyroidism A reduction in the production of thyroid hormones caused by underactivity of the thyroid gland.

Idiopathic Of unknown cause.

Immune complexes Antigen and antibody complexes which can be soluble or insoluble. This depends on the size of the complex and the presence of complement.

Immune paresis Suppression of normal immunoglobulin production by a malignant bone marrow plasma cell clone.

Immunodeficiency Defects in the immune system resulting in gaps in the bodies body's defence against pathogens.

Immunofixation Process in which a specific antibody is used to 'fix' antigens within a gel after electrophoresis by means of the formation of antibody–antigen complexes. After removing unfixed molecules by washing and then staining the fixed complexes, the presence or absence of specific molecules in the original sample can be demonstrated.

Immunological memory is the ability of the immune system to 'recall' a previous encounter with an antigen, resulting in a stronger immunological response.

Immunosuppression A suppression of the immune system with a reduction in number, reactivity, expansion, or differentiation of T and/or B lymphocytes.

Infectious mononucleosis The disease caused by a severe infection of Epstein–Barr virus (EBV). Symptoms include extreme fatigue, fever, sore throat, swollen lymph nodes, and an increase of lymphocytes in the blood. Patients with weakened or suppressed immune systems are at risk of serious complications of infectious mononucleosis.

Inflammation A characteristic physiological response of tissues to injury. The signs of inflammation are heat, redness, swelling, and pain.

Innate immunity The natural immunity that exists prior to sensitization from an antigen. It is often nonspecific.

Lambert–Eaton myasthenic syndrome Muscle weakness, fatigue, difficulty swallowing, and vision changes.

Lectin pathway A means of activation of complement on bacterial and other microorganism surfaces. It is antibody-independent and shares C2, C3, and C4 with the classical pathway, to which it is highly analogous.

Limbic encephalitis Inflammation of the brain leading to memory loss, drowsiness, confusion, disorientation, and seizures.

Lipodystophy The progressive loss of fat. Lipodystrophy may be congenital or acquired, and may affect all of the body (generalized lipodystrophy) or just parts of the body (partial lipodystrophy).

Lupus anticoagulant An autoantibody which interferes with blood coagulation, as well as *in vitro* tests of clotting function, causing elevation in the partial thromboplastin time.

Lymphocytes A type of white blood cell of which there are three subtypes: B cells, which give rise to humoral immunity, and T cells, which give rise to cellular immunity, and Natural killer cells.

Macrocytic anaemia An anaemia in which the red blood cells are larger in volume than normal (increased mean cell volume, MCV).

Macrophages Phagocytic cells found in the tissues that ingest, kill, and digest bacteria, foreign cells, and tissue debris. These cells also play a role in antigen presentation in the immune system.

Major histocompatibility complex (MHC) A group of genes that code for cell-surface histocompatibility antigens and are the principal determinants of tissue type and transplant compatibility.

Membrane attack complex (MAC) A large transmembrane pore formed from the terminal complement components which can cause lysis of the target cell by allowing free diffusion of molecules in and out of the cell.

Membranoproliferative glomerulonephritis (MPGN) A disorder of the kidney caused by immune complex deposition in the glomerular basement membrane. Complement activation results in inflammation of the glomeruli, causing disrupted kidney function, and can progress to chronic renal failure.

Microcytic anaemia An anaemia in which the red blood cells are smaller in volume than normal (reduced mean corpuscular volume, MCV).

Mitosis Division of a somatic cell to form two genetically identical daughter cells.

Monoclonal antibodies Antibodies produced from a single clone of cells, consisting of identical molecules.

Monoclonal gammopathy Disease characterized by the finding of monoclonal immunoglobulin in the serum and/or urine.

Monoclonal gammopathy of undetermined significance (MGUS) Monoclonal gammopathy in which the monoclonal quantification and clinical features do not meet the diagnostic criteria for any specific disease.

Mononuclear cells White blood cells with only one nucleus; includes monocytes and lymphocytes.

Multidisciplinary team A group of professionals (i.e. doctors, nurses, scientists) who meet to discuss individual patients, using the knowledge from each discipline to work towards effective diagnosis and treatments.

Multisystem disease A disease affecting more than one component of the body. An example is rheumatoid arthritis, which can affect the joints, lungs, kidneys, and blood vessels.

Myasthenia gravis Weakness and rapid fatigue of voluntary muscles.

Necrosis Unprogrammed cell death.

Negative selection T-cell recognition of self-antigen in the thymus, resulting in deletion by apoptosis.

Neoantigen A newly acquired and expressed antigen; often present after a cell is infected by an oncogenic virus.

Neuromyotonia Abnormal nerve impulses from peripheral motor neurons causing twitching, stiffness, cramps, and slowed movement.

Neuropathy Disorder of peripheral nervous system involving motor, sensory, and/or autonomic nerves.

Neutrophils Phagocytic white blood cells that ingest and destroy bacteria as part of the innate immune response. These cells rapidly accumulate, in large numbers, at sites of infection and inflammation.

Oesophangeal motility Involvement of the oesophagus in scleroderma.

Opsoclonus–myoclonus (OM) Rapid, irregular eye movements (opsoclonus) coupled with quick involuntary muscle jerks (myoclonus).

Opsonization The binding of complement and antibodies to the surface of a pathogen or foreign substance to aid phagocytosis.

Overflow proteinuria Proteinuria caused by glomerular filtration of levels of protein which exceed the reabsorption capacity of the renal tubules.

Paraprotein An abnormal (usually monoclonal) protein seen in a monoclonal gammopathy such as MGUS or myeloma.

Pathogenesis The origination and development of a disease.

Plasmoblast A precursor cell of the plasmocyte which constitutes 1% of the nucleated white blood cells. Not commonly seen in the peripheral blood of normal people, but can be seen is chronic infections, granulomatous and allergic diseases, and plasma cell myeloma.

Polymorphism Variations in a gene locus at a frequency greater than 1% (adj. **polymorphic**)

Positive selection The survival of a T cell through the TCR binding to MHC with weak affinity, ensuring that T cells can recognize antigen in the context of self.

Prodrome An early symptom of disease.

Protein electrophoresis The separation of the protein molecules within a solution (usually serum, urine, or cerebrospinal fluid) as a result of their differing motilities within an electric field.

Proteinuria The presence of protein in the urine. Proteins filtered through the kidney glomeruli should be actively reabsorbed in the tubules and so proteinuria should normally be absent or minimal.

Raynaud's phenomenon Spasm of the tiny artery vessels supplying blood to the extremities during periods of low ambient temperature.

Scanning densitometry (densitometry) Determination of the density of stain along a protein electrophoresis strip by means of light absorption. If the stain density has a linear relationship to the amount of protein present, the densitometric scan can be used to determine the amount of protein in a given area, e.g. within a monoclonal band.

Sclerodactyly Localized thickening and tightness of the skin of the fingers or toes.

Sensitivity The ability of an assay to correctly identify disease. The number of false negatives.

Seroconversion The detection of antibodies in response to an antigen (infectious organism). In HIV infection, the conversion from an antibody-negative to an antibody-positive state can take from 1 week to several months.

Somatic hypermutation The introduction of mutations into the variable region of an antibody, to increase the antibody affinity.

Specificity Lack of interference from other elements other than the analyte being measured. The number of false positives.

Stiff person syndrome Progressive, severe muscle stiffness or rigidity, mainly in spine and legs.

Synovial membrane The thin membrane that lines the inside of a joint. Its function is to lubricate the joint and produce synovial fluid.

Telangiectasias Dilated capillaries that form tiny red areas, frequently on the face.

Thrombosis The formation of a blood clot (thrombus) within the blood vessels.

Thyrotoxicosis The condition resulting from an excess of thyroid hormones.

Vasculitis Inflammation of the blood vessels.

Abbreviations

AAE	Acquired angioedema		EAACI	European Academy of Allergology and Clinical Immunology
ACE	Angiotensin converting enzyme		ECP	Eosinophil cationic protein
AChR	Acetylcholine receptor antibody		EGTA	Ethylene glycol tetra-acetic acid
ACTH	Adenocorticotrophic hormone		ELISA	Enzyme-linked immunosorbent assay
ADCC	Antibody-dependent cell-mediated cytotoxicity		ENA	Extractable nuclear antigens
AGA	Anti-ganglioside antibodies		ESR	Erythrocyte sedimentation rate
AIDS	Acquired immune deficiency syndrome		EUROEQAS	European External Quality Assessment Service
AIRE	Autoimmune regulator gene		FBC	Full blood count
ALBIA	Addressable laser bead immunoassay		FPIA	Fluorescent polarization immunoassay
ALTM	All laboratories trimmed mean		FTT	Failure to thrive
AMPAR	α-Amino-3-hydroxy-5-methyl-4-isoxazole propionic acid receptor		G6PD	Glucose-6-phosphate dehydrogenase
ANNA-1	Anti-neuronal nuclear antibody type 1 (Hu is an alternative name)		GAD	Glutamic acid decarboxylase
			GINA	Global Initiative for Asthma
ANNA-2	Anti-neuronal nuclear antibody type 2 (Ri is an alternative name)		HAE	Hereditary angioedema
			HbA_{1c}	Glycosylated haemoglobin
APC	Antigen-presenting cell		HCV	Hepatitis C virus
APECED	Autoimmune polyendocrinopathy, candidiasis, ectodermal dystrophy		HIDS	Hyper IgD syndrome
			HIV	Human immunodeficiency virus
APS	Autoimmune polyglandular syndrome *also* anti-phospholipid syndrome		HLA	Human leukocyte antigen
			HUVS	Hypocomplementaemic urticarial vasculitis
AQP4	Aquaporin 4 antibody (NMO is an alternative name)		IA-2	Insulinoma-like antigen-2
			ICA	Islet cell antibody
ATP	Adenosine triphosphate		IgA	Immunoglobulin A
CCD	Cross-reactive carbohydrate determinants		IgD	Immunoglobulin D
CD	Cluster of differentiation		IgE	Immunoglobulin E
CLR	Collagen-like region		IgG	Immunoglobulin G
CNS	Central nervous system		IgM	Immunoglobulin M
CPD	Continuing professional development		IL	Interleukin
CRD	Component-resolved diagnosis		IFCC	International Federation of Clinical Chemistry
CRMP-5	Collapsin response-mediator brain proteins		IUIS	International Union of Immunological Societies
CRP	C-reactive protein			
CSF	Cerebrospinal fluid		JDF	Juvenile Diabetes Foundation
CTLA	Cytotoxic T-lymphocyte antigen		LADA	Latent autoimmune diabetes of adults
CV-2	Alternative name for CRMP-5 antibody		LEMS	Lambert–Eaton myasthaenic syndrome
CZE	Capillary zone electrophoresis		LFT	Liver function test
DAF	Decay-accelerating factor		MAC	Membrane attack complex
DBPCC	Double-blind placebo-controlled challenge		MAG	Myelin-associated glycoprotein antibodies
DNP	Deoxyribonucleoprotein		MASP	MBL-associated serine protease
DTT	Dithiothreitol			

MBL	Mannan-binding lectin		PCR	Polymerase chain reaction
MCP	Membrane cofactor protein		PEG	Polyethylene glycol
MCTD	Mixed connective tissue disease		PEM	Paraneoplastic encephalomyelitis
MCV	Mean cell volume		PLE	Paraneoplastic limbic encephalitis
MDT	Multidisciplinary team		PNA	Paraneoplastic neurological antibody
MG	Myasthenia gravis		PNH	Peripheral nerve hyperexcitability
mGluR1	Anti-metabotropic glutamate receptor 1		PNS	Paraneoplastic neurological syndrome
MGUS	Monoclonal gammopathy of undetermined significance		POM	Paraneoplastic opsoclonus–myoclonus
			RAST	Radioallergosorbent test
MHC	Major histocompatibility complex		RF	Rheumatoid factor
MICA	MHC class 1-related gene A		RNP	Ribonucleoproteins
MKD	Mevalonate kinase deficiency		RSV	Respiratory syncitial virus
MPGN	Membranoproliferative glomerulonephritis		SCLC	Small-cell lung cancer
MPO	Myeloperoxidase		SDBIS	Standard deviation of the bias index score
MRBIS	Mean running bias index score		SEP	Serum electrophoresis
MRI	Magnetic resonance imaging		sIgE	Allergen-specific immunoglobulin E
MRVIS	Mean running variance index score		SIT	Specific immunotherapy
MS	Multiple sclerosis		SLE	Systemic lupus erythematosus
MuSK	Muscle-specific kinase		SPS	Stiff person syndrome
NIDG	UK Neuroimmunology Discussion Group		T_3	Tri-iodothyronine
NK	Natural killer (cells)		T_4	Thyroxine
NMDAR	N-methyl D-aspartate receptor		TCC	Terminal complement complex
NMJ	Neuromuscular juction		TNF	Tumour necrosis factor
NMO	Neuromyelitis optica		TPO	Thyroid peroxidase
NMT	Neuromyotonia		TSH	Thyroid-stimulating hormone
NSAID	Nonsteroidal anti-inflammatory drug		TSHRAB	TSH receptor antibody
OM	Opsoclonus-myoclonus		tTG	Tissue transglutaminase
OMRVIS	Overall mean running variance index score		U&E	Urea and electrolytes (test)
PAD	Peptidylarginine deiminase		UKNEQAS	United Kingdom National External Quality Assessment Service
PCA-1	Purkinje cell cytoplasmic antibody type 1 (Yo is an alternative name)		UEP	Urine electrophoresis
PCA-2	Purkinje cell cytoplasmic antibody type 2		VGCC	Voltage-gated calcium channel antibody
PCA-Tr	Purkinje cell cytoplasmic antibody type Tr (Tr is an alternative name)		VGKC	Voltage-gated potassium channel antibody
PCD	Paraneoplastic cerebellar degeneration		WAO	World Allergy Organization
PCNA	Proliferating cell nuclear antigen		WHO	Word Health Organization

Hints and tips for discussion questions

Chapter 1

1.1

- Good knowledge of more than one discipline.

- Ability to interpret results from different disciplines, as results from one discipline should be considered together with those from the other disciplines for meaningful interpretation and diagnosis.

- Biomedical scientists usually specialize in one discipline but they need to have at least a basic understanding and to be aware of the scope of the other disciplines.

- Greater opportunity for career progression, as trained in more than one discipline.

1.2

- An internationally recognized benchmark of quality and excellence.

- Biomedical scientists can register as a Chartered Scientists if they have achieved the level of qualification required, show evidence of continuing professional development, and have the minimum level of work experience required.

- Demonstration of practicing science at the full professional level.

Chapter 2

2.1 Immunoglobulin molecule subunits are called domains and are named according to their location in the immunoglobulin molecule, e.g. constant region heavy chain domain 1 is CH1. Within each domain the polypeptide chain is folded into beta-pleated sheets held by intrachain disulphide bonds.

2.2 (a) CH2; (b) CH3; (c) VH.

2.3 IgG1: Complement activation ++, IgG Fc receptor II & III binding ++++, placental transfer ++, produced to peptide antigens.

IgG2: Complement activation +, IgG Fc receptor II & III binding +, placental transfer +, produced to polysaccharide antigens.

IgG3: Complement activation +++, IgG Fc receptor II & III binding +++, placental transfer ++, produced to peptide antigens.

IgG4: Complement activation 0, IgG Fc receptor II & III binding +, placental transfer +, produced to peptide antigens.

2.4 As a fixed amount of antibody is combined with increasing amounts of antigen, the larger is the immune complex that is formed. When antigen exceeds available antibody, the large complexes break apart, leaving small or single-antibody immune complexes which generate a small optical signal similar to that generated by low concentrations of antigen. This is described by the Heidelberger–Kendall curve.

Chapter 3

3.1

- Natural extracts should contain the relevant allergenic components.

- Extraction processes may destroy the allergenicity of the final product.

- There can be problems with reproducibility of reagents and variability between commercial suppliers.

- Recombinant technology allows the production of single proteins with defined allergenic epitopes.

- Recombinant allergens can be used as diagnostic tools to supplement natural extracts or as single reagents.

- Testing with recombinant allergens can lead to component-resolved diagnosis.

- Reagents which are based on recombinant allergens may not cover the complete repertoire of allergenic epitopes.

3.2

- Internal quality control using sera and/or commercial preparations of known sIgE concentrations in the assay.

- Assay verification undertaken by monitoring Levy–Jennings plots and by applying Westgard rules.

- It is impractical to undertake internal quality control for every allergen. Therefore, choose most appropriate and test at relevant sIgE concentrations.

- Undertake external quality assessment, e.g. EUROEQAS scheme.

- Compare performance with peer group because of potential variability in allergen preparations.

- Enrol in web-based educational programmes.

3.3

- Most common approach is in assessing basophil activation.

- Applicable in situations where specific IgE tests are unavailable or have poor diagnostic sensitivity or specificity, e.g. drug allergy.

- May be useful when skin/challenge testing cannot be undertaken.

- May provide diagnostic evidence when sIgE results are equivocal, as the method may more accurately reflect the *in vivo* pathophysiological pathway.

Chapter 4

4.1

- Opsonization.
- Stimulation of an inflammatory response.
- Activation of endothelium.
- Recruitment and activation of phagocytes.
- Lysis of target cells by membrane attack complex.

4.2

- C1 esterase inhibitor.
- Autosomal dominant inheritance.
- Symptoms: episodes of angioedema which can affect any part of the body; intra-abdominal swellings can lead to obstruction; airway swellings can lead to death by asphyxiation.
- Treatments: tranexamic acid (which may inhibit some of the proteases which cleave C1 inhibitor); androgenic steroids danazol or stanozolol (which increase transcription of many genes, including the normally functioning copy of C1 inhibitor); C1 esterase inhibitor concentrate (a blood product); bradykinin inhibitors.

4.3

- Activation is different: antibody antigen complexes for the classical pathway and bacterial cell membrane components for the lectin pathway.

- The initial proteins are different. However, there is homology between them with C1q, C1r, and C1s being structurally similar to MBL, MASP1, and MASP2.
- Subsequently the pathways converge, with cleavage of C4 and C2 leading on to the production of C3 convertase and C5 convertase and formation of the membrane attack complex.

Chapter 5

5.1 Four out of the following eleven criteria need to be present for the diagnosis to be made:

- Malar rash
- Discoid rash
- Photosensitivity
- Oral ulcers
- Nonerosive arthritis involving >2 peripheral joints
- Pleuritis or pericarditis
- Renal disorder: persistent proteinuria or cellular casts
- Neurological disorder: seizures or psychosis in the absence of drugs or known metabolic disorders
- Haemotological disorder: haemolytic anaemia or leucopenia or lyphopenia or thrombocytopenia
- Immunological disorder: antibodies to dsDNA or Sm or positive finding of antiphospholipid antibodies (anti-cardiolipin, lupus anticoagulant or a false positive syphilis test)
- Positive anti-nuclear antibodies.

5.2

Method	Advantages	Disadvantages
Indirect immunofluorescence	Good screening test to eliminate negative sera Low-cost Semi-quantitative (titration)	Antibody specificity not identified Will detect other nonclinically relevant autoantibodies Requires experienced staff to read accurately
ELISA/FPIA/bead immunoassay	Antibody specificity identified Automatable tests Quantitative measurement	
Western blot	Antibody specificity identified	Qualitative test Not useful for monitoring
Dot blot	Antibody specificity identified	Qualitative test Not useful for monitoring

5.3

- Proliferation of cells within the synovial membrane.
- Migration of immune cells to site of inflammation.
- Release of pro-inflammatory cytokines and chemokines within the fluid of the joint.
- Autoantibodies in the circulation of patients with RA, including rheumatoid factor and antibodies to citrullinated proteins.

- The presence of cryoglobulins.
- Increase of proteins associated with an acute phase response such as fibrinogen and C-reactive protein.
- Increase complement breakdown products (C3d or C4d).
- Presence of circulating immune complexes.

Chapter 6

6.1

Method	Advantages	Disadvantages
Indirect immunofluorescence	Good screening test to eliminate negative sera Low cost	Antibody specificity not identified Will detect other autoantibodies, e.g. ANA Requires experienced staff to read accurately Semi-quantitative (titration)
ELISA/FPIA/bead immunoassay	Antibody specificity identified Automatable tests Quantitative measurement	
Western blot	Antibody specificity identified	Qualitative test Not useful for monitoring
Dot blot	Antibody specificity identified	Qualitative test Not useful for monitoring

6.2

General:

- Weight loss.
- Night sweats.
- Fatigue.
- Arthritis.

Specific:

- Changes in blood biochemistry indicating decreasing kidney function: increased urea, increased creatinine.
- Haemoptysis.
- Haematuria.
- Kidney biopsy showing damage to glomeruli with crescent formation. Immunochemistry shows no immunoglobulin or complement present (in ANCA-associated diseases) or liner IgG staining of the glomerular basement membrane sometimes accompanied by associated complement deposition (anti-GBM disease).
- Radiograph showing infiltrates (granulomas).

6.3

- Antibody titres in many patients show a direct relationship to disease activity.
- They are capable of binding to primed neutrophils and initiate a respiratory burst, which leads to degranulation and the release of proteolytic enzymes, which are capable of causing damage to surrounding tissues.
- The antibodies may also bind directly to endothelial cells and thus render them susceptible to damage by cell-mediated or complement-mediated cytotoxicity.

Chapter 7

7.1

- First, the patient needs to be genetically susceptible to the disease. Also within this sphere are endogenous factors such as hormone balance.
- Secondly, the patient requires some form of trigger to break tolerance. Often this trigger is unknown, but infections are commonly thought to be involved (sometimes called 'molecular mimicry').
- Finally, the patient requires an element of bad luck, as even identical twins brought up in the same environment do not always both get the disease.

7.2

- Autoantibodies may be detected in some members of the normal, healthy population.
- Also note that the transient appearance of autoantibodies, particularly during and after a viral infection, is a common occurrence.
- Most patients do not go on to develop autoimmune disease, although some do.
- Where this balance is not restored, the patient may go on to develop autoimmune disease.
- Those with persistent antibody on retesting are more likely to develop the associated autoimmune disease in the future.

7.3

- Hypothyroidism: Hashimoto's thyroiditis, atrophic thyroiditis, postpartum thyroiditis, subclinical hypothyroidism, focal thyroiditis. juvenile lymphocytic thyroiditis.
- Hyperthyroidism: Grave's disease.

7.4

- IgA responses predominate and are the more important in diagnosis. However, IgA deficiency is about 10 times more common in patients with coeliac disease than in the general population. If a patient is IgA deficient, then IgA tests for coeliac disease will be negative.

7.5

- The destruction of parietal cells in the stomach leads to a lack of intrinsic factor, which is necessary for efficient vitamin B_{12} absorption.

- Intrinsic factor autoantibodies can further impair the absorption of vitamin B_{12}, either preventing B_{12} binding to intrinsic factor or by interfering with the binding of intrinsic factor to receptors in the ileum.

Chapter 8

8.1

- All the variables that constitute the assay; the serum screening dilution1/10, in line with international consensus document as the antibody may be present in very low concentration; the use of appropriate control sera; choice and dilution of FITC conjugate (must do chequerboard titration to ensure optimum performance); optimization of microscope optics and light source; competence of the observers (there should be two experienced observers); use of an antigen-specific based assay to confirm microscopic findings; participation in external quality assurance scheme.

8.2

- Result suggests AMA-negative PBC, or is IIF not sufficiently sensitive? Use an anti-M2 specific ELISA or immunoblot. Better still, use a recombinant ELISA with three target M2 antigens to increase sensitivity. If these are negative then sample is probably anti-M2 negative. However, there are ANAs associated with PBC, rim, MND, and centromere. Test the sample on HEp-2 cells or one of the derivative cell lines to look for these autoantibodies. Ultimately, the liver biopsy will confirm or deny presence of PBC.

8.3

- A high-titre anti-M2 will mask the presence of other autoantibodies of lower titre. The use of HEp-2 cells may reveal ANA but F actin SMA will probably be lost in the M2 fluorescence of the HEp-2 cytoplasm. Anti-LKM 1 and anti-LC 1 are unlikely in PBC/AIH overlap and again would be lost in the anti-M2 pattern. Use alternative techniques; ELISA and/or immunoblot for liver disease-related autoantibodies. The blots are easy to use and provide all the potential autoantigen targets (more efficient than using four separate ELISAs).

- Also the blots contain an SLA antigen which is not detectable in IIF even in the absence of anti-M2. In this scenario anti-SLA was detected along with the expected anti-M2 on immunoblot. This is not an infrequent pair of autoantibodies to find in PBC/AIH overlap.

Chapter 9

9.1

- Infiltration of immune mediators in the affected areas of the brain and antibodies from patients with PNS can be shown to bind to the brain tissue.

9.2

- Neuronal antigens expressed in the tumour cause immune response against tumour and brain cell (neuron) antigens.

9.3

- A diagnosis of paraneoplastic neurological syndrome is confirmed if the classical neurological syndrome and a well-characterized PNA are present together.

9.4

- Irreversible neurological damage. The objective is usually to stabilize the syndrome and improve quality of life; death can occur from tumour burden or associated severe neurological problems.

Chapter 10

10.1

- They enable B cells to class switch, i.e. make IgG (without T cells' help they would only make IgM).

- Activate macrophage killing of pathogens.

- CD4⁺ T cells help CD8⁺ T cells to kill cells infected with virus.

10.2

- XLA and B-SCID.

- Set up a lymphocyte panel including HLA-DR.

- XLA would have normal T cells, i.e. normal CD4/CD8 ratio and normal activation.

- SCID would have no T cells (MFE or Omenn's; T cells would be very activated).

10.3

- Lymphadenopathy/hepatosplenomegaly, autoimmune cytopenias.

- Defect in apoptosis.

- Look for the presence of increased numbers of double-negative TCR $\alpha\beta$ T cells.

10.4

- (SCID) SCID, nonrandom X inactivation of the T cells.

- (XLA) Normal BTK in all B cells, 50:50 normal/abnormal BTK in the monocytes.

- (CGD) Two populations of neutrophils, one with normal and one with abnormal oxidative burst.

Chapter 11

11.1 HIV infection is usually determined using an ELISA which combines the testing of p24 antigen and anti-HIV antibodies, together with other HIV-1 antigens, such as gp160, gp41. Some

HIV tests differentiate between HIV-1 and HIV-2, although confirmation is usually by western blot or line probe assays—reactivity to gp120 and gp41 indicative of HIV-1 infection while samples positive for HIV-2 would react with gp105 and gp36, but not with gp120 and gp41. In developing countries, point-of-care or rapid screening tests may be offered.

11.2 Yes. Most ELISAs differentiate between HIV-1 and HIV-2, although as discussed above, confirmation of HIV-1 or HIV-2 infection is usually by western blot.

11.3 The term seroconversion refers to the development of antibodies following infection or immunization, i.e. the change from an antibody-negative to antibody-positive state. In HIV-1 infection, however, individuals are said to have 'sero-converted' following a 'seroconversion illness' which may precede the development of antibodies and may be marked by a significant viraemia.

11.4 During seroconversion illness patients may experience flu-like symptoms, myalgia, pyrexia, and lymphadenopathy. Occasionally patients present with a morbilliform rash.

11.5 Long-term nonprogressors or elite controllers (those who maintain a viral loads of <50 copies/mL) are individuals who have been infected with HIV virus but have sustained low-level viraemia and normal CD4 counts in the absence of antiretroviral therapy.

11.6 Disease progression and/or therapy efficacy can be determined by monitoring CD4 counts and HIV viral load. In treatment-naive patients, approximately one-third will present with a CD4 count of <200 cells/μL. These patients, even after commencing antiretroviral therapy, will have a significantly higher risk of disease progression or death than those starting with higher CD4 counts. Patients presenting with low CD4 counts may have contracted the disease a long time ago and the CD4 count may be a reflection of the progressive damage to the immune system over time. Predictions may be made about possible disease progression from initial CD4 count and viral load.

11.7 Treatment failure may occur for a number of reasons: development of resistant strains, suboptimal absorption, or may be due to patient noncompliance.

11.8 If mutations are not detected following genotypic resistance testing, a failure in antiretroviral therapy may be due to noncompliance or poor absorption—therapeutic drug monitoring may be useful in this circumstance.

11.9 The failure to produce an effective HIV-1 vaccine is in part down to the high mutation rate of the HIV-1 virus and inability of the immune system to produce a broad spectrum of cross-neutralizing antibodies capable of recognizing a range of target envelope antigens.

Index